DATE DUE

Obesity and Diabetes

Other titles in the Wiley *Diabetes in Practice* Series

Diabetic Nephropathy
Edited by Christoph Hasslacher   (0 471 48992 1)

Diabetes in Pregnancy: An International Approach to Diagnosis and Management
Edited by Anne Dornhorst and David R. Hadden   (0 471 96204 X)

Diabetic Complications Second Edition
Edited by Ken Shaw   (0 470 86597 2)

Childhood and Adolescent Diabetes
Edited by Simon Court and Bill Lamb   (0 471 97003 4)

Hypoglycaemia in Clinical Diabetes
Brian M. Frier and B. Miles Fisher   (0 471 98264 4)

Exercise and Sport in Diabetes
Edited by Bill Burr and Dinesh Nagi   (0 471 98496 5)

Psychology of Diabetes Care
Edited by Frank Snoek and T. Chas Skinner   (0 471 97703 9)

The Foot in Diabetes Third Edition
Edited by Andrew J. M. Boulton, Henry Connor and Peter R. Cavanagh   (0 471 48974 3)

Nutritional Management of Diabetes Mellitus
Edited by Gary Frost, Anne Dornhorst and Robert Moses   (0 471 49751 7)

Obesity and Diabetes

Editors

Anthony H. Barnett

Department of Medicine, University of Birmingham and Birmingham Heartlands and Solihull NHS Trust (Teaching), UK

Sudhesh Kumar

Professor of Medicine, Diabetes & Metabolism, Warwick Medical School, University of Warwick, UK

John Wiley & Sons, Ltd

Other Wiley Editorial Offices

John Wiley & Sons Inc., 111 River Street, Hoboken, NJ 07030, USA

Jossey-Bass, 989 Market Street, San Francisco, CA 94103-1741, USA

Wiley-VCH Verlag GmbH, Boschstr. 12, D-69469 Weinheim, Germany

John Wiley & Sons Australia Ltd, 33 Park Road, Milton, Queensland 4064, Australia

John Wiley & Sons (Asia) Pte Ltd, 2 Clementi Loop #02-01, Jin Xing Distripark, Singapore 129809

John Wiley & Sons Canada Ltd, 6045 Freemont Boulevard, Mississauga, Ontario, Canada, L5R 4J3

Wiley also publishes its books in a variety of electronic formats. Some content that appears
in print may not be available in electronic books.

Library of Congress Cataloging-in-Publication Data

Obesity and diabetes / editors, Anthony H. Barnett, Sudhesh Kumar.
     p. ; cm. – (Wiley diabetes in practice series)
  Includes bibliographical references and index.
  ISBN 0-470-84898-7 (cloth : alk. paper)
  1. Obesity. 2. Non-insulin-dependent diabetes.
  [DNLM: 1. Diabetes Mellitus, Type II – etiology. 2. Obesity – complications. 3.
Diabetes Mellitus, Type II – epidemiology. 4. Diabetes Mellitus, Type II – therapy. 5.
Obesity – therapy.] I. Barnett, A. H. (Anthony H.), 1951– II. Kumar, Sudhesh. III.
Diabetes in practice.
  RC628.O2263 2004
  616.3′98 – dc22

                                         2004011558

British Library Cataloguing in Publication Data

A catalogue record for this book is available from the British Library

ISBN 0-470-84898-7

Typeset in 10.5/13pt Times by Laserwords Private Limited, Chennai, India
Printed and bound in Great Britain by Antony Rowe Ltd, Chippenham, Wiltshire
This book is printed on acid-free paper responsibly manufactured from sustainable forestry
in which at least two trees are planted for each one used for paper production.

Contents

Foreword

Type 2 diabetes has become a major worldwide public health problem with an exponential rise in numbers in recent decades. There are presently around 200 million people who have the condition, with numbers expected to reach 300 million by 2025. The reasons for this staggering increase include an ageing population, but particularly the explosion in the numbers of people with obesity that has been seen in many parts of the world in recent years. Globally, there are more than 1 billion overweight adults, at least 300 million of them obese. In England, most adults are now overweight and one in five is obese. The associated costs are substantial. The UK National Audit Office estimated that obesity accounted for 18 million days of sickness absence and 30,000 premature deaths in 1998. On average, each person whose death could be attributed to obesity lost nine years of life. Treating obesity costs the NHS at least half a billion pounds per year. The wider costs to the economy in lower productivity and lost output could be a further £2 billion each year.

Obesity is not just a problem of the developed world but also of the developing world. Indeed, there are now more people suffering the consequences of over-nutrition than malnutrition. Adoption of a Western-type lifestyle has resulted in populations changing to diets high in saturated fat and sugar, coincident with dramatic reductions in activity levels. The result has been an epidemic of what has been termed "diabesity". Obesity rates have risen three-fold or more since 1980 in some areas of Eastern Europe, the Middle East, the Pacific Islands, Australasia and China. In most Latin American countries, the prevalence of overweight, which may lead to obesity, is very high and the rate of obesity in children is increasing. Often coexisting in developing countries with under-nutrition, obesity is a complex condition, with serious social and psychological dimensions, affecting virtually all ages and socioeconomic groups.

Childhood obesity is already epidemic in some areas and on the rise in others. An estimated 17.6 million children under five are estimated to be overweight worldwide. According to the US Surgeon General, in the USA the number of overweight children has doubled and the number of overweight adolescents has trebled since 1980. The problem is global and increasingly extends into the developing world; for example, in Thailand the prevalence of obesity in 5-to-12 year old children rose from 12.2% to 15-6% in just two years.

Obesity and diabetes are intimately interlinked. Obesity is frequently accompanied by a state of insulin resistance, which may develop into full-blown diabetes. The degree of insulin resistance is roughly proportional to body fat mass but the distribution of body fat is also important. These two conditions have become major public health issues of modern times. The problem though is not just the numbers of cases but also the long-term complications in terms of cardiovascular disease, obesity-related cancers, osteoarthritis and much else. In addition, diabetes remains the single commonest cause of blindness and renal failure in many countries and a major reason for non-traumatic lower limb amputation. Around 80% of type 2 diabetic patients will die from cardiovascular disease, many prematurely.

For the above reasons, it is almost impossible to overstate the importance of obesity and diabetes. In this book, the editors, Tony Barnett and Sudhesh Kumar, have brought together an internationally recognised group of experts to discuss these issues. The emphasis is very much on management, treatment and prevention, with the target audience being the doctors, nurses and other health-care professionals who deal with these patients on a daily basis. The opening chapters describe the changing epidemiology of obesity and its implications for diabetes and the genetic causes of obesity. However, genetic influences are being swamped by the effects of modern lifestyles and this is where preventive and therapeutic efforts must be focused. The book contains chapters on therapies based on diet, changes in food intake, behavioural modification and increasing physical activity. The evidence base and therapy implications for diabetes, obesity and cardiovascular disease are discussed, together with specific drug therapy options for the obese diabetic patient. Other chapters include a discussion of childhood obesity and type 2 diabetes, this association being increasingly recognised in many parts of the world. There is also consideration of obesity and polycystic ovary syndrome and finally discussion of the multidisciplinary approach to diabesity management in primary care.

This book should appeal to all health professionals with an interest in obesity and diabetes. Each chapter stands in its own right but there is also a clear thread linking each of them. The book can be used for reference, but is also well written and can be read as individual chapters or from cover to cover. The editors have done an excellent job in bringing together so many experts in their respective fields to produce a book which should remain topical for years to come.

Paul Zimmet
Foundation Director of the International Diabetes Institute
and Professor of Diabetes,
Monash University, Australia
May 2004

List of Contributors

Anthony H. Barnett

Professor of Medicine and Consultant Physician, Dept of Medicine/Diabetes/Endocrinology, Birmingham Heartlands Hospital, Birmingham, UK

Timothy Barrett

Senior Lecturer in Paediatric Endocrinology, Dept of Endocrinology, Diabetic Home Care Unit, The Children's Hospital NHS Trust, Steelhouse Lane, Birmingham B4 6NH, UK

Iain Broom

Consultant in Clinical Biochemistry and Metabolic Medicine, The Robert Gorden University, School of Life Sciences, St. Andrew Street, Aberdeen, AB25 1HG, UK

Ian W. Campbell

Park House Medical Centre, 61 Burton Road, Carlton, Nottingham NG4 3DQ, UK

Tahseen A. Chowdhury

Consultant Physician, Department of Metabolic Medicine, The Royal London Hospital, London, UK

Richard N. Clayton

Dept of Endocrinology, School of Medicine, Keele University, Thornburrow Drive, Hartshill, Stoke-on-Trent, Staffs ST4 7QB, UK

Carlton B. Cooke

Professor of Sport and Exercise Research, Centre for Leisure and Sport Research, Leeds Metropolitan University, Leeds, UK

James Evans

Specialist Registrar for General Surgery, University Hospital, Aintree, Liverpool, UK

Paul J. Gately   Principal Lecturer in Exercise Physiology and
                               Health, Centre for Leisure and Sport Research,
                               Leeds Metropolitan University, Leeds, UK

Susan A. Jebb   MRC Human Nutrition Research, Elsie
                               Widdowson Laboratory, Fulbourn Road,
                               Cambridge CB1 9NL, UK

David D. Kerrigan   Consultant Surgeon, University Hospital,
                               Aintree, Liverpool L9 7AL, UK

Jeremy Krebs   Wellington Clinical School of Medicine,
                               University of Otago, P.O. Box 7343,
                               Wellington South, New Zealand

Sudhesh Kumar   Professor of Medicine, Diabetes & Metabolism,
                               Warwick Medical School, University of
                               Warwick, Coventry CV4 7AL, UK

Victor J. Lawrence   Wellcome Trust Research Training Fellow,
                               Department of Diabetes and Metabolic
                               Medicine, Barts and The London School of
                               Medicine & Dentistry, London, UK

Jaana Lindström   National Public Health Institute, Department of
                               Epidemiology and Health Promotion, Finland

Krystyna A. Matyka   Senior Lecturer in Paediatrics, Birmingham
                               Heartlands Hospital, Bordesley Green East,
                               Birmingham B9 5SS, UK

Phillip McTernan   Division of Clinical Sciences, Warwick Medical
                               School, Coventry, UK

John Pinkney   Senior Lecturer in Diabetes and Endocrinology,
                               University Hospital Aintree, Liverpool, UK

Diana Raskauskiene   Dept of Endocrinology, School of Medicine,
                               Keele University, Thornburrow Drive,
                               Hartshill, Stoke-on-Trent, ST4 7QB, UK

Jayadave Shakher   Associate Specialist, Diabetes and
                             Endocrinology, Birmingham Heartlands and
                             Solihull NHS Trust (Teaching), Birmingham,
                             UK

Karri Silventoinen   Department of Public Health, University of
                             Helsinki, and Diabetes and Genetic
                             Epidemiology Unit, Department of
                             Epidemiology and Health Promotion, National
                             Public Health Institute, Helsinki, Finland

Jaakko Tuomilehto   Department of Public Health, University of
                             Helsinki, and Diabetes and Genetic
                             Epidemiology Unit, Department of
                             Epidemiology and Health Promotion, National
                             Public Health Institute, Helsinki, Finland

Brent Van Dorsten   Associate Professor, Department of
                             Rehabilitation Medicine, University of
                             Colorado Health Sciences Center, Box 1650,
                             Mail Stop F-713, Anschutz Outpatient
                             Pavilion, Aurora, CO 80010, USA

Jonathan Webber   Consultant Diabetologist, Diabetes Centre, Selly
                             Oak Hospital, Birmingham, B29 6JD, UK

John P.H. Wilding   Reader in Medicine, Clinical Sciences Centre,
                             University Hospital Aintree, Longmoor Lane,
                             Liverpool L9 7AL, UK

1

Changing Epidemiology of Obesity – Implications for Diabetes

Jonathan Webber

Introduction

It is clear that there is a global epidemic of obesity (World Health Organization, 2000) and the implications for diabetes of this epidemic are now starting to be realized (Mokdad *et al.*, 2003). A large number of co-morbidities are associated with obesity, but it is type 2 diabetes that is most closely linked with increasing adiposity (Willett *et al.*, 1999) and even within the normal weight range diabetes prevalence begins to rise with increasing adiposity (Chan *et al.*, 1994; Colditz *et al.*, 1995). There are currently about 110 million patients with diabetes on a worldwide basis, with this number projected to increase to 180 million by 2010 (King *et al.*, 1998). Being overweight or obese with an abdominal fat distribution probably accounts for 80–90 per cent of all patients with type 2 diabetes (Astrup and Finer, 2000).

Assessment of obesity in epidemiological studies

Most current epidemiological studies of body weight use body mass index (BMI) to define degrees of obesity. BMI is calculated as the subject's weight in kilograms divided by the square of their height in metres ($kg\,m^{-2}$). Cut-offs for underweight, normal weight, overweight and obesity are shown in Table 1.1.

BMI correlates well with total adiposity (Webster *et al.*, 1984) and with morbidity and mortality from many diseases (Willett *et al.*, 1999), although for a

Obesity and Diabetes. Edited by Anthony H. Barnett and Sudhesh Kumar
© 2004 John Wiley & Sons, Ltd ISBN: 0-470-84898-7

Table 1.1   World Health Organization classification of obesity

WHO classification	BMI $(kg\,m^{-2})$
Underweight	<18.5
Healthy weight	18.5–24.9
Overweight (grade 1 obesity)	25–29.9
Obese (grade 2 obesity)	30–39.9
Morbid/severe obesity (grade 3 obesity)	>40

number of co-morbidities, including type 2 diabetes, the relationship is closer with abdominal body fat distribution than total body fat (Ohlson *et al.*, 1985). In epidemiological studies intra-abdominal fat is most commonly estimated using measurements of waist and hip circumference and these can be used to identify increased risk of diabetes and other cardiovascular risk factors (Han *et al.*, 1995).

Prevalence of obesity

The prevalence of obesity is increasing throughout the world at an unprecedented rate. To be a healthy BMI, as defined by the World Health Organization (WHO), is now to be in a minority in much of western Europe as well as the United States. Indeed, in many developing countries overweight and obesity are now so common that they are replacing more traditional problems such as undernutrition and infectious diseases as the most significant causes of ill-health (World Health Organization, 2000). In 1995, there were an estimated 200 million obese adults worldwide and another 18 million under-5 children classified as overweight. As of 2000, the number of obese adults has increased to over 300 million. This obesity epidemic is not restricted to industrialized societies; in developing countries, it is estimated that over 115 million people suffer from obesity-related problems (World Health Organization, 2000). As the proportion of the population with a low BMI decreases, there is an almost symmetrical increase in the proportion with a BMI above 25. The WHO MONICA project compares obesity rates in 48 populations spread throughout the world (Berrios *et al.*, 1997). In the period 1983 to 1986 these rates varied from less than 5 per cent in Beijing in China to about 20 per cent in Malta. Recent data suggests that the BMI distribution is moving upwards in China as in the rest of the world. From 1989 to 1997 overweight (BMI $25-29.9\,kg\,m^{-2}$) doubled in females (from 10.4 to 20.8 per cent) and almost tripled in males (from 5.0 to 14.1 per cent) (Bell *et al.*, 2001). Some of the highest prevalence figures come from the Pacific region where in urban Samoans obesity has increased from 38.8 per cent in men in 1978 to 58.4 per cent in 1991 (World Health Organization, 2000).

Within the developed world the United States has led the obesity epidemic. In the adult population in the United States the prevalence of obesity, as determined from the National Health and Nutrition Examination Survey (NHANES), has increased from 22.9 per cent in the period 1988–1994 to 30.5 per cent in

1999–2000 (Flegal *et al.*, 2002). Corresponding increases have also occurred in overweight and in morbid obesity. Self-reported data (Behavioural Risk Factor Surveillance System) from much larger numbers of subjects confirm these worrying trends in the United States (Mokdad *et al.*, 1999, 2003). Indeed, if weight gain continues at the current rate in the United States by 2008 39 per cent of the population will be obese (Hill *et al.*, 2003). The overall data on obesity prevalence masks other differences, including higher rates of overweight and obesity in non-Hispanic black women and in a number of minority ethnic groups. In the UK a number of surveys have documented the changes in obesity from 1980 to the current day (Prescott-Clarke and Primatesta, 1999; Figure 1.1). There has been a tripling in obesity prevalence even in this relatively short period of time, with the likelihood that the UK rates will continue to rise to attain those already existing in the United States.

The age of onset of obesity is getting progressively younger (McTigue *et al.*, 2002). This is reflected in the trends in overweight and obesity in children. In the US the prevalence of overweight (defined as at or above the 95th centile of BMI for age) increased from 10.5 to 15.5 per cent of 12–19-year olds between 1994 and 2000 and in the 2–5-year age group period the increase was from 7.2 to 10.4 per cent in this 6-year timespan (Ogden *et al.*, 2002). In England 9.0 per cent of boys aged between 4 and 11 years were overweight in 1994 compared with 5.4 per cent in 1984 (Chinn and Rona, 2001). The corresponding figures for girls were 13.5 per cent (1994) and 9.3 per cent (1984). Though not all obese children become obese adults, a considerable proportion will do so (Kotani *et al.*, 1997). The continuing rise in childhood obesity is likely to lead to a massive increase in the prevalence of those co-morbidities linked to obesity.

The epidemiological link between obesity and diabetes

The link between obesity prevalence and rates of diabetes in different populations was demonstrated by West with an increase in the prevalence of type 2

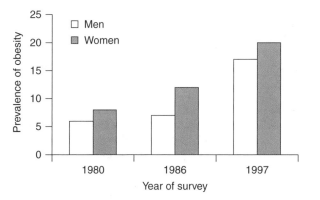

Figure 1.1 Prevalence of obesity in the UK from 1980 to 1997 from Joint Health Surveys Unit on behalf of the Department of Health 1999.

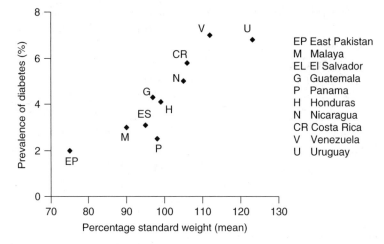

Figure 1.2 Graph showing the relationship between the prevalence of diabetes (predominantly type 2 diabetes) and body weight in 10 representative populations. Body weight is expressed as the population mean, relative to a 'standard' weight that is given an arbitrary score of 100. Reproduced from West 1978 by permission of Elsevier Science.

diabetes as the population becomes more obese (West, 1978; Figure 1.2). Whilst there are changes in the incidence of type 1 diabetes, it is type 2 diabetes that is largely responsible for the global epidemic of diabetes.

Within populations there is clear evidence of a strongly positive relationship between obesity and the risk of diabetes. Data in the United States from the Health Professionals' Follow-up Study in men (Chan *et al.*, 1994) and the Nurses' Health Study in women (Colditz *et al.*, 1995) graphically illustrates the increasing risk of diabetes that obesity brings (Figure 1.3). Compared with those of a BMI less than 21, women with a BMI greater than 35 had a 93-fold excess risk of developing diabetes. The risk of developing type 2 diabetes rises progressively with increasing adiposity (whether assessed by BMI, or percentage of ideal body weight). Data from NHANES shows that for each kilogram increase in weight of the population the risk of diabetes increases by 4.5 per cent (Ford *et al.*, 1997). More recent examination of diabetes trends in the US showed an even steeper increment of diabetes risk with weight gain, with a 9 per cent increased risk of diabetes for each kilogram of body weight gain (Mokdad *et al.*, 2000). Whether this large difference is a real phenomenon, or is explained by increased public awareness of diabetes is not clear, as the later study depended on telephone surveys.

Where populations have changed their lifestyle and become more obese (e.g. Pima Indians of Arizona, Micronesian Nauruan Islanders) an epidemic of type 2 diabetes has followed on. Groups that were previously lean and had a low incidence of diabetes have become obese diabetics. 80 per cent of adult Pima Indians are now obese and 40 per cent of this population now has type 2 diabetes (Zimmet, 1982). In comparison, a genetically almost identical Pima Indian population in Mexico has been described who are lean and whose incidence of

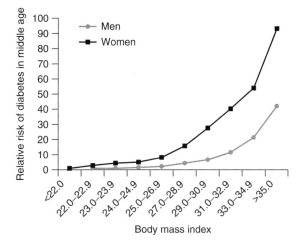

Figure 1.3 Relative risk of type 2 diabetes with increasing BMI. Drawn from data in Chan *et al.*, 1994 (reproduced by permission of American Diabetes Association) and Colditz *et al.*, 1995 (reproduced by permission of American College of Physicians).

type 2 diabetes is virtually zero (Ravussin *et al.*, 1994; Esparza *et al.*, 2000). The importance of obesity in the development of diabetes is clearly demonstrated.

Amongst patients with type 2 diabetes excess adiposity is almost the rule. In the Diabetic Clinic in Dundee about 80 per cent of patients attending are either overweight or obese (Jung, 1997). Increasing obesity in the general population is now reflected in patients with diabetes. Of those patients newly presenting with diabetes in a clinic in Minnesota in the 1970s 33 per cent were obese, whereas 49 per cent of those diagnosed in the late 1980s were obese (Leibson *et al.*, 2001). Thus, not only are we likely to see more patients with diabetes, but also to see more obese patients amongst our diabetic patients with the additional difficulties that accompany their clinical management.

In tandem with the rise in childhood obesity there is now marked rise in type 2 diabetes in children and adolescents. There has been a 10-fold increase in type 2 diabetes amongst children between 1982 and 1994 in the USA (Pinhas-Hamiel *et al.*, 1996). Diabetes in this age group is clearly linked with obesity, although genetic and environmental factors also play a role with many such subjects having a family history of type 2 diabetes and belonging to minority populations (Fagot-Campagna *et al.*, 2000). In place of type 1 diabetes type 2 diabetes may soon become the more common form of childhood diabetes (Zimmet *et al.*, 2001).

Factors modifying the relationship between obesity and diabetes

A large number of factors influence the relationship between obesity and diabetes and many of them are closely inter-related. That obesity on its own is not sufficient to cause diabetes is apparent from the observation that 20 per cent of patients with type 2 diabetes are not obese and even in the highest risk group with high BMI and high waist–hip ratio over 80 per cent will escape type 2 diabetes (Colditz et al., 1995). Other factors include body fat distribution, duration of obesity, weight gain, age, physical activity, diet, the in utero environment, childhood stunting and genetic factors. Methodological issues are also important in examining the relationship between obesity and diabetes. Some of the observed increase in diabetes prevalence attributed to obesity could be related to more awareness and detection of type 2 diabetes, rather than a true increase in numbers (previous Diabetes UK estimates are that 50 per cent of patients do not know they have type 2 diabetes). The change in the diagnostic criteria for diabetes introduced by the American Diabetes Association in 1997, with less use of the oral glucose tolerance test and more emphasis on the fasting glucose, appear to underestimate the prevalence of diabetes in obese subjects who may have a relatively normal fasting blood glucose in the presence of a high post-load glucose (Melchionda et al., 2002; Richard et al., 2002).

Abdominal obesity may be an even better predictor of the development of type 2 diabetes than BMI (Larsson et al., 1984; Ohlson et al., 1985). The predictive value of high waist–hip ratios and high waist circumferences in mediating the risk of diabetes appears to be of most importance in those in the highest quintile of these measures (Chan et al., 1994) and perhaps in leaner subjects. For a given BMI many Asian populations have a much higher risk of type 2 diabetes, even at a BMI well within the normal range (Mather and Keen, 1985). WHO is currently studying the use of a more limited range of normal BMI ($18.5–22.9\,\mathrm{kg\,m^{-2}}$) in these groups together with use of waist circumference (James et al., 2001). The duration of exposure to obesity is an important modulator of the risk of diabetes. In Pima Indians, subjects whose BMI was greater than $30\,\mathrm{kg\,m^{-2}}$ for more than 10 years had over twice the risk of type 2 diabetes compared with those who had been obese for less than 5 years (Everhart et al., 1992). The epidemic of childhood obesity allied with the influence of obesity duration suggests both increasing frequency of diabetes and its earlier onset.

Weight gain during adult life acts in addition to BMI per se to modify the risk of diabetes. In the Health Professionals' Follow-up Study men who gained more than 13.5 kg over the five years of the study had a 4.5-fold increased risk of diabetes in comparison with those men who remained within 4.5 kg of their weight at entry to the study (Chan et al., 1994). Similar findings apply to women as described in the Nurses' Health Study where the relative risk of diabetes was 2.7 in those who gained 8–10.9 kg compared with those who were weight stable over a 14-year period (Colditz et al., 1995).

Alongside the epidemic of childhood obesity and diabetes there is also an epidemic of diabetes related to the ageing population. The prevalence of type 2 diabetes increases progressively with age peaking at 16.5 per cent in men and

12.8 per cent in women at age 75–84 years (Wilson and Kannel, 2002). Obesity rates plateau about 20 years earlier (Prescott-Clarke and Primatesta, 1999), but the age-related increases in total body fat and visceral adiposity make BMI a less good marker of adiposity in older age groups. Indeed, many normal weight elderly men and women are at high risk of type 2 diabetes due to increased visceral abdominal fat (Goodpaster et al., 2003). In the UK it is projected that due to population ageing by 2036 there will be 20 per cent more cases of type 2 diabetes than in 2000 (Bagust et al., 2002).

Decreasing levels of physical activity are undoubtedly implicated in the epidemic of obesity, but physical activity also has independent protective effects on the risk of diabetes. In the British Regional Heart Study, whilst BMI was the dominant risk factor for diabetes, men engaged in moderate levels of physical activity had a substantially reduced risk of diabetes, relative to the physically inactive men, even after adjustment for age and BMI (Perry et al., 1995). Similar data in women demonstrate a relative risk of type 2 diabetes of 0.67 in those who engaged in vigorous exercise at least once a week compared with women who did not exercise weekly (Manson et al., 1991). At least in terms of reducing the risk of type 2 diabetes it is probably better to be overweight and physically active, than to be normal weight and inactive (Wei et al., 1999).

Dietary factors appear to have effects independent of those on obesity on the development of type 2 diabetes. Increasing fat in the diet is associated with both obesity and the development of diabetes (West, 1978), but much of this link is explained simply by the high energy intake that accompanies high fat diets. However, some populations with high-fat diets (e.g. Eskimos and the Japanese) have a relatively low prevalence of diabetes compared with that expected from their obesity rates and this may be explained by a high intake of omega-3 polyunsaturated fatty acids (Malasanos and Stacpoole, 1991). A recent large prospective study of diet in women aged 34 to 59 years without diabetes at baseline and followed for 14 years found that total fat intake was not associated with risk of type 2 diabetes, but for a 5 per cent increase in energy from polyunsaturated fat, the relative risk was 0.63 and for a 2 per cent increase in energy from trans fatty acids the relative risk was 1.39 (Salmeron et al., 2001). The authors estimated that replacing energy derived from trans fatty acids with polyunsaturated fat would lead to a 40 per cent lower risk of type 2 diabetes.

Whilst the vast majority of studies either show diabetes rates rising as obesity prevalence climbs, or project such a rise in diabetes from the observed obesity prevalence, one Swedish population survey has not demonstrated this (Eliasson et al., 2002). From 1986 to 1999 the mean BMI in adults in northern Sweden increased from 25.3 to 26.2 kg m^{-2} and the prevalence of obesity rose from 11 to 15 per cent. However, in spite of the marked increase in obesity there was no increase in the prevalence of known diabetes. Dietary factors may account for some of this discrepant finding, with the diet over this period containing less saturated fat and having a lower glycaemic index. One additional observation was a decrease in waist–hip ratio (representing reduced visceral adiposity), perhaps also contributing to the absence of a BMI effect on diabetes. Findings such as these may mean that the gloomy picture of the diabetes epidemic painted by many authors is not quite as inevitable an outcome as projected.

In contrast, data from Australia show a dramatic increase in diabetes over the last 20 years, with a doubling of diabetes prevalence to its current value of 7.4 per cent (Dunstan et al., 2002). An additional 16.4 per cent had abnormal glucose tolerance. Although obesity rates in this population have increased, neither obesity nor changes in the age profile of the population fully explain the extent of the diabetes epidemic. It is likely that some of the other factors discussed above, including body fat distribution, duration of diabetes and physical activity account for this adverse pattern.

Whilst obesity is clearly important, other factors appear to influence the susceptibility both to weight gain and to the development of diabetes. The 'thrifty' gene hypothesis (Neel, 1962) suggests that the obese-type 2 diabetes mellitus genotype may have had some survival advantage, perhaps by favouring fat storage at times when food was abundant, so leading to improved survival during famines. However, this hypothesis remains an epidemiological explanation, with the exact genetic factors remaining unclear and no prospective data showing a survival advantage in subjects felt to have a thrifty genotype. Much recent discussion has centred on the potential importance of the *in utero* environment in the causation of later type 2 diabetes (Hales and Barker, 2001). This hypothesis, the 'thrifty' phenotype hypothesis suggests that the epidemiological associations between poor fetal and infant growth and the subsequent development of type 2 diabetes results from the effects of poor nutrition in early life, which produces permanent changes in glucose and insulin metabolism. These changes lead to reduced insulin secretion and increased insulin resistance and hence predispose to type 2 diabetes. The relative contribution of thrifty genes, a thrifty phenotype and later environmental factors (e.g. physical activity and diet) to obesity-related diabetes is not clear. Perhaps the trend for average birth weights to gradually increase in many populations indicates that the *in utero* environment is improving and this may mean reduced susceptibility to later diabetes. However, the explosion in childhood obesity is likely to outweigh the potentially beneficial birthweight effect in most populations.

One further adverse early life effect on susceptibility to obesity and probably also to later diabetes is childhood stunting. This remains common in lower income countries. Surveys in a number of countries show a significant association between stunting and overweight status in children of all countries (Popkin et al., 1996). With the transition from a lower income developing country to a more affluent developed one it is likely that the increased early stunting-mediated susceptibility to obesity will be compounded by later economic and social changes driving up obesity and diabetes rates.

Conclusions

There is no doubt that obesity is at present the major player in the increasing prevalence of type 2 diabetes. The current epidemic of obesity shows little sign of abating in most parts of the world and in contrast is still accelerating, particularly in children. Global predictions of the diabetes epidemic with 300 million patients with type 2 diabetes by 2025 are well on course (King *et al.*, 1998). Many of the factors that modify the relationship between obesity and diabetes, such as duration of obesity and physical activity levels are also changing adversely and are exacerbating the diabetes epidemic. The challenge for society is to reverse the ever-increasing prevalence of obesity.

References

Astrup A and Finer N (2000) Redefining type 2 diabetes: 'diabesity' or 'obesity dependent diabetes mellitus'? *Obes Rev* **1**, 57–9.

Bagust A, Hopkinson PK, Maslove L and Currie CJ (2002) The projected health care burden of Type 2 diabetes in the UK from 2000 to 2060. *Diabet Med* **19**, 1–5.

Bell AC, Ge K and Popkin BM (2001) Weight gain and its predictors in Chinese adults. *Int J Obes* **25**, 1079–86.

Berrios X, Koponen T, Huiguang T *et al.* (1997) Distribution and prevalence of major risk factors of noncommunicable diseases in selected countries: the WHO Inter-Health Programme. *Bull World Health Org* **75**, 99–108.

Chan JM, Rimm EB, Colditz GA *et al.* (1994) Obesity, fat distribution, and weight gain as risk factors for clinical diabetes in men. *Diabetes Care* **17**, 961–9.

Chinn S and Rona RJ (2001) Prevalence and trends in overweight and obesity in three cross sectional studies of British Children, 1974–94. *Br Med J* **322**, 24–6.

Colditz GA, Willett WC, Rotnitzky A and Manson JE (1995) Weight gain as a risk factor for clinical diabetes mellitus in women. *Ann Intern Med* **122**, 481–6.

Dunstan DW, Zimmet PZ, Welborn TA *et al.* (2002) The rising prevalence of diabetes and impaired glucose tolerance: the Australian Diabetes, Obesity and Lifestyle Study. *Diabetes Care* **25**, 829–34.

Eliasson M, Lindahl B, Lundberg V and Stegmayr B (2002) No increase in the prevalence of known diabetes between 1986 and 1999 in subjects 25–64 years of age in northern Sweden. *Diabet Med* **19**, 874–80.

Esparza J, Fox C, Harper IT, *et al.* (2000) Daily energy expenditure in Mexican and USA Pima Indians: low physical activity as a possible cause of obesity. *Int J Obes* **24**, 55–9.

Everhart JE, Pettitt DJ, Bennett PH and Knowler WC (1992) Duration of obesity increases the incidence of NIDDM. *Diabetes* **41**, 235–40.

Fagot-Campagna A, Pettitt DJ, Engelgau MM, *et al.* (2000) Type 2 diabetes among North American children and adolescents: an epidemiologic review and a public health perspective. *J Pediatr* **136**, 664–72.

Flegal KM, Carroll MD, Ogden CL and Johnson CL (2002) Prevalence and trends in obesity among US adults, 1999–2000. *JAMA* **288**, 1723–7.

Ford ES, Williamson DF and Liu S (1997) Weight change and diabetes incidence: findings from a national cohort of US adults. *Am J Epidemiol* **146**, 214–22.

Goodpaster BH, Krishnaswami S, Resnick H, *et al.* (2003) Association between regional adipose tissue distribution and both type 2 diabetes and impaired glucose tolerance in elderly men and women. *Diabetes Care* **26**, 372–9.

Hales CN and Barker DJ (2001) The thrifty phenotype hypothesis. *Br Med Bull* **60**, 5–20.

Han TS, van Leer EM, Seidell JC and Lean MEJ (1995) Waist circumference action levels in the identification of cardiovascular risk factors: prevalence study in a random sample. *Br Med J* **311**, 1401–1405.

Hill JO, Wyatt HR, Reed GW and Peters JC (2003) Obesity and the environment: where do we go from here? *Science* **299**, 853–5.

James PT, Leach R, Kalamara E and Shayeghi M (2001) The worldwide obesity epidemic. *Obes Res* **9**, 228S–233S.

Jung RT (1997) In *Textbook of Diabetes*, Pickup JC and Williams G (eds), Blackwell Science Ltd, Oxford, pp. 19.4–19.5.

King H, Aubert RE and Herman WH (1998) Global burden of diabetes, 1995–2025: prevalence, numerical estimates, and projections. *Diabetes Care* **21**, 1414–31.

Kotani K, Nishida M, Yamashita S *et al.* (1997) Two decades of annual medical examinations in Japanese obese children: do obese children grow into obese adults? *Int J Obes* **21**, 912–21.

Larsson B, Svardsudd K, Welin L *et al.* (1984) Abdominal adipose tissue distribution, obesity, and risk of cardiovascular disease and death: 13 year follow up of participants in the study of men born in 1913. *Br Med J* **288**, 1401–4.

Leibson CL, Williamson DF, Melton LJ 3rd *et al.* (2001) Temporal trends in BMI among adults with diabetes. *Diabetes Care* **24**, 1584–9.

Malasanos TH and Stacpoole PW (1991) Biological effects of omega-3 fatty acids in diabetes mellitus. *Diabetes Care* **14**, 1160–79.

Manson JE, Rimm EB, Stampfer MJ *et al.* (1991) Physical activity and incidence of non-insulin-dependent diabetes mellitus in women. *Lancet* **338**, 774–8.

Mather HM and Keen H (1985) The Southall Diabetes Survey: prevalence of known diabetes in Asians and Europeans. *Br Med J* **291**, 1081–4.

McTigue KM, Garrett JM and Popkin BM (2002) The natural history of the development of obesity in a cohort of young U.S. adults between 1981 and 1998. *Ann Intern Med* **136**, 857–64.

Melchionda N, Forlani G, Marchesini G *et al.* (2002) WHO and ADA criteria for the diagnosis of diabetes mellitus in relation to body mass index. Insulin sensitivity and secretion in resulting subcategories of glucose tolerance. *Int J Obes* **26**, 90–6.

Mokdad AH, Ford ES, Bowman BA *et al.* (2000) Diabetes trends in the US: 1990–1998. *Diabetes Care* **23**, 1278–83.

Mokdad AH, Ford ES, Bowman BA *et al.* (2003) Prevalence of obesity, diabetes, and obesity-related health risk factors, 2001. *JAMA* **289**, 76–9.

Mokdad AH, Serdula MK, Dietz WH *et al.* (1999) The spread of the obesity epidemic in the United States, 1991–1998. *JAMA* **282**, 1519–22.

Neel J (1962) Diabetes mellitus: a thrifty genotype rendered detrimental by progress? *Am J Hum Genet* **14**, 353–62.

Ogden CL, Flegal KM, Carroll MD and Johnson CL (2002) Prevalence and trends in overweight among US children and adolescents, 1999–2000. *JAMA* **288**, 1728–32.

Ohlson LO, Larsson B, Svardsudd K *et al.* (1985) The influence of body fat distribution on the incidence of diabetes mellitus. 13.5 years of follow-up of the participants in the study of men born in 1913. *Diabetes* **34**, 1055–8.

Perry IJ, Wannamethee SG, Walker MK *et al.* (1995) Prospective study of risk factors for development of non-insulin dependent diabetes in middle aged British men. *Br Med J* **310**, 560–4.

Pinhas-Hamiel O, Dolan LM, Daniels SR *et al.* (1996) Increased incidence of non-insulin-dependent diabetes mellitus among adolescents. *J Pediatr* **128**, 608–15.

Popkin BM, Richards MK and Montiero CA (1996) Stunting is associated with overweight in children of four nations that are undergoing the nutrition transition. *J Nutr* **126**, 3009–16.

Prescott-Clarke P and Primatesta P (1999) *Health Survey for England 1997*. HMSO, London.

Ravussin E, Valencia ME, Esparza J *et al.* (1994) Effects of a traditional lifestyle on obesity in Pima Indians. *Diabetes Care* **17**, 1067–74.

Richard JL, Sultan A, Daures JP *et al.* (2002) Diagnosis of diabetes mellitus and intermediate glucose abnormalities in obese patients based on ADA (1997) and WHO (1985) criteria. *Diabet Med* **19**, 292–9.

Salmeron J, Hu FB, Manson JE *et al.* (2001) Dietary fat intake and risk of type 2 diabetes in women. *Am J Clin Nutr* **73**, 1019–26.

Webster JD, Hesp R and Garrow JS (1984) The composition of excess weight in obese women estimated by body density, total body water and total body potassium. *Hum Nutr Clin Nutr* **38**, 299–306.

Wei M, Gibbons LW, Mitchell TL *et al.* (1999) The association between cardiorespiratory fitness and impaired fasting glucose and type 2 diabetes mellitus in men. *Ann Intern Med* **130**, 89–96.

West K (1978) *Epidemiology of Diabetes and its Vascular Lesions*. Elsevier, New York.

Willett WC, Dietz WH and Colditz GA (1999) Guidelines for healthy weight. *N Engl J Med* **341**, 427–34.

Wilson PW and Kannel WB (2002) Obesity, diabetes, and risk of cardiovascular disease in the elderly. *Am J Geriatr Cardiol* **11**, 119–23,125.

World Health Organization (2000) Obesity: preventing and managing the global epidemic. Report of a WHO consultation. WHO, Geneva.

Zimmet P (1982) Type 2 (non-insulin-dependent) diabetes – an epidemiological overview. *Diabetologia* **22**, 399–411.

Zimmet P, Alberti KG and Shaw J (2001) Global and societal implications of the diabetes epidemic. *Nature* **414**, 782–7.

2

The Genetics of Human Obesity

Victor J. Lawrence and **Tahseen Chowdhury**

Introduction

In recent years there has been rapid progress in our understanding of single gene disorders. The genetic basis of the more important diseases of the 21st century, such as obesity and diabetes, however, remains elusive.

The rapidly changing field of obesity genetics renders any 'State of the Art' review obsolete even before publication. Fortunately, rapidly updated information on specific genes and syndromes is readily available by searching on-line databases such as the Online Mendelian Inheritance in Man (OMIN; http://www.ncbi.nlm.nih.gov/omim/) or http://obesitygene.pbrc.edu/

In this chapter, we intend to illustrate some of the major challenges facing research in this area, to describe some of the methods and their limitations currently available and how, in principle, they may be used to advance our understanding of this heterogeneous condition.

Why has the genetics of obesity been difficult to study?

Defining the phenotype

One of the first problems faced in attempting to define a genetic basis for obesity is deciding what kind of effect (phenotype) we seek to examine. Obesity is a heterogeneous clinical disorder. Whilst it can be conveniently defined and clinically measured in terms of elevated body mass index (BMI), this is a definition chosen to define people or populations thought to be most at risk from its complications. It is a composite measure of body mass in relation to height, and

Obesity and Diabetes. Edited by Anthony H. Barnett and Sudhesh Kumar
© 2004 John Wiley & Sons, Ltd   ISBN: 0-470-84898-7

is dependant on fat mass, lean tissue, bone and fluid mass, all of which may be subject to independent genetic or environmental influence. As BMI is not based on any specific pathophysiological process, it is an inherently unsatisfactory endpoint when looking for the effects of single genes or gene clusters.

For this reason, some studies have investigated genetic influence on more specific measures of body composition such as percentage body fat, total fat mass, visceral fat mass, subcutaneous fat mass or waist–hip ratio. These variables can be measured by bioelectrical impedance, computed tomography, magnetic resonance imaging, dual-energy X-ray absorbimetry scanning or underwater weighing. Whilst there is often a reasonable correlation with BMI (e.g. 0.83 between BMI and fat mass in one recent study; Deng *et al.*, 2002), the strength of such relationships varies unpredictably according to sex and age. Furthermore, these variables are not easy to measure in the large populations required for genetic study and even then may result from complex individual interrelationships between factors such as energy intake, age, sex, resting, voluntary and diet-induced energy expenditure and environmental (e.g. dietary, psychological and sociopolitical) influences.

Some researchers have attempted to examine the effects of putative genes on basic 'intermediary' biological measures such as resting metabolic rate, which may be affected by 'candidate' genes such as those encoding mitochondrial uncoupling proteins (UCPs) or elements of the sympathetic nervous system such as the β_3-adrenoceptor. This approach also has drawbacks; subjects with established obesity tend to have high rather than low resting metabolic rates, for example. Using more complex constructs such as the difference between predicted and measured metabolic rate is possible but moving away from the clinical phenotype may mean that people displaying abnormalities are not obese.

Gene interactions

Having chosen an appropriate phenotype upon which to build a specific hypothesis, it is then necessary to consider the potential for a range of temporal and other para-genetic factors to influence gene expression and effect. These include the potential for genes to act at critical periods during different developmental stages, the effect that age related fat accretion will have on phenotype and sexual dimorphism of lipid storage (e.g. 'gynoid versus android' distributions and total body fat differences between males and females). Epistasis between genes, whereby the effect of one gene may be modified by other genes and interactions between genes and environment may further complicate the picture. Conversely, 'phenocopies' of obesity may exist without possessing the genotype sought by any particular study hypothesis thus reducing the power to detect genetic influence.

Thus, despite the fascinating physiological (and pharmacological) insights into the pathways involved in body weight regulation provided by unravelling the aetiology of some forms of monogenic obesity, it is increasingly clear that ultimate genetic understanding of common forms of human obesity will rely upon dissection of many small effects of multiple genetic variants superimposed on a permissive environment.

Many of these principals are illustrated by recent progress in understanding the genetics of Bardet–Biedl syndrome (BBS). First, more accurate phenotyping has permitted this syndrome to be separated from the Lawrence–Moon syndrome, which appears to be a distinct entity. Second, it is apparent that more than one genetic abnormality may be responsible for the observed abnormalities in this condition; at the time of writing, at least six loci (BBS 1–6) on different chromosomes have been identified with subtly different effects on phenotype such as stature, body weight or pattern of polydactyly (Iannello *et al.*, 2002). Third, in at least some forms of the disease, it may be necessary to have up to three distinct mutations (tri-allelic inheritance) for full disease expression, illustrating the principle of epistasis between disease alleles (Katsanis *et al.*, 2001).

How much of obesity is genetic?

Given that the explosion in obesity prevalence over the past 20 years is likely to have taken place against a background of relatively constant population genetic structure, the question of to what extent obesity is subject to genetic influence is one that merits careful consideration. Many studies have attempted to resolve the population variance of a specific obesity phenotype into genetic, environmental and unknown (or residual) effects. In principle, the total observed phenotypic variance, V_p may be considered to be due to the sum of genetic variance (V_g), shared environmental variance (V_c) and an unknown residual (unshared environmental) variance (V_e) such that $V_p = V_g + V_c + V_e$. The percentage genetic inheritability of the trait in question is represented by the term V_g/V_p. Modifications of this simple model to attempt detection of gene–gene and gene–environment interactions and the application of complex multivariate computational modelling in different study populations are reviewed in detail elsewhere (Bouchard *et al.*, 1998).

Twin studies

Twin studies allow separation of genetic and environmental components of variance since monozygotic (MZ) twins share 100 per cent of their genes whilst non-identical dizygotic (DZ) twins share 50 per cent on average. The fact that there is discordance in the prevalence of obesity between MZ and DZ twins raised together supports the concept of genetic heritability of obesity if it is assumed that twins share exactly the same environmental influences (although it has been suggested that MZ twins may share more environmental influences than DZ twins; Hebebrand *et al.*, 2001). Total genetic variance may then be subdivided into two components; *additive variance*, which results from the sum of contributions of many alleles at different loci and *non-additive* effects, which are principally determined by the dominance of one allele over another at the same locus. It follows that an additive model is suggested when intrapair correlations of DZ twins are half that of MZ twins and a non-additive model is suggested when DZ twins have substantially less than half the intrapair correlations of variance of MZ twins.

Comparison of MZ twins raised together with MZ twins raised apart probably represent the ideal study group. However, such study populations are difficult to find and, even then, twins will have shared the same intra-uterine environment (which may be important on the basis of the Barker hypothesis; Hales and Barker, 1992). Furthermore, there may be indirect genetic effects in operation and the effect of environment may be underestimated as certain environmental conditions are likely to be common to both twins (e.g. the general availability of fast foods).

One study (Stunkard *et al.*, 1986) assessed body mass index in a sample of 1974 MZ and 2097 DZ male twin pairs and found concordance in MZ twins to be around 0.8. This was twice as high as that in DZ twins both at age 20 and at 25 year follow up. Others (Fabsitz *et al.*, 1992), however, report an age-specific effect such that only 40 per cent of the genetic factors that influence body weight at the age of 20 continue to do so by the age of 48.

One of the best estimates of obesity heritability, accounting for 67 per cent of variance, is derived from the Virginia cohort of 30 000 twins, their parents, siblings, spouses and children (McLaughlin, 1991). Overall, weighted mean BMI correlations have been calculated to be 0.74 for MZ twins, 0.32 for DZ twins, 0.25 for siblings, 0.19 for parent–offspring pairs, 0.06 for adoptive relatives and 0.12 for spouses (Maes *et al.*, 1997) and the overall relative risk of siblings lies within the approximate range 3–7 (Allison *et al.*, 1996).

The heritability of gene–environment interactions thought capable of leading to obesity has also been demonstrated using MZ twin populations (Bouchard *et al.*, 1998). The principle of this approach lies in the variability of individual response to environmental perturbation (in this case, weight change in response to either overfeeding or to increasing exercise with energy intake held constant). Where the response differs more between than within pairs of MZ twins, it may be assumed that genetic factors are responsible. These studies have demonstrated considerably more variance (in some cases by up to a factor of 3–6 depending on the variable studied) between rather than within twin pairs for a number of measures of body fat accumulation, distribution and energy expenditure. This supports the hypothesis that individual responses to diet and exercise have a substantial genetic component and may go some way to explaining the observation of increasing obesity prevalence on the background of a relatively constant gene pool. To what extent there is a genetic basis for the fact that obese people of similar BMI may be variably subject to obesity-related complications such as type 2 diabetes (independent of other risk factors) is unclear.

Adoption studies

Adoption studies rely on the assumption that differences between adopted children and their adoptive parents/siblings are due to genetic differences and differences between them and their biological families are due to environmental influences. However, adoption studies are complicated by problems relating to ascertainment of the biological father (false paternity being found in some 8 per cent of individuals in many studies), the effects of selective or late placement of the child and the inherent inability of such studies to assess gene–environment interactions.

Thus there has been considerable heterogeneity in published estimates of the heritability of obesity depending for the large part on the type of study and population used. Whereas twin studies are thought in general to overestimate the true heritability, adoption studies are thought to underestimate it. Thus, estimates for obesity heritability from adoption studies are lower than those from twin studies and range from around 0.2–0.6 with two very large family studies providing estimates of 0.3–0.4 (Maes *et al.*, 1997).

Is there a major gene for obesity?

Several large population studies using segregation techniques predicted the existence of one or more 'major' recessive gene effects independent of the discovery of any specific obesity gene (Rice *et al.*, 1996; Borecki *et al.*, 1998). Studies based on candidate genes or obesity syndromes have reported concentration of mutations thought capable of contributing to the obese phenotype amongst the obese population at large.

Segregation studies

Segregation studies test the hypothesis that there exist one or more (uncharacterized) recessive genes with major effects on a specific obesity phenotype. Support for a putative large (recessively inherited) genetic component of obesity was initially suggested by observations that the obese proband in many studies often demonstrates a far greater degree of obesity than either their parents or siblings. If it is hypothesized that the parents carry heterozygous mutations, one would expect that the frequency of transmission of a recessive allele from a homozygous dominant, homozygous recessive or heterozygous parent would be close to 0, 100 and 50 per cent, respectively. Evidence for one or more major recessive genes accounting for some 45 per cent of the variance in fat mass being so transmitted has been reported in 6 per cent of individuals in one study population (Rice *et al.*, 1993). In addition, reports of major gene effects accounting for some 37–42 per cent of the variance in regional fat distribution have raised the intriguing possibility of one major gene effect subtending total and visceral fat accumulation with another influencing subcutaneous fat topography elsewhere (Bouchard *et al.*, 1998).

It has been suggested recently that 2.9 per cent of the general obese population are heterozygotes for at least one of the six autosomal recessive genetic defects present in BBS (Croft *et al.*, 1995) and mutations in the gene coding for the MC-4 receptor may be present in up to 4 per cent of the obese (Vaisse *et al.*, 2000). However, it remains to be seen whether these mutations are biologically important in the sense of leading to alterations in protein function and their true significance is currently debated (Jacobson *et al.*, 2002).

How to identify obesity genes

The ultimate goal of obesity genetics is to identify a gene defect found exclusively in obese patients producing a functional variant (for example with altered or absent protein function, the so-called 'smoking gun'). The approaches that may be used in the attempt to identify such mutations depend to a large extent on what is known *a priori* about the function of the normal protein product.

The candidate gene approach

If there is knowledge that an abnormal protein product is capable of causing obesity (or counteracting it), evidence for the presence of mutations in the responsible 'candidate gene' may be sought in the population at large and related to measures of adiposity. In general, a gene may be considered a candidate gene for obesity based either on knowledge of its physiological role or because it becomes implicated in one or more forms of experimental or naturally occurring animal or human obesity.

Candidate genes based on physiological function

The candidate gene approach has been applied directly to examine the role of a number of polymorphisms in genes known to encode proteins with a role in energy homeostasis including the Trp64Arg mutation of the β_3-adrenoceptor, mutations of the mitochondrial UCPs1-3 and lipoprotein lipase. Unfortunately, the results of this direct approach have often been confusing. Two meta-analyses published in the same year of the Trp64Arg β_3-adrenoceptor mutation, with data from over 40 studies of 7000 subjects, have concluded with rather different assessments of its significance (Allison *et al.*, 1998; Fujisawa *et al.*, 1998). A common reason for discordant results is that differences in polymorphism frequency in different populations may give rise to population stratification effects. Furthermore, the presence of a polymorphism may not necessarily lead to alterations in protein structure or function and even if the protein product is altered, this may not always lead to obesity (an effect seen with certain null mutations of the MC-4 receptor; Hirschhorn and Altshuler, 2002). In addition, publication bias towards positive results may overestimate the strength of an association. Conversely, true candidate gene effects may be missed if they are modulated by the presence of gene–environment interactions (such as those reported to occur between exercise and polymorphisms in the β_2-adrenoceptor gene; Macho-Azcarate *et al.*, 2002) or have effects specific to certain ethnic groups or sexes.

At the time of writing, there have been positive reports in human populations of significant association between some 58 candidate genes and various measures of body weight/body composition/energy expenditure/serum leptin and temporal changes in body weight, although the evidence is somewhat conflicting for a number of these associations (e.g. leptin receptor, β_3-adrenoceptor, lipoprotein lipase, UCP-1–3, pro-opiomelanocortin (POMC) tumour necrosis factor and peroxisome proliferator-activated receptor-γ; Rankinen *et al.*, 2002).

The search for candidate genes amongst animal and human forms of monogenic or syndromic obesity has often been more illuminating.

Single gene defects

Following the identification of the leptin gene mutation in *ob/ob* mice, three highly obese children from two consanguineous but unrelated families who carried non-functioning mutations of the leptin gene were identified from a study population characterized by extreme obesity. The defect in both pedigrees was a homozygous deletion of a single guanine nucleotide at codon 133 of the leptin gene which resulted in a frameshift mutation and truncated protein (Montague *et al.*, 1997). Although immunoreactive leptin concentrations are typically increased rather than decreased in obesity suggesting that this defect *per se* is certainly not a common cause of obesity in the general population, this discovery led to intensification of the search amongst other forms of both syndromic and non-syndromic forms of obesity for other candidate genes. Mutations of six genes have been characterized in human forms of monogenic obesity (Table 2.1). It is noteworthy that five of these six human monogenic obesity genes encode proteins involved in the leptin pathway of appetite regulation (see Figure 2.1). Whether this is because this pathway is the dominant pathway of weight regulation, or whether it results from poor understanding of alternative regulatory pathways is not yet clear.

Syndromic obesity

Prader–Willi syndrome   Long known to result from the deletion of a paternally inherited 4–4.5-Mb segment of chromosome 15, Prader–Willi syndrome

Table 2.1   Monogenic forms of human obesity

Gene product	Human phenotype	Linkage with common human obesity	Association with common human obesity
Leptin	1. Hypogonadotrophic hypogonadism 2. Immune dysfunction 3. Hypothalamic–pituitary–thyroid abnormalities 4. Hyperinsulinaemia (in proportion to fat mass in humans) 5. Possible peripheral effects of leptin (e.g. vascular) 6. Increased glucocorticoid production in animals but not in man	Yes	Yes
Leptin receptor	1. Leptin deficiency phenotype described above 2. Growth retardation 3. Secondary hypothyroidism	Yes	Conflicting results
POMC	1. Adrenocortical insufficiency 2. Abnormal pigmentation	Yes	No
MC4 Receptor	1. Non-syndromic obesity of widely varying extent 2. Hyperinsulinaemia	Yes	Conflicting results
Pro-hormone convertase 1	1. abnormal glucose homeostasis 2. hypogonadotrophic hypogonadism 3. hypocortisolism 4. elevated plasma proinsulin and POMC concentrations 5. low insulin levels	No	No
Sim1	1. Massive overeating with normal energy expenditure 2. Likely to be due to developmental abnormalities of hypothalamic PVN	No	No

POMC, pro-opiomelanocortin; PVN, paraventricular nucleus.

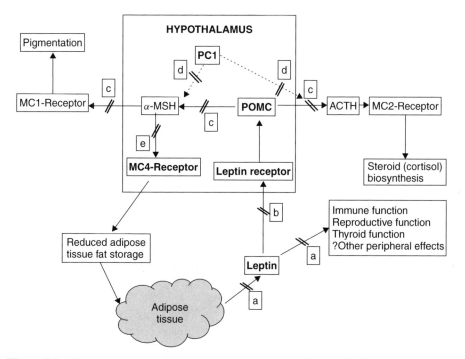

Figure 2.1 Protein products of genes known to be associated with human monogenic forms of obesity are shown in bold (see also Table 2.1). POMC, pro-opiomelanocortin; α-MSH, α-melanocyte stimulating hormone; PC-1, pro-hormone convertase-1; MC-1, 2 and 4, melanocortin-1, 2 and 4 receptors. The *ob* gene mutation causing an absence of leptin is represented by (a) and leptin receptor mutations by (b). POMC mutations (c) disrupt cortisol biosynthesis and α-MSH-induced pigmentation as well as appetite regulation whereas PC-1 mutations (d) do not appear to have a major effect on pigmentation but instead lead to hypogonadism and glucoregulatory abnormalities. MC-4 mutations (e) are notable for causing little disturbance to regulatory pathways other than appetite and thus best represent common forms of non-syndromic obesity.

(PWS) exhibits the interesting phenomenon of 'genetic imprinting'; when the deletion is inherited from the mother, Angelman syndrome (which does not have obesity as a cardinal feature) results but when the deletion is inherited from the father, loss of expression of one or more of the many C/D box, small nucleolar RNAs (snoRNAs) encoded within the paternally expressed small nuclear riboprotein N (SNRPN) locus permits the PWS phenotype to be expressed. Generalized disruptions to the normal paternal expression of genes in this region (such as maternal uniparental disomy 15, imprinting centre mutations and specific balanced translocations with breakpoints within the paternally expressed SNRPN locus have also been reported to lead to PWS phenotype expression (Nicholls and Knepper, 2001). The precise cellular function of snoRNAs has yet to be determined but they are thought to play a part in the cellular localization and processing of RNA transcripts. To date, no link between common forms of human obesity and these abnormalities has been reported.

BBS   This syndrome, until recently considered to be autosomal recessive in nature and frequently confused with the Lawrence–Moon syndrome, is diagnosed on the basis of the presence of a constellation of major and minor features of which obesity (in 72–96 per cent of cases, preferentially distributed in the trunk and proximal limbs), retinal dystrophy, polydactyly, learning disabilities, male hypogonadism and renal abnormalities are most characteristic (Katsanis *et al.*, 2001). BBS prevalence varies widely, ranging from as little as 1:160 000 in ethnic Europeans to as much as 1:13 000 in populations such as Kuwait and Newfoundland where a founder effect has been postulated. Diagnostic difficulty has been compounded by a high degree of phenotypic variability, as much within as between families segregating the condition.

Since 1993, a combination of genome wide linkage scans in affected pedigrees and pooled sample homozygosity approaches have led to identification of the approximate position of six loci on chromosomes 16 (BBS2), 11 (BBS1), 3 (BBS3), 15 (BBS4), 2 (BBS5) and 20 (BBS6) with at least one further putative locus (BBS7) accounting for the 19–42 per cent of cases not explained by any of the above loci. BBS6 was first to be directly implicated in 2000 (Katsanis *et al.*, 2000; Slavotinek *et al.*, 2000) following its cloning as the gene responsible for a rather similar condition, the much rarer McKusick–Kaufman syndrome (MKKS). This knowledge, applied with increasingly detailed phenotyping, has permitted reclassification of some individuals previously thought to have MKKS as actually having BBS. Positional cloning of the BBS1, 2 and 4 loci has followed apace. Whereas BBS1 mutations appear sufficient for the development of classical BBS (Mykytyn *et al.*, 2002), it has been suggested that three specific mutations at the other loci may be necessary for disease expression, at least in some cases (tri-allelic inheritance). Intense effort is currently underway to elucidate the precise function of these gene products in the hope that they may shed light on new mechanisms of body weight regulation.

New candidate genes may be identified by detailed 'expression profiling' whereby expression is found to be qualitatively (e.g. in appropriate tissues) or quantitatively (e.g. variable gene expression under different nutrient or energy balance conditions) consistent with a role in body weight regulation. Alternatively, loci which become implicated in obesity by the use of 'positional' genetic approaches may then be further investigated using the candidate gene approach.

Positional approaches

Positional genetic techniques require no special previous knowledge of the function of an individual genomic region but implicate it in the causation of obesity purely on the grounds that identifiable markers in the region are found in obese phenotypes more frequently than would be expected by chance (i.e. they *segregate* in obesity and are identified in families by linkage or in populations by genetic association).

In practice, there is often a sequence of investigation using positional (described below) and then candidate approaches termed the 'positional candidate approach'. After identification of a region of interest using linkage studies in families, the genomic area of interest may be 'fine mapped' using techniques such as linkage disequilibrium (LD) to an area a few tens or hundred thousand base pairs in length (Figure 2.2). Subsequent association studies may attempt direct detection of an increased prevalence of a mutation (signalled either by a marker close to the mutation or a specific mutation itself) in affected individuals (probands) relative to unaffected population controls. Candidate studies then focus on genes with a plausible role in body weight regulation in the genomic region thus identified.

This 'positional candidate' approach may become more productive in its application to complex polygenic disease following publication of the human genome sequences. Functional annotation of the human genome sequence, now underway, may speed identification of possible candidate genes in stretches of genomic DNA identified by positional approaches. Furthermore, recent enhancements of single nucleotide polymorphism maps (Sachidanandam *et al.*, 2001) will provide many more identifiable genetic markers than have been available hitherto and may thus confer greater precision to gene mapping.

Once identified, further evidence for the potential role of a particular candidate gene in regulation of body weight may be sought from manipulation of the gene in animal models (e.g. transgenic or knockout models). Indeed, where the

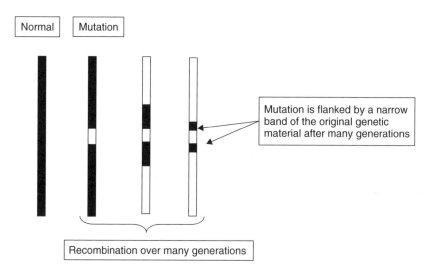

Figure 2.2 Linkage disequilibrium. A disease mutation initially arising on an ancestral haplotype becomes flanked by progressively smaller remnants of the original haplotype that are in LD with it and thus tend not to become separated from it by recombination events. These remnants may contain sequences which can be used to mark the position of the disease locus in a later generation. Although the detection of sequences derived from the ancestral haplotype may become more difficult after many generations, the precision of localization may be increased.

function of a locus revealed in association or LD studies is poorly understood, this may be vital in order to show that the proposed mutation is causative rather than simply being itself in linkage equilibrium with the real disease locus.

Linkage studies

Linkage is said to occur if two different alleles are passed to a subsequent generation in a proportion different to that expected by chance alone and is therefore a technique applied to family pedigrees rather than to cases and population controls. If two loci are completely linked (which usually means that they are very close together on the same chromosome), they will nearly always be passed together via the gametes to the offspring. Thus no new combinations of these two alleles will be found to have occurred during meiosis in the transmitted chromosome. Where similar alleles at the two loci are completely unlinked, the alleles assort independently in meiosis and 50 per cent of the offspring will have chromosomes with combinations not found in the parental strain. In practice, the proportion of new genotypes will be between 0 and 50 per cent depending on the recombination percentage present (the number of gametes with a recombination that separates two particular parental alleles divided by the total number). Clearly, the closer the two gene loci (or a gene and a marker locus), the less likely it is for a recombination event to separate them. By convention, a 1 per cent recombination frequency implies a distance of 1 centimorgan (cM) at least for differences less than 10 cM and this equates (depending on the region of the genome) to some 1 million base pairs in distance. By detecting linkage with polymorphic markers whose location is known, it is possible to use this technique to infer the approximate location of a disease susceptibility gene.

In principle, genetic linkage may be sought between a particular marker variant and phenotype or throughout the entire genome, the latter requiring no assumptions to be made about gene function. However, the sheer scale of this endeavour must be appreciated. Typically, a genome scan might utilize some 300–400 polymorphic markers to localize linkage (with a given confidence interval, say 95 per cent) to an area spanning approximately 10–20 cM (typically around 10–20 million base pairs). This genomic region may contain more than 200 genes, 60 000 common variants and many other rarer variants in intronic, exonic and regulatory sequences (McCarthy, 2002). It is clear from this that finer mapping techniques must then be used if there is to be any realistic prospect of cloning a specific gene.

The statistical significance of a linkage signal is denoted by the log odds likelihood ratio difference (LOD) score, which is the logarithm of the likelihood of the odds that two loci are linked compared with the likelihood of the odds for independent assortment. Correct interpretation of linkage signals relies critically on understanding the precise meaning of a LOD score to avoid inadvertent type 1 error. Whilst a LOD score of 3 for the effect of a single genotype on a single phenotype denotes a nominal p value of less than 0.0001, when repeated for multiple markers in a typical genome linkage scan, this equates to a true p value of around 0.09 and thus fails to reach classically defined statistical significance. It has been recommended that adopting LOD score thresholds of 3.3–3.8 to define definite linkage will result in less than 5 per cent probability of type 1 error over a whole genome scan comprising 300–400 marker loci whilst linkage signals with LOD scores between 1.9 and 3.3 are best considered 'suggestive' and worthy of further investigation (Lander and Kruglyak, 1995).

Limitations of traditional linkage analysis include its reliance on assumptions about disease transmission (genetic architecture) and the fact that linkage signals may be hard to detect when the gene in question contributes only marginally to the phenotype. The use of special relationships such as discordant sibling pairs has been used to circumvent these problems to some extent but, even with the advent of more complex study designs and elaborate computational methods (including models robust to assumptions about mode of inheritance such as non-parametric linkage analysis) it is still not possible to model the involvement of more than two disease loci and this is especially problematic in human obesity where disease susceptibility may depend more on particular configurations of more than one variant (as with calpain 10 in type 2 diabetes; Altshuler *et al.*, 2000) than on the presence or absence of a single variant.

At the time of writing, human genome scans in various ethnic populations have uncovered obesity loci on chromosomes 2 (containing the POMC gene), 5, 10 (confirmed in multiple ethnic populations), 11 and 20 (Clement *et al.*, 2002). To date, and probably for all the reasons discussed above, none of these linkage signals has led to the identification of a specific polymorphism that is associated with obesity in the general population.

Association studies

In contrast to linkage studies, association studies aim to detect co-segregation of a marker with a specific obesity phenotype in closely matched samples of affected and non-affected individuals who need not be related.

The simplest application of association is its use in testing the hypothesis that a specific polymorphism in a candidate gene is present in obese probands at a frequency greater than would be expected by chance (using χ^2 or similar tests) and is thus either causal or at least capable of conferring susceptibility to the development of obesity. It is clearly essential that controls and probands are from closely matched populations so that the overall population polymorphism frequency is similar, otherwise a positive result may occur due to population stratification. Where there is no obvious candidate gene, controls and obese probands may be genotyped for the presence of one or more marker alleles and differences in respective frequencies are compared to determine whether particular markers are significantly associated with the phenotype of interest.

Association studies have traditionally been used further to evaluate signals detected by linkage methods and the greater *a priori* likelihood of a true association confers additional statistical confidence in a positive result. As they are usually more convenient to perform and can localize genes with only moderate or small effects on phenotype, association studies are increasingly being used as a first line of investigation, significant association suggesting that the allele either affects the phenotype of interest or at least is close enough to be in linkage disequilibrium with the allele that is actually responsible.

As with linkage studies, there are considerable inherent problems in determining the significance of an apparently positive finding and the literature is littered with uncorroborated reports of significant association, many of which are likely to prove spurious. Factors that have led to poor replication in association studies include latent population stratification, lack of detailed and accurate ascertainment of phenotype and lack of power to confirm or refute an association especially where there may be multiple single nucleotide polymorphisms (SNPs) in intronic, exonic, regulatory and upstream regions of the locus all of which require investigation in multiple populations before disease relevance may confidently be excluded (Hirschhorn and Altshuler, 2002).

Linkage disequilibrium

Linkage disequilibrium (Figure 2.2) is defined as the non-random association between two alleles at two different loci on the same chromosome. Although similar to linkage and based on the same fundamental genetic principles, the method is population rather than pedigree based and has the distinct advantage of being able to localize a linkage signal with far greater precision than is possible with traditional linkage alone (Jorde, 2000). When a gene mutation first occurs in an individual, it forms part of a unique haplotype, which tends to dissipate over many successive generations as recombination events dislodge alleles at loci on the same chromosome (Figure 2.2). As with linkage, loci situated furthest away from the disease gene are most subject to separation from it during meiosis. After many generations (assuming non-lethality and lack of effect on reproductive potential) all that is left of the original chromosome in descendents is the disease gene flanked by a few alleles from the original haplotype which can be used to mark its position. The ideal circumstances for fine LD mapping are encountered in founder communities (e.g. North-American Hutterites, Amish, Finnish or French-Canadian populations) because it is likely that the disease mutation was introduced by a single individual, producing the potential for a strong association between the disease and a specific haplotype in the current generation. Thus LD in such a population may be somewhat analogous to a family linkage study over many generations with an ancestral haplotype replacing a parental one. The ability to study many more 'offspring' (i.e. the present-day population) for linkage after many recombination events thus confers greater statistical power and much more precise localization than is possible with traditional linkage based methods.

The degree of LD depends on time elapsed since the mutation arose: in 'older' founder populations, the degree of LD often diminishes but due to more recombination events elsewhere, the ability to fine map a mutation may often be greater. Important constraints of LD based methods include the fact that they depend on the disease of interest existing in suitable founder populations in a way not obscured by marker mutation within the population, new disease mutations, genetic drift, locus heterogeneity, population admixture or the existence of multiple disease susceptibility loci. Problems related to population structure may also yield false positive results, that is, association without true linkage. Thus, assortive mating causing the eventual emergence of discrete genetic subpopulations (population stratification) and population admixture (where two genetically diverse populations have recently merged) may both lead to the association of unlinked loci.

Thus, additional studies are often required to determine whether a positive association is truly the result of genetic linkage between disease and marker loci. The transmission disequilibrium test determines the transmission frequency of marker alleles from a heterozygous parent to an affected offspring. In the absence of true linkage, both alleles of a two allele marker locus will be transferred with equal frequency to an affected offspring. However, transmission of allele combinations with a frequency greater than that expected by chance is taken as evidence of true linkage.

It is hoped that in the future it will be possible to perform whole genome LD scans but there are conceptual as well as practical difficulties to be overcome before this is likely to become a routine tool (Kruglyak, 1999).

Quantitative trait loci (QTL)

QTL are loci which individually have a small but measurable influence on a continuous phenotype such as body weight rather than giving rise to discrete disease present or absent phenotypes. The principal advantage of this methodology is that interactions between loci each having only a small phenotypic effect may be investigated, particularly where the sum of more than one such effect is large. The principle of attempting to define QTL as a tool for gene mapping relies on the fact that rodents may be selectively inbred to produce strains that differ widely in body weight and fat deposition under the influence of polygenic loci. Breeds with opposite poles of a phenotypic extreme may then be crossbred to produce F1 progeny whose phenotype will depend on the exact genotype inherited from each parental strain (Brockmann and Bevova, 2002). The resultant F1 generation may then be back-crossed to a parent or permitted to bred with siblings to generate a back-cross or sib-mated F2 population containing a number of allele combinations (and phenotypes) not encountered in either of the parental or F1 strains. Provided the two breeds differ in one or more molecular markers associated with each locus (e.g. restriction fragment length polymorphisms, microsatellites or single nucleotide polymorphisms), the F2 generation may be genotyped and phenotyped to associate genetic markers (and thus specific allele combinations) with the resulting phenotype.

Over 165 QTL spanning the entire genome (except the Y chromosome) have been mapped in animals (mainly mice) to date (Rankinen *et al.*, 2002). Many appear to exert rather modest effects on phenotype (as may be expected in a complex polygenic disorder) although some do appear to have more major effects. Following identification of QTL in mice, loci of interest may be mapped to the homologous (syntenic) region in man and the region further tested for association with obesity in a human population. Thus, the many benefits of performing genetic studies in mice may be reaped whilst maintaining relevance to human populations. These advantages include stable environmental conditions, pure breeding strains, the ability to perform sibling and back-cross mating, rapid breeding (generation) times and the ability to obtain accurate phenotypical data. At present, the use of this method has identified QTL having effects on intermediary phenotypes such as thermogenesis, serum leptin levels and insulin resistance, gene–environment interactions such as susceptibility to diet-induced obesity and with time of obesity onset and gender-specific susceptibility to obesity (Brockmann and Bevova, 2002).

Because this technique examines the effects of many combinations of more than one allele, the opportunity to examine gene–gene interactions is presented. For example, the mouse strains M. Spretus and C57BL/6 are relatively lean as are the F1 progeny resulting from crossing these parental strains. However, back-crossed progeny (with allelic combinations not found in the parental or F1 strains) vary in percentage body fat content from about 1 to 60 per cent. Significant association (LOD score >3.3) was found in the back-crossed F2 progeny between a number of intermediary phenotypes and four genomic regions (designated as mob1–4 on chromosomes 7, 6, 12 and 15, respectively). A further association with percentage body fat, accounting for some 7 per cent of the observed variance of this trait, was considered 'suggestive' rather than statistically significant (Warden *et al.*, 1995; Warden and Fisler, 1998). These loci include a number of plausible candidate genes including *IGFR-1* (mob1), *ob* (mob2) and GH receptor (mob4). It is of interest that M. Spretus-derived alleles appear to promote obesity at chromosomes 6, 7 and 12, whereas C57BL/6-derived alleles promote obesity only when present on chromosome 15 and then only when the loci at 6, 7, and 12 are heterozygous, providing a clear demonstration of the complexities of epistasis in the aetiology of complex polygenic disorders such as obesity.

Animal models with altered genetic expression

Transgenic techniques involve introduction of genes (or regulatory sequences) into the germline of mice so that target gene expression may be either introduced *de novo* or alternatively up or downregulated whereas knockout techniques involve elimination of endogenous gene expression. These genetic manipulations have provided a powerful tool for the study of gene function in the intact animal but have led in some instances to the publication of confusing or unexpected results. Thus, animals lacking dopamine β-hydroxylase are completely unable to synthesize catecholamines but do not develop obesity (Thomas and Palmiter, 1997). Also, animals carrying a knock-out version of the Y5 form of the NPY receptor are phenotypically normal until they develop a late onset form of obesity due to overfeeding rather than the underfeeding which might be expected from the known physiology of this receptor system (Erickson *et al.*, 1996; Palmiter *et al.*, 1998). Another problem is the fact that some germ line mutations are incompatible with foetal development and, with rare exceptions such as the intrauterine rescue of dopamine β-hydroxylase knockout mice with temporary provision of a downstream metabolite (Thomas and Palmiter, 1997), it has not been possible to produce an adult animal model of such mutations.

It is likely that recent refinements of these techniques to permit both temporal activation/de-activation of the gene, and tissue specific modulation of gene activity will greatly enhance the usefulness of this research tool. Thus inserted or wild-type gene expression may be linked to a tissue specific promoter or to an inducible regulatory sequence (e.g. a tetracycline response element) so that, in this case, gene expression is either enabled or inhibited by the presence or absence of tetracycline in the animal's blood. However, even with advanced conditional (as opposed to classical germ line) gene expression targeting, there still remain problems of interpretation caused by factors such as the redundancy evident in the control of energy homeostasis leading to compensation for the failure of one regulatory component by up-regulation of another.

Summary and conclusions

In writing this chapter, we set out to illustrate some of the problems that have beset the study of obesity genetics, to evaluate some of the techniques currently available and to provide some examples of the progress made to date and future prospects for this rapidly moving field. In the past few years alone, fascinating and specific new lines of investigation have been suggested by unravelling the genetic and molecular basis of elements of the leptin pathway and of syndromic forms of obesity such as the BBS.

In the future, continuing refinements to genetic tools for the identification of new candidate genes as well as functional analysis and exploration of gene–gene and gene–environment interactions offer the potential for insights into complex polygenic inheritance scarcely thinkable only a few years ago. The tempo of significant discovery will doubtless increase following publication of the human and mouse genomic DNA sequences together with increasingly precise functional annotation of these sequences. Improvements in the characterization and promulgation of common SNPs throughout the genome are likely to facilitate the study of genetic association and it may now only be a matter of time before the possibility of conducting studies of LD throughout large areas of the human genome becomes realized. Combined with routine access to huge, almost 'real-time' on-line data repositories, better computational tools and the increasing ease of collaborative study, we are now able to look forward with much greater hope than has hitherto been possible to the achievement of fundamental insight into the genetic biology of obesity in coming years.

References

Allison DB, Faith MS and Nathan JS (1996) Risch's lambda values for human obesity. *Int J Obes Relat Metab Disord* **20**, 990–9.

Allison DB, Heo M, Faith MS and Pietrobelli A (1998) Meta-analysis of the association of the Trp64Arg polymorphism in the beta3 adrenergic receptor with body mass index. *Int J Obes Relat Metab Disord* **22**, 559–66.

Altshuler D, Daly M and Kruglyak L (2000) Guilt by association. *Nat Genet* **26**, 135–7.

Bouchard C, Perusse L, Rice T and Rao DC (1998) The genetics of human obesity. In *Handbook of Obesity*. Marcel Dekker, New York, pp. 157–190.

Borecki IB, Blangero J, Rice T *et al.* (1998) Evidence for at least two major loci influencing human fatness. *Am J Hum Genet* **63**, 831–8.

Brockmann GA and Bevova MR (2002) Using mouse models to dissect the genetics of obesity. *Trends Genet* **18**, 367–76.

Clement K, Boutin P and Froguel P (2002) Genetics of obesity. *Am J Pharmacogenomics* **2**, 177–87.

Croft JB, Morrell D, Chase CL and Swift M (1995) Obesity in heterozygous carriers of the gene for the Bardet–Biedl syndrome. *Am J Med Genet* **55**, 12–15.

Deng HW, Deng W, Liu YJ *et al.* (2002) A genomewide linkage scan for quantitative-trait loci for obesity phenotypes. *Am J Hum Genet* **70**, 1138–51.

Erickson JC, Clegg KE and Palmiter RD (1996) Sensitivity to leptin and susceptibility to seizures of mice lacking neuropeptide Y. *Nature* **381**, 415–21.

Fabsitz RR, Carmelli D and Hewitt JK (1992) Evidence for independent genetic influences on obesity in middle age. *Int J Obes Relat Metab Disord* **16**, 657–66.

Fujisawa T, Ikegami H, Kawaguchi Y and Ogihara T (1998) Meta-analysis of the association of Trp64Arg polymorphism of beta 3-adrenergic receptor gene with body mass index. *J Clin Endocrinol Metab* **83**, 2441–4.

Hales CN and Barker DJ (1992) Type 2 (non-insulin-dependent) diabetes mellitus: the thrifty phenotype hypothesis. *Diabetologia* **35**, 595–601.

Hebebrand J, Sommerlad C, Geller F *et al.* (2001) The genetics of obesity: practical implications. [Review] [70 refs]. *Int J Obes Relat Metabol Dis* **25**(Suppl 1), S10–S18.

Hirschhorn JN and Altshuler D (2002) Once and again-issues surrounding replication in genetic association studies. *J Clin Endocrinol Metab* **87**, 4438–41.

Iannello S, Bosco P, Cavaleri A *et al.* (2002) A review of the literature of Bardet–Biedl disease and report of three cases associated with metabolic syndrome and diagnosed after the age of fifty. *Obes Rev* **3**, 123–35.

Jacobson P, Ukkola O, Rankinen T *et al.* (2002) Melanocortin 4 receptor sequence variations are seldom a cause of human obesity: the Swedish Obese Subjects, the HERITAGE Family Study, and a Memphis cohort. *J Clin Endocrinol Metab* **87**, 4442–6.

Jorde LB (2000) Linkage disequilibrium and the search for complex disease genes. *Genome Res* **10**, 1435–44.

Katsanis N, Ansley SJ, Badano JL *et al.* (2001) Triallelic inheritance in Bardet–Biedl syndrome, a Mendelian recessive disorder. *Science* **293**, 2256–9.

Katsanis N, Beales PL, Woods MO *et al.* (2000) Mutations in MKKS cause obesity, retinal dystrophy and renal malformations associated with Bardet–Biedl syndrome. *Nat. Genet.* **26**, 67–70.

Katsanis N, Lupski JR and Beales PL (2001) Exploring the molecular basis of Bardet–Biedl syndrome. *Hum Mol Genet* **10**, 2293–9.

Kruglyak L (1999) Prospects for whole-genome linkage disequilibrium mapping of common disease genes. *Nat Genet* **22**, 139–44.

Lander E and Kruglyak L (1995) Genetic dissection of complex traits: guidelines for interpreting and reporting linkage results. *Nat Genet* **11**, 241–7.

Macho-Azcarate T, Calabuig J, Marti A and Martinez JA (2002) A maximal effort trial in obese women carrying the beta^2-adrenoceptor Gln^{27}Glu polymorphism. *J Physiol Biochem* **58**, 103–8.

Maes HH, Neale MC and Eaves LJ (1997) Genetic and environmental factors in relative body weight and human adiposity. *Behav Genet* **27**, 325–51.

McCarthy MI (2002) Susceptibility gene discovery for common metabolic and endocrine traits. [Review] [111 refs]. *J Mol Endocrinol* **28**, 1–17.

McLaughlin J (1991) The inheritance of body mass index in the Virginia 30 000. *Behav Genet* **21**, 581.

Montague CT, Farooqi IS, Whitehead JP *et al.* (1997) Congenital leptin deficiency is associated with severe early-onset obesity in humans. *Nature* **387**, 903–908.

Mykytyn K, Nishimura DY, Searby CC *et al.* (2002) Identification of the gene (BBS1) most commonly involved in Bardet–Biedl syndrome, a complex human obesity syndrome. *Nat. Genet.* **31**, 435–438.

Nicholls RD and Knepper JL (2001) Genome organization, function, and imprinting in Prader–Willi and Angelman syndromes. *Annu Rev Genomics Hum Genet* **2**, 153–75.

Palmiter RD, Erickson JC, Hollopeter G *et al.* (1998) Life without neuropeptide Y. *Recent Prog Horm Res* **53**, 163–99.

Rankinen T, Perusse L, Weisnagel SJ *et al.* (2002) The human obesity gene map: the 2001 update. *Obes Res* **10**, 196–243.

Rice T, Borecki IB, Bouchard C and Rao DC (1993) Segregation analysis of fat mass and other body composition measures derived from underwater weighing. *Am J Hum Genet* **52**, 967–73.

Rice T, Tremblay A, Deriaz O *et al.* (1996) A major gene for resting metabolic rate unassociated with body composition: results from the Quebec Family Study. *Obes Res* **4**, 441–9.

Sachidanandam R, Weissman D, Schmidt SC *et al.* (2001) A map of human genome sequence variation containing 1.42 million single nucleotide polymorphisms. *Nature* **409**, 928–33.

Slavotinek AM, Stone EM, Mykytyn K *et al.* (2000) Mutations in MKKS cause Bardet–Biedl syndrome. *Nat Genet* **26**, 15–16.

Stunkard AJ, Foch TT and Hrubec Z (1986) A twin study of human obesity. *JAMA* **256**, 51–54.

Thomas SA and Palmiter RD (1997) Thermoregulatory and metabolic phenotypes of mice lacking noradrenaline and adrenaline [see comments]. *Nature* **387**, 94–7.

Vaisse C, Clement K, Durand E *et al.* (2000) Melanocortin-4 receptor mutations are a frequent and heterogeneous cause of morbid obesity. *J Clin Invest* **106**, 253–62.

Warden CH and Fisler JS (1998) Molecular genetics of obesity. In *Handbook of Obesity* Marcel Dekker, New York, pp. 223–42.

Warden CH, Fisler JS, Shoemaker SM *et al.* (1995) Identification of four chromosomal loci determining obesity in a multifactorial mouse model. *J Clin Invest* **95**, 1545–52.

3

Lifestyle Determinants of Obesity

Susan A. Jebb and Jeremy Krebs

The importance of energy balance

Body weight is the integrated product of a lifetime's energy intake, offset by energy needs. Throughout the last century there has been a trend towards increased body weight and increases in body mass index, a measure of weight relative to height. Data from the annual Health Survey for England (Department of Health, 2002) shows that the average gain in weight of the adult population over the last 10 years has been approximately 0.35 kg/year, which is primarily adipose tissue, with modest concomitant increases in lean tissue. At an individual level, excess weight gain may occur gradually, almost imperceptibly, over many years or, in intermittent episodes of more pronounced positive energy balance, perhaps related to holidays or festive periods when usual diet and activity habits are distorted. However, spontaneous weight loss is rare, except in association with pathological processes. This asymmetry in energy balance is underpinning the rise in obesity.

Energy balance is the product of both innate and discretionary processes. Energy expenditure consists predominately of three components; resting energy expenditure, thermogenesis and physical activity (Jebb, 1997). Resting energy expenditure is a product of an individuals size, shape and body composition and accounts for 50–80 per cent of energy needs. Additional energy (approximately 10 per cent) is expended in the thermogenesis accompanying digestion and processing of food, or for thermoregulation. Only the energy expended in physical activity is discretionary and thus modifiable. Energy intake is more complex.

Obesity and Diabetes. Edited by Anthony H. Barnett and Sudhesh Kumar
© 2004 John Wiley & Sons, Ltd ISBN: 0-470-84898-7

Undoubtedly there is a complex regulatory system in place that underpins eating behaviour, but this is an imperfect system, easily disrupted by specific food properties, social or environmental cues and subject to a high degree of cognitive control.

The nature of these various mechanisms to control energy balance is the subject of intensive research. With a day-to-day coefficient of variation of energy intake of around 23 per cent and physical activity about 8 per cent (Goldberg *et al.*, 1991), it is readily apparent that most humans do not regulate energy balance on a daily basis. Indeed some, for example in The Gambia, regulate their weight across an entire annual agricultural cycle as a period of plenty following the annual harvest is gradually followed by diminishing food reserves and escalating physical activity during the production of the new crop, a process driven by climatic imperatives (Prentice *et al.*, 1992). Yet despite this innate capacity to cope with fluctuations in energy balance the rising tide of obesity throughout the world suggests that these mechanisms are increasingly failing to constrain excess weight gain in children and young people and to maintain a stable body weight in adults.

In situations where changes in lifestyle are imposed there are profound effects on body weight. Obesity is almost unknown in animals in the wild, but rapidly develops in captivity. Small animals housed in laboratories, fed standard chow are able to maintain a healthy body weight, yet when given access to highly palatable, refined diets, rich in fat and sugar, they rapidly gain excess weight and become obese. In humans living in economically developed societies dietary choices and physical activity are discretionary components of an individual or family lifestyle. This chapter will consider how these lifestyle habits can determine the risk of obesity.

Physical activity

A comparison of contemporary living with historical accounts quickly reveals that habitual physical activity has declined, but data on secular trends using objective measures is lacking. Cross-sectional analyses of measures of activity and the risk of obesity consistently report a reduced weight or body mass index (BMI) with higher categorical levels of physical activity (DiPietro, 1995). This is particularly true for vigorous activity, which may reflect improved reporting of such activities in questionnaires relative to the lower intensity of activities of daily living. However, the interpretation of these cross-sectional analyses is limited due to difficulties in dissecting the directionality of the association. Physical activity may influence weight, but weight may also influence the intensity or nature of physical activity.

Prospective studies provide evidence that physical activity may attenuate weight gain, but there is no consistent evidence to suggest that activity can fully prevent or reverse age-associated increases in body weight (DiPietro, 1999). For example in the US Health Professionals Follow-up of almost 20 000 men those in the lowest activity category at baseline and follow up gained 1.1 kg compared to those in the highest activity category at the two time points who gained only 0.8 kg (Coakley *et al.*, 1998). Data from individuals who have recently lost weight, and therefore represent a group at high risk of weight gain also shows that increases in physical activity can significantly reduce, but not prevent, weight regain. For example in a 3-year follow-up of 192 patients who had initially lost an average of 22 kg using a very-low-energy-diet programme, weight regain averaged 19 kg (Grodstein *et al.*, 1996). There was however considerable inter-individual variability. Multivariate regression analysis showed that each hour per week spent watching TV was associated with an increase in weight of 0.3 kg (95 per cent CI 0.1–0.5 kg) whereas each hour of exercise per week resulted in a decrease of 2.0 kg (95 per cent CI −3.0–1.0 kg).

Randomized controlled interventions with prescribed increases in physical activity or exercise have yielded little evidence of effectiveness in halting the rise in excess weight, but it is acknowledged that compliance to such interventions is poor (Hardeman *et al.*, 2000). Increased activity requires a personal lifestyle commitment that only well-motivated individuals are prepared to make. Thus, subjects in the intervention arm are diluted by those unwilling to make the necessary changes, while the control group may be contaminated by highly motivated individuals who respond to the generic public health education messages to increase activity, thus diluting the difference between the groups.

In spite of these limitations in the scientific case there is sufficient evidence that low levels of physical activity are an important lifestyle determinant of obesity. Together with the positive benefits with respect to a range of other aspects of ill-health this evidence has underpinned the development of public health strategies to promote activity. The lack of quantitative information on the contribution of specific components of activity to obesity has resulted in a rather broad approach which includes recommendations to reduce sedentary pursuits, especially television viewing, increase activities of daily living and vigorous exercise sessions. Nonetheless such initiatives are likely to make a positive contribution to public health.

Energy intake

Analysis of the dietary factors associated with obesity is confounded by the difficulties in assessing food intake and eating behaviour. Dietary surveys are increasingly beset by the problem of underreporting, probably related to the increased awareness of nutrition issues and concern over body weight, which leads individuals to consciously or sub-consciously mis-report their food intake. In 1986 Prentice *et al.* demonstrated that obese women under-reported energy intake relative to energy needs by a mean of 3.5 MJ/day, while among lean women the two measures agreed to within 0.14 MJ/day (Prentice *et al.*, 1986).

This observation has been repeatedly reconfirmed, although it is now recognized that there is a spectrum of mis-reporting of food intake across the population, the nature of which is not easily predicted on the basis of individual phenotype or demographic statistics. Others may alter their dietary habits during periods of food recording, usually leading to a record of undereating (Goris *et al.*, 2000).

Analysis of the dietary determinants of obesity is also confounded by the problems of post-hoc changes in consumption in response to increasing body weight. This makes it difficult to draw quantitative conclusions from cross-sectional or even prospective studies of food intake and body weight. Nonetheless increasingly refined recording tools and statistical analysis are seeking to understand more about the broader context of eating behaviour with targeted questions about the location and social context of eating episodes and using factor analysis to identify types of dietary patterns, which may inform future strategies to prevent and treat obesity (Whichelow and Prevost, 1996).

Instead much of our understanding of the relationship between dietary factors and the risk of obesity comes from experimental studies in the laboratory or highly controlled intervention studies in the community. These may not truly mimic eating behaviour in a naturalistic setting, but they provide useful insights into the response to imposed dietary manipulations under standardized conditions.

Energy density

Energy density is a critical component in the regulation of human appetite and plays an important role in determining total energy intake. In one of the most robust experimental studies Stubbs *et al* showed that lean, young healthy men, allowed to eat *ad libitum*, consumed significantly more energy as the fat content of the food was increased (Stubbs *et al.*, 1995a, b). Careful measurements of fat balance over one week in a whole body indirect calorimeter showed that body fat decreased by 0.86 ± 0.61 kg on the 20 per cent fat diet, while increasing by 0.39 ± 0.59 kg and 2.24 ± 0.94 kg on the 40 and 60 per cent fat diets respectively. These studies provided no evidence of any physiological compensation or cognitive 'learning' associated with sustained consumption of foods of differing fat content even after a week or more of sustained over-consumption. Importantly, when the energy density of the food was equalized, through careful experimental manipulation of the recipes, the high fat hyperphagia was abolished (Stubbs *et al.*, 1996) (Figure 3.1). This strongly suggests that excess energy was consumed by a process of 'passive over-consumption', in which changes in food quality, not quantity, were the driving force beyond the disruption in the previously accurate regulation of body weight. This phenomenon implies that the bulk of food consumed is an important determinant of energy intake.

In the 'real world' energy-dense diets are frequently high in fat, since fat (37 kJ/g) contains more than twice as much energy gram-for-gram as protein

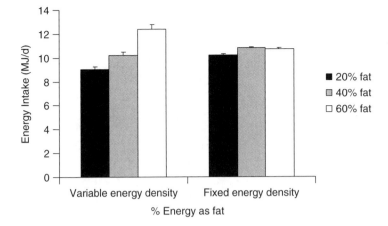

Figure 3.1 Impact of the proportion of dietary energy as fat on spontaneous energy intake of lean young men under conditions of variable or fixed energy density of food. Data from Stubbs *et al.* 1995a, b and 1996.

(17 kJ/g) or carbohydrate (16 kJ/g). Many low-fat foods, especially dairy products, contain substantially less energy than their full-fat equivalent, allowing consumers to maintain the bulk of food in the diet, while constraining energy intake. However, recent advances in food technology have resulted in some food ranges that are low in fat but where the energy content is similar to traditional equivalents. These foods, such as biscuits, cakes and desserts often contain large quantities of added sugars and might be expected to lead to similar passive over-consumption as high-fat foods of similar energy density.

Foods served in most 'fast-food' chains such as burger and chicken outlets are characterized by a particularly high energy density. These foods are frequently high in fat and have a low water content. A recent analysis has shown that the energy density of foods offered in a selection of these outlets has an energy density of over 1000 kJ/100 g relative to the typical energy density of the diet of a woman in the UK of 670 kJ/100 g (Prentice and Jebb, 2003). This implies that for regular consumers the total quantity of food which can be consumed without exceeding energy needs must be constrained to accommodate this increase in the energy density of the diet in regular consumers. The high energy density of these foods provides a plausible biological explanation for the epidemiological associations between 'fast-food' consumption and obesity. However this is likely to be compounded by large portion size and specific marketing strategies to encourage further consumption of these products.

Portion size

The size of portions of food commonly served is increasing (Neilson and Popkin, 2003). This trend, previously observed only in the USA, has rapidly swept across restaurants throughout the world as part of the process of globalization. It has been exploited by marketeers and now also affects household food from ready-meals to items such as crisps, confectionery and soft drinks.

A series of studies in both laboratory and free-living settings have demonstrated that large portions foster increased consumption in both adults and children of both genders and irrespective of adiposity (Rolls, 2003). For example, when faced with increasing portions of amorphous foods such as pasta individuals consumed 30 per cent more when the portion of food served was doubled (Rolls *et al.*, 2002) (Figure 3.2). There were no differences in reported hunger or satiety post-ingestion and less than half the participants recognized that the portion size varied on each occasion. Foods served in single units may be even more likely to prompt over consumption since the resistance to 'wasting' food is still strongly embedded in most cultures. For example, studies have shown that consuming increasingly large packets of crisps or sandwiches is associated with significant increases in consumption with no compensatory decrease in food intake at a subsequent meal (Ello-Martin *et al.*, 2002; Kial *et al.*, 2002). Together these studies suggest that individuals adjust their appetite regulation system to accommodate the larger portion. This may be compounded by cognitive adjustments that lead to long-term entrainment of portion size.

Snacking

There is a clear secular decline in traditional three-meal-a-day eating patterns and a rise in more frequent, less formal eating occasions, commonly described as snacking. Epidemiological associations between eating frequency and obesity yield mixed results and are heavily confounded by under-reporting of energy

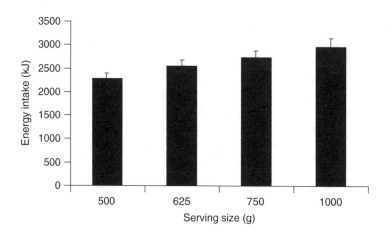

Figure 3.2 Increases in energy intake with increasing serving size of a macaroni cheese dish. Data from Rolls *et al.* (2002). Intakes in all conditions were significantly different from each other ($P < 0.05$) except 625 g and 750 g ($P = 0.097$).

intake and hence potentially under-reporting of eating episodes too (Bellisle *et al.*, 1997). Indeed a study involving covert observation of food consumption in a metabolic facility while volunteers were allowed free access to food showed that volunteers specifically under-reported food consumed between formal meal eating episodes when asked to recall the food consumed (Poppitt *et al.*, 1998).

Studies in the laboratory have shown that under isoenergetic conditions there is no effect of eating frequency on energy expenditure (Dallosso *et al.*, 1982). In conditions of *ad libitum* consumption imposed snacking does tend to lead to modest increases in total daily energy intake with the greatest impact observed in those who do not habitually eat between meals and vice versa (Green and Blundell, 1996). It is however extraordinarily difficult within experimental paradigms to mimic the social context and environmental cues to snacking that may prompt consumption in daily life. In day-to-day life the impact on body weight is likely to be determined by the quantity and quality of snacks consumed rather than by eating frequency *per se*.

Soft drinks

The emphasis on dietary fat as an important determinant of energy density has tended to divert attention from sugar-rich foods and drinks. However, it is important to recognize the energy density theory of appetite control cannot be equally applied across solid and liquid foods alike. Liquids have a lower energy density than solids because of their high water content, yet there is poorer energy compensation following isoenergetic liquids relative to solid food, perhaps due to differences in viscosity (Mattes and Rothacker, 2001).

It is evident that increases in soft drink consumption, as part of broader diet and lifestyle changes, have paralleled the rise in obesity. The increase has been marked, even among relatively young children. For example, in 4-year-olds in Britain the consumption of soft drinks and juices has increased from only 13 g/week in 1950 to 446 g/week in 1992/3 (Prynne *et al.*, 1999). In adults comparison of two nationally representative dietary surveys shows an increase from 669 g/week to 1050 g/week in soft drinks (excluding diet varieties and juices) from 1986 to 2000/1 (Gregory *et al.*, 1990; Henderson and Gregory, 2002). However, the greatest consumers of soft drinks are young people where, in 1997, boys aged 15–18-years reported consuming 6692 g/week and girls 4317 g/week of soft drinks (excluding diet varieties and juices) (Gregory and Low, 2000). Soft drinks are the single largest contributor to reported sugar intake in young people, representing 26 per cent of total energy, with 85 per cent of young people (4–18 years) consuming in excess of the recommended maximum of 11 per cent energy as sugar.

Sugar-rich drinks are frequently alleged to be a determinant of obesity risk but within cross-sectional surveys there is little evidence of an association. However, interpretation of the data is confounded by a number of laws in the evidence.

There is a secular trend towards increased under-reporting, especially of food and drinks consumed between traditional meal-eating episodes. Moreover, the extent of under-reporting is not evenly distributed across the population and is more pronounced in obese versus lean subjects. These errors tend to diminish the likelihood of observing an association. One prospective study, which avoids the post-hoc confounding caused by obesity, has shown that each additional serving of soft drinks was associated with a 1.6-fold increase in the risk of obesity but the data is far from perfect for the purpose (Ludwig *et al.*, 2001).

Highly controlled experimental studies, often using a preload paradigm, provide indirect evidence that soft drinks are an unhelpful addition to the diet of a nation prone to excess consumption since they tend to supplement rather than substitute for food (Spitzer and Rodin, 1987; Foltin *et al.*, 1993; Wilson, 2000). However these short-term studies preclude the possibility of longer-term physiological or cognitive compensation which may develop in regular consumers of sugar-rich drinks. Two free-living studies have tested the effects on sugar-rich drinks on body weight. In the first, daily consumption of 1150 g soda sweetened with a high-fructose corn syrup (530 kcal/day) versus aspartame (3 kcal/day) or no beverage, over 3 weeks each, showed that the high-fructose corn syrup drink significantly increased energy intake and body weight relative to both the aspartame and control treatments (Figure 3.3) (Tordoff and Alleva, 1990). Secondly, a 10-week trial examined the impact of sugar-rich versus artificially-sweetened foods and drinks in which >80 per cent of all intervention foods were beverages (Raben *et al.*, 2002). Over 10 weeks, weight increased by 1.6 kg in the high sugar group and decreased by −1.0 kg in the group in whom sugar rich foods and beverages were replaced by artificially sweetened varieties ($P < 0.001$). Overall, this data supports the hypothesis that consumption of sugar-rich drinks is a risk factor for obesity.

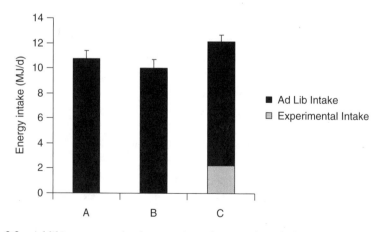

Figure 3.3 *Ad libitum* energy intake over three three-week periods (solid bars) plus intake from a prescribed beverage (hatched bars): A = no beverage, B = artificially sweetened, C = sweetened with high fructose corn syrup. Data from Tordoff and Alleva (1990).

Environmental impacts on lifestyle

The world we live in has changed and this transition has occurred at a rate far greater than man is able to evolve and adapt. Our genetic makeup has been moulded by an environment in which food was scarce and the physical demands for survival were high (Peters *et al.*, 2002). Today the decline in manual occupations, motorized transport and the rise in sedentary leisure pursuits such as television, computers and electronic toys have reduced our energy needs to a level below which innate appetite control systems are no longer able to precisely match energy intake to energy needs. A huge variety of highly palatable foods are more available to us than ever before, and we spend a smaller proportion of our disposable income on food than ever before. There has been a marked increase in the proportion of food consumed outside the home which contains a greater proportion of fat and is frequently more energy dense than household food. Consumption is encouraged through a variety of marketing strategies including advertisements and economic incentives to purchase larger or additional items. Portion sizes are standardized and not tailored to personal needs, and individuals have limited understanding of the composition of food items, which impairs any cognitive control over food intake. It has been argued that excess weight gain is a predictable response to this changed environment (Prentice, 1997), yet some individuals, families and sub-groups of the population are remaining lean. But how is this achieved?

Many individuals report using cognitive strategies to control their weight. For example, participants in the US National Weight Control Registry who have successfully lost at least 13 kg and maintained this loss for at least 1 year, report much lower intakes of fat and higher levels of exercise than the population average (Klem *et al.*, 1997). In a comprehensive review Campbell and Crawford (2001) identify a series of contributory factors through which the family environments may modulate the risk of obesity. These include the development of food preferences, household food availability, parental role-modelling of lifestyle behaviours, social interactions in relation to food and eating, media exposure and parental response to advertising. Economic circumstances may contribute to the increased risk of obesity among low-income families in the developed world. Energy-dense foods are frequently some of the best value (cost/calorie) and access to some active leisure opportunities can be disproportionately expensive.

Schools are frequently used as the setting for interventions to prevent the rise in obesity in children, reflecting the potential of school practices to impact on both diet and physical activity habits (Mueller *et al.*, 2001; Sahota *et al.*, 2001). Local communities may also provide micro-environments that may either foster the development of obesity or promote, facilitate and support lifestyles conducive to effective weight control. This is a potentially important element given the link between low socio-economic status (SES) and obesity and the clustering of SES by region. An interesting ecological analysis of the geographical association between fast-food outlets and area socio-economic status demonstrated that in the two highest SES areas, each fast-food outlet served a population of 14 256, whilst in the two lowest SES areas there was one outlet per 5641 head of population (Reidpath et al., 2002). Whether this reflects consumer demand or industrial opportunism is unclear, but the association exemplifies the impact of environmental factors on dietary habits of communities.

An integrated analysis

Secular increases in mean body weight show that at a population level there is a sustained small positive energy balance. Evidence cited previously suggests that this is driven by the two discretionary components of energy balance, namely food intake and physical activity. In the past too much emphasis has been placed on the study of each factor in isolation, but there is growing awareness of important interactions between these two lifestyle determinants of obesity at both a physiological and behavioural level.

In 1995 an ecological analysis of the relationship between diet, physical activity and obesity demonstrated that during the period 1970–1990, reported energy intake declined, while the rise in sedentary lifestyles closely paralleled the increase in obesity (Prentice and Jebb, 1995). This has been widely quoted to support the hypothesis that physical inactivity is the major determinant of weight gain. However, this misses the central tenet of the argument. Inactivity per se does not cause obesity. Obesity only develops when energy intake is not precisely downregulated to match the low energy needs of modern living. It is the coupling between intake and expenditure that is at the heart of the obesity epidemic (Prentice and Jebb, 2004).

The physiological coupling between intake and expenditure across the intermediary range of energy needs is clearly demonstrated in a study in laboratory animals, dating from the 1950s (Figure 3.4) (Mayer, 1966). Here animals were required to exercise for progressively increasing periods of time, increasing energy needs. Spontaneous energy intake increased in parallel and body weight was maintained. However, at extremely high levels of exercise, insufficient food was consumed and weight was gradually lost, while at very low levels of activity the animals were unable to constrain their consumption to match their excessively low energy needs and weight increased.

Detailed analysis of the interactions between intake, activity and obesity in humans is difficult because of the flaws in the assessment of lifestyle behaviours. However, a study conducted under controlled conditions in a whole-body calorimeter provides a quantitative insight into the vulnerability of the homeostatic mechanisms which regulate body weight. Here, a group of lean young men were exposed to a low or high fat diet, together with sufficient exercise to maintain habitual activity levels or required to remain sedentary in a 2 × 2 design (Murgatroyd et al., 1999). The results show that energy balance was close

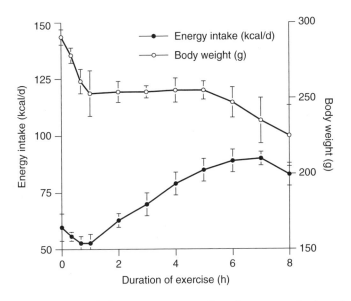

Figure 3.4   Energy intake relative to energy expenditure in a group of rats undergoing different levels of imposed exercise. Reproduced from Prentice and Jebb (2004) with permission from the International Life Sciences Institute.

to zero on the low-fat diet with habitual activity. The imposition of a sedentary behaviour pattern or the provision of a high-fat diet each created net energy gains (of +2.55 and +1.07 MJ/day, respectively). However, when imposed together, the two effects appeared to be more than additive, creating a positive imbalance of +5.13 MJ/d. This amounts to almost 50 per cent of the subjects' total daily energy requirement and equivalent to a fat gain of around 130 g/day.

Understanding the integrated effects of these two aspects of human behaviour is critical to our understanding of the lifestyle determinants of obesity, since poor dietary habits and low levels of physical activity frequently co-exist. Television viewing is frequently observed to be strongly associated with an increased risk of obesity (Crespo *et al.*, 2001). This may be mediated either through prolonged periods of sedentary activity, or through associated eating habits. For example among young people in Great Britain a survey in 1997 showed that there is a significant positive association between sedentary pastimes (outside school) and consumption of savoury snacks, and a negative association with fruit consumption (Rennie and Jebb, 2004). Television viewing may be causally linked to such eating habits through programme content or advertising, or it may simply act as an objective marker of a broader family lifestyle including eating habits.

Conclusions

Obesity is a complex heterogeneous disease. It is well accepted that there is an underlying genetic susceptibility to disease, but this is modified by environmental

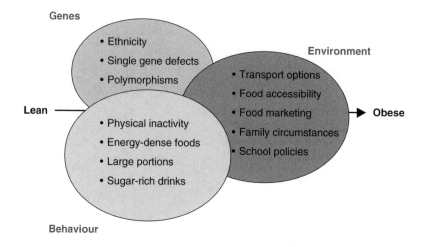

Figure 3.5   Integrated impact of genes, behaviour and environmental factors on the risk of obesity.

circumstances and individual lifestyle choices. Figure 3.5 indicates some of the many facets of the problem. Ultimately the risk of obesity is determined by energy balance, but the critical exposures (diet and activity) are difficult to measure reliably. In this scenario it is not surprising that direct, incontrovertible evidence of the specific lifestyle determinants of excess weight gain is lacking. However this integrated analysis of data from diverse sources points towards a number of factors that are likely to be important. These include energy-dense foods, large portions, excessive consumption of soft drinks and physical inactivity. Importantly a number of these factors may come together in an additive, or possible even synergistic manner, to influence the risk of obesity. Together they provide a compelling case for lifestyle interventions to tackle the epidemic of obesity.

However, there is a striking disparity in the national and international attitudes towards changes in physical activity versus eating habits. In both cases the evidence base is incomplete but the proposed lifestyle changes to prevent obesity are consistent with the prevention of chronic diseases such as coronary heart disease, diabetes and some cancers. It seems there is far greater willingness to embark on public health campaigns to increase activity than to alter dietary habits. This imbalance needs to be addressed if we are to effectively use our understanding of the lifestyle determinants of obesity to develop rational intervention strategies to prevent and treat obesity.

References

Bellisle F, McDevitt R and Prentice AM (1997) Meal frequency and energy balance. *Br J Nutr* **77**: S57–S70.

Campbell K and Crawford D (2001) Family food environments as determinants of preschool-aged children's eating behaviours: implications for obesity prevention policy. A review. *Aust J Nutr Dietet* **58**: 19–25.

Coakley EH, Rimm EB, Colditz G, *et al.* (1998) Predictors of weight change in men: Results from The Health Professionals Follow-Up Study. *Int J Obes* **22**: 89–96.

Crespo CJ, Smit E, Troiano S *et al.* (2001) Television watching, energy intake and obesity in US children: result from the Third National Health and Nutrition Examination Survey, 1988–1994. *Arch Pediatr Adolesc Med* **155**: 360–5.

Dallosso HM, Murgatroyd PR and James WPT (1982) Feeding frequency and energy balance in adult males. *Hum Nutr Clin Nutr* **36C**: 25–39.

Department of Health (2002) *Health Survey for England*. London, The Stationery Office.

DiPietro L (1995) Physical activity, body weight and adiposity: an epidemiologic perspective. *Exerc Sports Sci Rev* **23**: 275–303.

DiPietro L (1999) Physical activity in the prevention of obesity: current evidence and research issues. *Med Sci Sports Exerc* **31**: S542–S546.

Ello-Martin JA, Roe LS, Meengs JS *et al.* (2002) Increasing the portion size of a unit food increases energy intake. *Appetite* **39**.

Foltin RW, Kelly TH and Fischman MW (1993) Ethanol as an energy source in humans: comparison with dextrose-containing beverages. *Appetite* **20**: 95–110.

Goldberg GR, Black AE, Jebb SA, *et al.* (1991) Critical evaluation of energy intake data using fundamental principles of energy physiology. *Eur J Clin Nutr* **45**: 569–81.

Goris HC, Westerterp-Plantenga MS and Westerterp KR (2000) Undereating and underrecording of habitual food intake in obese men: selective underreporting of fat intake. *Am J Clin Nutr* **71**: 130–4.

Green SM and Blundell JE (1996) Effect of fat- and sucrose-containing foods on the size of eating episodes and energy intake in lean dietary restrained and unrestrained females: potential for causing over-consumption. *Eur J Clin Nutr* **50**: 625–35.

Gregory J, Foster K, Tyler H and Wiseman M (1990) *The Dietary and Nutritional Survey of British Adults*. London, HMSO.

Gregory J and Low S (2000) *National Diet and Nutrition Survey of young people aged 4–18 years Vol. 1 Report of the diet and nutrition survey*. London, HMSO.

Grodstein F, Levine R, Troy L *et al.* (1996) Three-year follow-up of participants in a commercial weight loss program. *Arch Intern Med* **156**: 1302–6.

Hardeman W, Griffin S, Johnston M *et al.* (2000) Interventions to prevent weight gain: a systematic review of psychological models and behaviour change methods. *Int J Obes* **24**: 131–43.

Henderson L and Gregory J (2002) The National Diet and Nutrition Survey: adults aged 19 to 64 years. *Types and quantities of foods consumed*. London, HMSO.

Jebb SA (1997) Aetiology of obesity. *Br Med Bull* **53**: 264–85.

Klem ML, Wing RR, McGuire MT *et al.* (1997) A descriptive study of individuals successful at long-term weight maintenance of substantial weight loss. *Am J Clin Nutr* **66**: 239–46.

Kral TVE, Meengs JS, Wall DE *et al.* (2002) Increasing the portion of a packaged snack increases energy intake. *Appetite* **39**: 86.

Ludwig DS, Peterson KE and Gortmaker SL (2001) Relation between consumption of sugar-sweetened drinks and childhood obesity. A prospective, observational analysis. *Lancet* **357**: 505–8.

Mattes RD and Rothacker D (2001) Beverage viscosity is inversely related to postprandial hunger in humans. *Physiol Behav* **74**: 551–7.

Mayer J (1966) Some aspects of the problem of regulation of food intake and obesity. *N Engl J Med* **274**: 610–16 and 722–31.

Mueller MJ, Asbeck I, Mast M *et al.* (2001) Prevention of obesity – more than an intention. Concept and first results of the Kiel Obesity Prevention Study (KOPS). *Int J Obes* **25**: S66–S74.

Murgatroyd PR, Goldberg GR, Leahy FE *et al.* (1999) Effects of inactivity and diet composition on human energy balance. *Int J Obes* **23**: 1269–75.

Nielsen SJ and Popkin BM (2003) Patterns and trends in food portion sizes 1977–1998. *JAMA* **289**: 450–3.

Peters JC, Wyatt HR, Donahoo WT and Hill JO (2002) Viewpoint: From instinct to intellect: the challenge of maintaining healthy weight in the modern world. *Obes Rev* **3**: 69–74.

Poppitt SD, Swann D, Black AE and Prentice AM (1998) Assessment of selective underreporting of food intake by both obese and non-obese women in a metabolic facility. *Int J Obes* **22**: 303–11.

Prentice AM, Jebb SA, Goldberg GR *et al.* (1992) Effects of weight cycling on body composition. *Am J Clin Nutr* **56** (suppl 1): 209S–216S.

Prentice AM and Jebb SA (1995) Obesity in Britain: Gluttony or Sloth? *Br Med J* **311**: 437–9.

Prentice AM (1997) Obesity – the inevitable penalty of civilisation? *Br Med Bull* **53**: 229–37.

Prentice AM, Black AE, Coward WA *et al.* (1986) High levels of energy expenditure in obese women. *Br Med J* **292**: 983–7.

Prentice AM and Jebb SA (2003) Fast foods, energy density and obesity – a possible mechanistic link. *Obes Rev* **4**: 187–94.

Prentice AM and Jebb SA (2004) Energy intake/physical activity interactions in the homeostasis of body weight regulation. *Nutr Rev* in press.

Prynne C, Paul MM, Price GM *et al.* (1999) Food and nutrient intake of a national sample of 4-year-old children in 1950: comparison with the 1990's. *Publ Health Nutr* **2**(4):537–47.

Raben A, Vasilaras TH, Moller AC and Astrup A (2002) Sucrose compared with artificial sweeteners: different effects on ad libitum food intake and body weight after 10 weeks of supplementation in overweight subjects. *Am J Clin Nutr* **76**: 721–9.

Reidpath DD, Burns C, Garrard J *et al.* (2002) An ecological study of the relationship between social and environmental determinants of obesity. *Health Place* **8**: 141–5.

Rennie K and Jebb SA (2004) Sedentary lifestyles are associated with being overweight and consumption of savoury snacks in young people (4–18 years). *Proc Nutr Soc* in press.

Rolls BJ, Morris EL and Roe LS (2002) Portion size of food affects energy intake in normal-weight and overweight men and women. *Am J Clin Nutr* **76**: 1207–13.

Rolls BJ (2003) The supersizing of America. *Nutr Today* **38**: 42–53.

Sahota P, Rudolf MCJ, Dixey R *et al.* (2001) Randomised controlled trial of primary school based intervention to reduce risk factors for obesity. *Br Med J* **323**: 1–5.

Spitzer L and Rodin J (1987) Effects of fructose and glucose preloads on subsequent food intake. *Appetite* **8**: 135–45.

Stubbs RJ, Harbron CG, Murgatroyd PR and Prentice AM (1995a) Covert manipulation of dietary fat and energy density: effect on substrate flux and food intake in men eating ad libitum. *Am J Clin Nutr* **62**: 316–29.

Stubbs RJ, Ritz P, Coward WA and Prentice AM (1995b) Covert manipulation of the ratio of dietary fat to carbohydrate and energy density: effect on food intake and energy balance in free-living men eating ad libitum. *Am J Clin Nutr* **62**: 330–7.

Stubbs RJ, Harbron CG and Prentice AM (1996) Covert manipulation of the dietary fat to carbohydrate ratio of isoenergetically dense diets: effect on food intake in feeding men ad libitum. *Int J Obes* **20**: 651–60.

Tordoff MG and Alleva AM (1990) Effect of drinking soda sweetened with aspartame or high fructose corn syrup on food intake and body weight. *Am J Clin Nutr* **51**: 963–9.

Wilson JF (2000) Lunch eating behaviour of preschool children: effects of age, gender and type of beverage served. *Physiol Behav* **70**: 27–33.

Whichelow MJ and Prevost AT (1996) Dietary patterns and their association with demographic, lifestyle and health variables in a random sample of British adults. *Br J Nutr* **76**: 17–30.

4

Pathogenesis of Obesity-Related Type 2 Diabetes

Philip McTernan and **Sudhesh Kumar**

Introduction

The profound changes in eating habits, agricultural capabilities and pattern of physical activity has fuelled today's epidemic of obesity, bringing with it a host of long-term complications. However, obesity has not always been regarded as a disadvantage. Statues dating from the Stone Age period appear to provide the earliest depictions of obesity. These Stone Age sculptures demonstrate not only the social importance attached to it, but also the survival advantage conferred by the ability to store energy (Bray, 1990). The most famous of these, the Venus of Willendorf, a 12-cm limestone figurine, demonstrates a woman with excessive body fat stores (Figure 4.1) whose habitus has been ascribed to a diet rich in fat and marrow and a sedentary lifestyle secondary to confinement in caves during the glacial period. These early depictions, however, not only highlight obesity as a phenomenon but also draw attention to the importance of body fat distribution. Whilst the lower body fat distribution of the Venus of Willendorf may have been symbolic of power and efficient fuel storage (Kissebah *et al.*, 1994) the concomitant hazards of obesity were, in fact, recognized as early as ~ 400 BC by Hippocrates who noted that 'sudden death is more common in those who are naturally fat than in the lean' (Bray, 1990). It is, however, only since the later half of the 20th century, that clinical obesity has emerged from the realm of sociology and a philosophical talking point to be recognized as a scientific discipline. This transformation can be most significantly attributed to the changing perception of adipose tissue as more than a mere site of lipid

Obesity and Diabetes.   Edited by Anthony H. Barnett and Sudhesh Kumar
© 2004 John Wiley & Sons, Ltd   ISBN: 0-470-84898-7

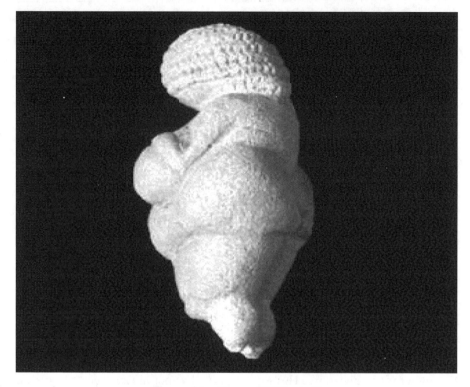

Figure 4.1   Venus of Willendorf.

storage and a recognition from epidemiological studies that fat distribution and accumulation alters the associated risk of disease (Vague, 1956).

Defining fat accumulation in terms of health risk

Due to the rising obesity in western society in the later part of the 20th Century and the predicted increasing obesity-related diseases for the 21st century the World Health Organization (WHO) published a set of definitions and guidelines on management of the obese state (WHO, 1998). These definitions were an attempt to determine the implications of obesity between individuals within a population as well as geographical and ethic populations to identify altered increased risk of mortality and morbidity. This publication classifies obesity using body mass index (BMI, weight (kg)/height^2 (m^2)) and its association with mortality, and defines obesity as 'a disease state in which excess fat has accumulated to an extent that health may be adversely affected' (Table 4.1) (WHO, 1998).

Definitions of obesity prior to the WHO classification were, however, based on studies carried out on Europeans and therefore failed to take account of the ethnic differences observed in body fat distribution and hence morbidity. In light of the biological implications of body fat distribution and the increasing ethnic diversity of the population this is of particular importance. The ethnic diversity was highlighted with studies indicating that while Caucasians may be at a low risk of obesity-related disease at a BMI of 23 kg m^{-2} this risk is significantly increased in the south Indian Asian population, where a higher mean waist–hip ratio reflects a more centralized body fat distribution for a given BMI (McKeigue *et al.*, 1991). In addition, a study with over 1500 Chinese people noted that the risk of diabetes, hypertension, and dyslipidaemia were observed to increase at a BMI of 23 kg m^{-2} as well (Ko *et al.*, 1999). This increase in morbidity and mortality observed at lower body mass index and smaller waist circumferences is reflected in the new guidelines published by the International Obesity Task Force (IOTF; IASO/IOTF 2000).

Implications of obesity-associated diabetes

The consequences of obesity are serious. Obese individuals are predisposed to a cluster of metabolic disturbances known as 'syndrome X' or the metabolic syndrome, which comprises glucose intolerance (the inability to metabolize glucose adequately), type 2 diabetes mellitus, hypertension, dyslipidaemia (high triglyceride levels accompanied by a raised concentration of low-density lipoproteins and diminished high-density lipoproteins), leading to an increased risk of stroke and cardiovascular disease (Ramirez, 1997; Reaven 1988, 1995; Walker 2001). In addition, obesity is also a risk factor for some malignancies such as endometrial cancer (Iemura *et al.*, 2000). The more life-threatening, chronic health problems have been categorized into four main areas by WHO. These include: cardiovascular problems including hypertension, stroke and coronary heart disease; conditions associated with insulin resistance, namely type 2 diabetes; certain types of cancer; as well as gall bladder disease.

Development of obesity-related type 2 diabetes

Weight increases, particularly in the adipose tissue depots when the amount of energy (calories) consumed exceed energy used for exercise and metabolic processes. This is known as 'positive energy balance' and the excess is stored as white adipose tissue (Frayn *et al.*, 1995; Gregoire *et al.*, 1998). It terms of the development of type 2 diabetes, this is largely observed as excessive consumption of nutrients, which are high in caloric content. Both excess consumption of macronutrients such as carbohydrates and lipids coupled with increasing adiposity lead to the progression of type 2 diabetes mediated principally via their negative influence on insulin action and intermediary metabolism (Hill and Peters, 1998;

Table 4.1 Summary of secreted factors from adipose tissue (AT), roles in the body and changes with obesity

Molecule	Function/effect	Normal distribution	Effect of obesity	References
Leptin	Satiety and appetite, signals to brain to regulate body fat mass	Subcutaneous (2.5×) > omental fat (adipocytes > pre-adipocyte cells)[a]	↑ in humans[b] ↓ in ob/ob mice	[a]Montague et al., 1997 [b]Lonnqvist et al., 1997
TNF-α	Interferes with insulin signalling and adipose tissue metabolism	Subcutaneous (1.67×)> omental fat[a]	↑ in humans[b], obese 2×.> lean[d1] ↓ adipose differentiation ↑ obese animals[d2]	[a]Hube and Hauner, 1999 [b]Montague et al., 1997 [c]Frübeck et al., 2001 [d1]Hotamisligil et al., 1995, [d2]1993b
IL-6	Glucose and lipid metabolism and host defence	1/3 of all circulating levels from fat		
PAI-1	Potent inhibitor of fibrinolytic pathway	Correlation with abd. Pattern of ATD[a]	↑ in humans to ↑ thromboembolic complications[b]	[a]Juhan-Vague and Alessi, 1997
Angiotensinogen	Precursor of AII, regulator of blood supply, induces differentiation of pre-adipocyte cells	mRNA omental fat > Subcutaneous fat[a]	↑ in humans[b]	[a]Van Harmelen et al., 2000 [b]Fried and Kral, 1998

				References
TGFβ	Varied role in proliferation, differentiation, apoptosis and development	Multifunctional, produced by variety of cells Inhibitor of differentiation	↑ ob/ob (obese) and db/db mice[a] ↑ pre-adipocyte cell proliferation, as with TNF-α ↑	[a]Samad and Loskuttof, 1996
Adipsin	Activation of complement system	Found in serum	↓ in rodent obesity[b]	[a]Mohamed-Ali et al., 1998 [b]Cook et al., 1986
ASP	Effects rate of TAG synthesis in AT	Subcutaneous> omental fat, male> female[a]		
GH	Regulation of body mass through life	[Deficiency = ↑ AT and ↓ Lean mass, GH = decreased AT mass, reversed with GH administration ∴ Stimulation of lipolysis in xs		Armellini et al., 2000 Ailhaud and Hauner, 1998
PPARγ	Regulate adipose cell differentiation	Subcutaneous Ad = Omental Ad (BMI < 28 kg/m²)[a]	↑ Subcutaneous (2×) WhT>Omental WhT (BMI < 30 kg/m²)[b]	[a]Montague et al., 1998 [b]Lefebvre et al., 1998
Adiponectin	Regulation of insulin sensitivity & Role in inflammation	Produced by adipose tissue[a]	↓ with adiposity (db/db)[b] and lower with obesity and type 2 diabetes[c]	[a]Maeda et al., 1996 [b]Fruebis et al., 2001 [c]Hotta et al., 2000

TNF-α, tumour necrosis factor alpha; IL-6 interleukin 6; PAI-1, plasminogen activator inhibitor-1; TGFβ, transforming growth factor beta; ASP, acylation stimulating protein; MIF, macrophage inhibitory factor; GH, growth hormone; PPARγ, peroxisome proliferator-activated receptor gamma; ATD, adipose tissue distribution; Ad, adipocytes; WhT, whole tissue. (Adapted from Frübeck et al., 2001.) Reproduced by permission of the American Physiological Society.

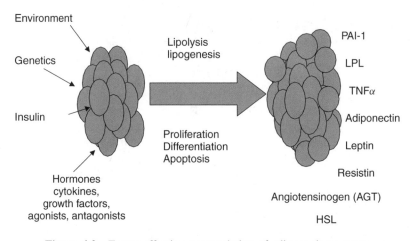

Figure 4.2   Factor affecting accumulation of adipose tissue mass.

Kopelman and Hitman, 1998; Woods *et al.*, 1998; Obici *et al.*, 2002). The number of adipocytes (mature fat cells) within an individual, which are not fixed, alters adiposity and such hyperplastic growth can occur at any time as a response to overfeeding. This activity is potentially controlled both at the hormonal and genetic level with key genes activating lipogenesis or lipolysis, therefore controlling the rate and intensity of fat deposition (Gregoire *et al.*, 1998). Adipose tissue accumulation is also thought to be under the control of a number of factors both neuronal and hormonal originating locally and at sites distant to the adipose tissue sites. Therefore, the aetiological link between obesity and type 2 diabetes lies in a multitude of factors, which include changes in adipose tissue distribution and metabolism, muscle metabolism, as well as alterations in levels of carbohydrates, fatty acids and adipocyte derived factors including leptin (Table 4.2), tumour necrosis factor-α (TNF-α), adiponectin and resistin (Figure 4.2).

Fat distribution

Increasing evidence has accumulated to demonstrate that regional adiposity plays a greater role in the development of diabetes, impaired glucose tolerance and atherosclerosis than generalized obesity. This concept is not entirely new – Vague first described it in 1956 (Vague, 1956).

Different patterns of obesity exist, central obesity in which there is an increase in intra-abdominal fat, particularly abdominal subcutaneous and omental fat; lower body obesity, which is characterized by fat stored predominantly in subcutaneous regions of hips, thighs and lower trunk (Abate, 1996). This fat

Table 4.2   Factors altering leptin expression

Factors increasing leptin expression	Factors decreasing leptin expression
Obesity	Weight reduction
Food intake	Fasting
Glucose	Insulin-dependent diabetes
Insulin	β-adrenoceptor agonists, cAMP elevating agents
Cortisol	TZDs

TZD, thiazolidinedione.

distribution can be readily identified between women and men. Vague proposed over 50 years ago that upper body obesity (i.e. central or abdominal) also known as either 'android' or 'male type obesity' correlated with increased mortality and risk for associated disease (such as type 2 diabetes and cardiovascular disease) compared with 'gynoid' or 'female type obesity' (lower body or gluteofemoral). In the female with increasing adiposity there is increased deposition in the lower part of the abdominal wall and the gluteofemoral area (Arner and Eckel 1998). It has been clearly shown that both an increase in fatness and a preferential upper-body accumulation of fat is independently related to insulin resistance (Clausen *et al.*, 1996). Obese women with a greater proportion of upper-body fat tended to be more insulin resistant, hyperinsulinaemic, glucose-intolerant and dyslipidaemic than obese women with a greater proportion of lower-body fat. Imaging techniques, such as magnetic resonance imaging (MRI) and computed tomography (CT), identified visceral-fat accumulation specifically associated with metabolic alterations of obesity in men and women (Despres *et al.*, 1995; Banerji *et al.*, 1995; Albu *et al.*, 1997, 2000). These data combined with the lipotoxicity effects (see lipid metabolism) led to the portal hypothesis which suggests that complications of obesity are attributable to increases in visceral adipose tissue with an associated rise in portal vein plasma non-esterified fatty acids (NEFA) concentrations (Bjorntorp, 1990.)

Evaluating obesity-related hypotheses for progression of type 2 diabetes

Although the portal hypothesis is associated with obesity, insulin resistance and the pathogenesis of type 2 diabetes associations between subcutaneous fat on the trunk and insulin resistance have been shown in obese non-diabetic men (Abate *et al.*, 1995; Goodpaster *et al.*, 1997) and in men with type 2 diabetes Abate *et al.*, 1996; Kelley and Mandarino, 2000; Smith *et al.*, 2001. As the present data suggests that subcutaneous fat, which accounts for 80 per cent of total adipose tissue, is a cause of insulin resistance this must occur via a non-portal mechanism as this fat depot does not drain into the portal vein. Furthermore, insulin resistance appears independently by an increased truncal subcutaneous adipose tissue and an increased visceral fat store (Albu *et al.*, 2000; Marcus *et al.*, 1999; Bavenholm *et al.*, 2003). Because of growing evidence that subcutaneous fat may play an important role in obesity-related type 2 diabetes with conflicting evidence for the role of the portal fat, changes in the model for the understanding of adipose tissue in the pathogenesis of type 2 diabetes have been proposed (Kuhn, 1962). The two emerging models are 'the ectopic fat storage syndrome' and to view the adipocyte as an endocrine organ (Ravussin and Smith, 2002).

Ectopic fat storage: fat content in obesity

Positive energy balance produces an excess of triglyceride with storage in the liver (Ryysy *et al.*, 2000) and skeletal muscle (Goodpaster and Kelley, 1998; Goodpaster *et al.*, 1997, 2000; Shulman, 2000) which is subsequently followed by insulin resistance, glucose, intolerance and diabetes. This similar effect is also observed in patients with lipodystrophy characterized by a severe reduction in adipose tissue with increased triglyceride storage in the liver and skeletal muscle (Robbins *et al.*, 1979, 1982) and subsequent type 2 diabetes disease. These observations suggest that in either the obese or lipodystrophic state, adipose tissue mass is unable to sequester dietary lipid away from the liver, skeletal muscle or the pancreas. As a result, too much or too little adipose tissue mass leads to ectopic fat storage and may further predispose individuals to insulin resistance and finally type 2 diabetes (Figure 4.3).

How does triglyceride become stored to account for ectopic fat? Deposition of triglyceride stored in unusual places, under normal physiological condition, may occur for several reasons, which will be discussed briefly as follows. Emerging evidence suggest that the mature adipocytes have a specific size capacity to efficient glucose uptake and therefore as rising adiposity correlates with enlarged adipocytes and insulin resistance this may effect systemic insulin resistance and triglyceride storage (Bjorntorp *et al.*, 1971; Czech, 1976). However adipose tissue only stores minimal glucose and therefore this is unlikely to have a profound effect to cause systemic insulin resistance (Ravussin and Smith, 2002). It has therefore been suggested that although large adipocytes are problematic in a lack of appropriate metabolic activity it may be the lack of further proliferating and differentiating of pre-adipocytes that give rise to enlarged adipocytes (Weyer *et al.*, 2000; Paolisso *et al.*, 1995). It is apparent that both commitment of stems cells into pre-adipocytes, proliferation and differentiation rely on complex mechanisms. Adipocytes develop from mesenchymal stem cells (Rangwala and Lazar, 2000), although mesenchymal cells can differentiate into several cell types including chondrocytes, osteocytes, tenocyte and adipocytes depending

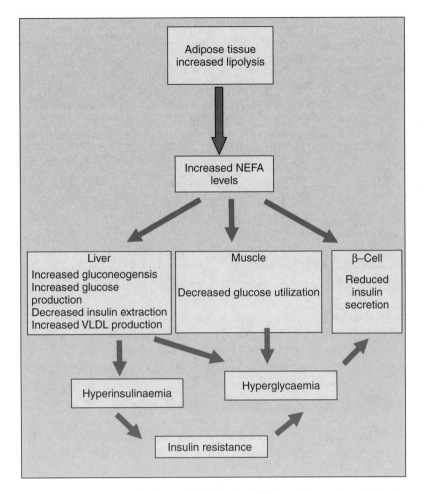

Figure 4.3   The exposure of the liver to high levels of FFA and glycerol results in increased VLDL production (not shown), reduced hepatic insulin clearance resulting in peripheral hyperinsulinaemia, which induces peripheral insulin resistance and increased hepatic gluconeogenesis. (Figure adapted from Jung).

on the balance of paracrine, endocrine and metabolic actions (Pittenger *et al.*, 1999). Adipocyte differentiation requires the coordinated actions of transcription factors to activate several genes necessary for lipid storage and insulin sensitivity (Nadler and Attie, 2001). These transcription factors are influenced by extracellular signals such as cytokines, hormones including insulin; therefore defects in any one of the steps can lead to failure in proliferation and or differentiation of adipocytes.

The failure of pre-adipocytes to proliferate and or differentiate may not account for ectopic fat storage; this may be due to impaired fat oxidation. Therefore, if fat oxidation is impaired while intracellular lipid rises this may lead to ectopic accumulation of intracellular lipid. In this situation metabolic oxidation of fat is insufficient to cope with the accumulation of dietary fat being presented to the body. Both human and rodent studies suggest evidence to support the impaired fat oxidation hypothesis, and together with increased intracellular lipid there is decreased fat oxidation and decreased insulin action (Zurlo et al., 1990; Seidell et al., 1992; Valtuena et al., 1997; Dobbins et al., 2001).

An additional hypothesis to account for ectopic fat may lie with the adipocytes' ability to respond and integrate hormonal and metabolic stimuli (Ramsay et al., 1989; Darimont et al., 1994; Serrero and Lepak, 1996; Ailhaud et al., 2000; Bruun et al., 2000; Lofgren et al., 2000; Berg et al., 2001; Berger, 2001; Yamauchi et al., 2001). Adipocytes, as detailed previously, produce a wide array of factors that have systemic, autocrine and paracrine effects. The balance of these effects may alter with enlarged adipocytes compared with the smaller adipocytes and result in systemic effects leading to ectopic fat storage (Ravissin and Smith, 2002). It may be by analysing clinical patient abnormalities that lead to ectopic fat storage that we may determine the cause of this problem. In reality, ectopic fat syndrome may present itself through a combination of these explanations, therefore understanding the pathophysiology of this occurrence is vital to understanding how to address therapy for it.

Non-alcoholic steatohepatitis (NASH), along with other forms of non-alcoholic fat liver disease, can often present its self as the first clinical indication of insulin resistance, with its complications of high blood pressure, coronary heart disease and type 2 diabetes (Scheen and Luyckx, 2003). NASH is relatively common with at least 20 per cent of obese adults or children with type 2 diabetes and in approximately 5 per cent of those who are overweight (Farrell, 2003). The prevalence and degree of severity of liver steatosis are related to BMI, waist circumference, hyperinsulinaemia, hypertriglyceridaemia and impaired glucose tolerance. The pathophysiology of NASH principally involves two steps: first, insulin resistance, which leads to steatosis, and second, oxidative stress, which causes lipid peroxidation and stimulates inflammatory cytokines (Farrell, 2003; Yki-Jarvinen, 2002). Identifying the progression of this two-stage disease is difficult and determining an appropriate therapy may also represent a challenge. It is important to note that studies indicate that substantial weight loss is associated with improvements in insulin sensitivity and components of the metabolic syndrome as well as regression of liver steatosis in most patients (Hickman et al., 2002; Nakao et al., 2002; Spaulding et al., 2003). Therefore, NASH may be considered another disease associated with the western lifestyle of reduced activity coupled with increased calorific intake.

Lipid metabolism in adipose tissue

It is apparent that one of the main factors in causing the progression from obesity to type 2 diabetes is the increase in the availability and oxidation of NEFA. With NEFA acting as a competitive energy source to glucose this can lead to resulting defects in both oxidative and non-oxidative pathways of glucose metabolism, affecting skeletal and adipose tissue metabolism The maintenance of triglyceride stores relies principally on two processes, lipolysis and lipogenesis, which remain pivotal in both health and disease.

Lipogenesis

Lipogenesis describes the process by which triglycerides circulating in the blood are hydrolysed to form NEFAs, which can be taken up by adipocytes and re-esterified in the form of intracellular triglycerides. NEFA are transported bound to albumin. However, cholesterol, triglycerides and phospholipids are transported as one of six different forms of lipoprotein complexes (three of which are the very-low density lipoproteins (VLDL), low-density lipoproteins (LDL) and high-density lipoproteins (HDL). Lipoproteins consist of a hydrophobic core of triglyceride and cholesteryl esters surrounded by phospholipids and proteins, these being apoproteins (the major ones being apoprotein E, C and B; Ganong, 1997). The most important pathway regulating the process for accumulating triglycerides in human tissue is the lipoprotein lipase (LPL) pathway.

Adipose tissue triglyceride depots are the major storage form for energy in the body and account for 10–30 per cent of body weight. In humans, the liver is the main anatomical site for lipogenesis, with the adipocyte making only a limited contribution. Dietary and hepatic sources form the main source of lipid for adipocytes with their uptake being regulated by LPL. LPL is a 55-kDa protein which is an evolutionarily conserved enzyme that catalyses the rate-limiting step in the lipogenic pathway (Wion et al., 1987).

The enzyme is activated by apolipoprotein C_{II} that is present different forms of lipoprotein complexes previously mentioned (Eckel, 1989). Upon activation, LPL hydrolyses the core triglyceride of the lipoproteins, including VLDL and chylomicrons. The VLDL particles contain the highest concentrations of triacylglycerol during the fasting state, whereas the chylomicrons predominantly carry triacylglycerols that have been absorbed following a meal and contain neutral fat. The hydrolysis of the lipoprotein results in the production of HDL that essentially contain the remnant particles of the chylomicrons. Although the process of hydrolysis of triglyceride takes place on the capillary luminal surface where LPL is attached to heparin sulphate proteoglycans, LPL is actually synthesized and secreted by adipocytes. In the cytoplasm of the cell, re-assembly into triglycerides occurs through the esterification of NEFA with glycerol-3-phosphate (Figure 4.2). Although glycerol-3-phosphate in adipocytes can be generated from glucose via glycolysis, there is little *de novo* lipogenesis in human adipose tissue with the lipid backbone of triglyceride almost exclusively coming from the imported NEFA rather than primarily synthesized from glucose. Although a previous study has highlighted that glycerol

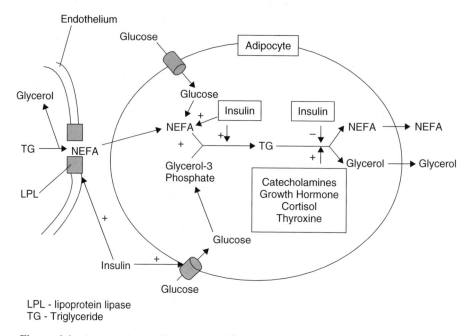

LPL - lipoprotein lipase
TG - Triglyceride

Figure 4.4   An overview of lipogenesis, lipolysis and some of the hormonal regulators.

itself cannot be used in triglyceride synthesis as adipocytes lack glycerokinase (Vaughan *et al.*, 1965) which converts glycerol to glycerol-3-phosphate, recent data indicates that adipocytes also express glycerokinase when treated with rosiglitazone (Guan *et al.*, 2002). Formation of triglycerides in adipose tissue involves several stages in which insulin has an important role although the regulation is not clearly understood (Figure 4.4). Insulin stimulates lipogenesis and acts partly by increasing the activities of lipogenic enzymes such as pyruvate dehydrogenase, and acetyl CoA carboxylase as well as stimulating glucose uptake, through glucose transporter 4 (GLUT-4), therefore increasing the availability of pyruvate for fatty acid synthesis and glycerol-3-phosphate for their esterification.

Previous studies have shown that LPL levels are higher in obese individuals than lean subjects. In addition LPL levels are observed to be higher in women than men and higher in femoral adipose tissue than abdominal subcutaneous tissue. LPL has been shown to be under the hormonal regulation of catecholamines, insulin, growth hormone, sex steroids, glucocorticoids and cytokines (Kern *et al.*, 1985; Fried *et al.*, 1993; Kruszynska, 1997; Arner and Eckel, 1998) influencing lipogenesis activity.

Lipolysis

The process by which fatty acids are hydrolysed from intracellular triglyceride moieties within adipose tissue ready for release into the blood stream is known as lipolysis. It is regulated by the enzymes hormone-sensitive lipase (HSL), the name reflecting the important role hormones play in its regulation, and monoacylglycerol. In contrast to HSL, monoacylglycerol does not appear to be hormonally regulated (Greenstein and Greenstein, 1996).

HSL is activated, with a concomitant 50-fold increase in activity, following cAMP-dependent protein phosphorylation at a single serine residue (Ser^{552}) and releases two fatty acids from triacylglycerol; the third is removed by mono-acylglycerol (Langin D *et al.*, 1996). The phosphorylation of a second site, the basal site, not only inactivates HSL but also prevents any further activation at Ser^{552}. Dephosphorylation of the basal residue reverses this process (Kruszynska, 1997; Arner and Eckel, 1998). Activation of HSL by phosphorylation occurs in response to hormone receptor binding. The primary lipolytic agents in human adipocytes are catecholamines with a more limited effect exerted by growth hormone whilst insulin, insulin-like growth factors I and II, adenosine, prostaglandin E_1 and neuropeptide Y, are all potent inhibitors of the process. The effects of the catecholamines are exerted through two types of adrenoreceptor–α and $\beta 1$, $\beta 2$ and $\beta 3$ (which activate adenylate cyclase and increase cAMP). The stimulation of α receptors inhibits lipolysis whereas the β receptors enhance lipolysis.

Effects of NEFA on hepatic insulin action

Circulating NEFA levels are raised in obese subjects, especially those with increased intra-abdominal fat or visceral obesity. It is well established that visceral adipose tissue is more metabolically active than subcutaneous fat, with high rates of triglyceride turnover and NEFA release. This situation may arise due to the close anatomical location with the liver, the dense vascular network, dense sympathetic innervation and increased levels of the β-adrenoceptor that mediates lipolysis (Rosell and Belfrage, 1979). NEFA generated from visceral fat enters the portal circulation and is delivered directly to the liver and is subsequently oxidized to acetyl CoA. Acetyl CoA stimulates pyruvate carboxylase and therefore the gluconeogenic production of glucose from pyruvate. Hepatic glucose production therefore increases. However, with increasing adiposity insulin resistance of visceral fat combined with a number of other metabolic characteristics, such as increase lipolytic response to catecholamines results in an accelerated rate of lipolysis (Richelsen *et al.*, 1991). This combined with the venous drainage of intraperitoneal fat, exposes the liver to high levels of NEFA and glycerol (Bjorntorp, 1990). This results in increased secretion of VLDL triglyceride, as NEFAs are the major substrate for hepatic triglyceride production, and as VLDL secretion is normally under the tonic inhibitory influence of insulin and this is lost in the insulin-resistant state (Durrington *et al.*, 1982). There is also reduced ApoB degradation; once again an insulin regulated process (Jackson *et al.*, 1990), with subsequent formation of small, dense atherogenic LDL. This high flux also reduces hepatic insulin clearance with subsequent peripheral hyperinsulinaemia and increases hepatic gluconeogenesis (Figure 4.3).

This situation is further exacerbated, as adipose LPL, an insulin-responsive hormone, which is normally responsible for triglyceride removal from VLDL, appears to be insulin resistant–a situation culminating in hypertriglyceridaemia. Unfortunately, studies looking at the fundamental question of whether insulin resistance precedes and worsens during obesity (Ludvil *et al.*, 1995), or whether it is a consequence of obesity (Campbell and Gerich, 1990), have to date provided conflicting epidemiological evidence, even when the same population has been studied (Swinburn *et al.*, 1991; Odeleeye *et al.*, 1995).

Adipose-tissue derived factors

Adipose tissue produces a large number of cytokines (Table 4.1) which include: leptin, the product of the *ob* gene (Zhang *et al.*, 1994), TNF-α (Hotamisligil *et al.*, 1993a; Kern *et al.*, 1995), resistin (Holcomb *et al.*, 2000; Steppan *et al.*, 2001a, b; McTernan *et al.*, 2002a), adiponectin (Maeda *et al.*, 1996; Hotta *et al.*, 2000) and interleukin-6 (IL-6) (Mora and Pessin, 2002; Spranger *et al.*, 2003), which may serve as important factors determining the pathogenesis of type 2 diabetes from obesity. This present chapter will discuss the regulatory effects of leptin, TNF-α, resistin, adiponectin, and IL-6 in the pathogenesis of obesity-related type 2 diabetes.

Leptin

Leptin is secreted and predominantly produced by adipose tissue, which circulates in the blood as a protein of 146 amino acids with a molecular mass of 16 kDa (Zhang *et al.*, 1994; Madej *et al.*, 1995). Leptin is presently viewed as a hormone that adapts and responds to metabolic effects on peripheral tissues as well as a satiety signal. Data presently suggests that leptin regulates energy expenditure mainly by acting on the brain. Leptin is actively transported across the blood–brain barrier and reaches the hypothalamus where it binds to specific leptin receptors located on the surface of neuropeptide Y, a tyrosine-containing peptide with powerful stimulatory effects on appetite. This leads to suppression of appetite, and ultimately activates the release of noradrenaline from the sympathetic nerve terminals that innervate adipose tissue and influence insulin actions in adipose tissue, liver, pancreas and potentially reproductive organs (Lönnqvist *et al.*, 1999). The central action of leptin was first demonstrated by studies carried out on mice that were induced to have a homozygous defective (*ob/ob*) gene. The mice became obese and developed diabetes but, upon treatment with recombinant leptin, they lost weight and their diabetes improved (Pelleymounter *et al.*, 1995). This generated intense interest and leptin was postulated to be the key mediator in the negative feedback loop from adipose tissue to the brain,

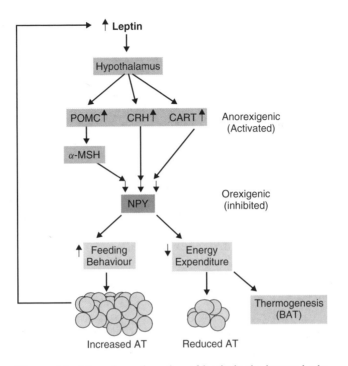

Figure 4.5   The schematic action of leptin in the human body.

enabling the central nervous system to sense the size of the body fat depot (Considine *et al.*, 1996; Van Gaal *et al.*, 1999; Figure 4.5).

The role of leptin has turned out to be far more complex than first thought as leptin mutations inducing obesity are rare and, conversely, plasma leptin concentrations are elevated in obese humans and other rodent models depot leptin (Considine *et al.*, 1996). Furthermore, there is a strong positive correlation between plasma leptin levels and fat mass (Zhang *et al.*, 1994). Consequently, it is suggested that the hyperleptinaemia found in obese subjects may be a consequence of leptin resistance in these individuals.

The receptors for leptin (OB-R) have been identified in the hypothalamus and surrounding brain regions–a finding that is consistent with its centrally mediated effects on appetite, metabolism and other endocrine systems involved in the starvation response (Tartaglia *et al.*, 1995; Schwartz *et al.*, 1996). However, leptin receptors have also been identified in many other tissues such as adipose tissue, skeletal muscle, the liver, the pancreas and tubular renal cells. Consequently leptin has several peripheral effects such as a possible role in the regulation of glucose uptake into skeletal muscle tissue and adipose tissue as well as being implicated in the development of insulin resistance (Muller *et al.*, 1997; Shimomura *et al.*, 1999; Yaspelkis *et al.*, 1999).

Circulating leptin concentrations appear to be in direct proportion to the amount of *ob* mRNA in the adipose tissue, which is increased in obese subjects.

(Considine and Caro, 1996). *ob* mRNA decreases with weight loss in both humans and rodents and increases with weight gain (Maffei *et al.*, 1995). Over-feeding has shown to increase *ob* mRNA in the absence of a significant weight gain in rats (Harris *et al.*, 1996).

In rodents, *ob* mRNA expression increased by insulin injection (Saladin *et al.*, 1995; Leroy *et al.*, 1996) while in humans insulin does not have an acute effect on *ob* mRNA but a chronic effect of insulin on *ob* mRNA, both from *in vivo* and *in vitro* studies has been described (Considine and Caro, 1997; Kolaczyn-ski *et al.*, 1996). The expression of leptin is also regulated by other factors such as the thiazolidinediones (TZD) a class of antidiabetic drug also known as insulin sensitizers that improve insulin sensitivity, decrease leptin mRNA in human and murine adipocytes (Zhang *et al.*, 1996; Nolan *et al.*, 1996). The effect is mediated via activation of adipose tissue-specific transcription factor peroxisome proliferator-activated receptor-γ (PPAR-γ), although a specific con-sensus sequence for the transcription factor on the *ob* gene promoter could not be identified. Other factors such as β-adrenergic receptor agonists reduce leptin mRNA and leptin release in isolated rat adipocytes (Slieker *et al.*, 1996). Other agents such as intracellular cyclic adenosine monophosphate (cAMP), isopro-terenol are also known to reduce weight gain while cortisol effects on leptin increases adiposity (De Vos *et al.*, 1995; Figure 4.6).

TNF-α

TNF-α is a multifunctional cytokine produced by a variety of cells that includes monocytes/macrophages, muscle cells and adipose tissue. Originally identified in its capacity to cause regression of tumours, it is now implicated as a pathogenic factor in the development of insulin resistance because of the multitude of effects it exerts on adipose tissue metabolism. Studies conducted in animal models and human subjects have demonstrated a positive correlation between TNF-α and obesity with regard to protein and mRNA expression in adipose tissue, as well as circulating levels of TNF-α (Hotamisligil *et al.*, 1993b, 1995). In addition to this, an association between elevated TNF-α expression in adipose tissue and features of insulin resistance has been described in obese and diabetic animal models (Hotamisligil *et al.*, 1995).

TNF-α is known to have a catabolic role in adipose tissue that has been demonstrated *in vitro* and *in vivo*. In 3T3-L1 cells, TNF-α has been shown to stimulate lipolysis (Hardardóttir *et al.*, 1992) and decrease activity of the lipogenic enzyme LPL via suppression at the mRNA and protein level (Beutler and Cerami, 1986). Furthermore, studies performed on murine cells *in vitro* show that TNF-α suppresses expression of the majority of adipocyte-specific genes, such as PPAR-γ, which is involved in adipocyte differentiation. The enhanced lipolysis may contribute to the glucose–fatty acid cycle that is consid-ered to be an important factor in the progression from insulin resistance to type 2

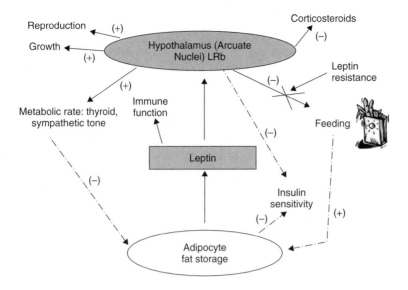

Figure 4.6   The multiple roles of leptin.

diabetes. This is supported by findings in TNF-α-deficient mice, which show improved insulin sensitivity and have decreased circulating levels of free fatty acids (FFAs). Furthermore, in studies by Gokhan and co-workers (Hotamisligil *et al.*, 1993), increased insulin sensitivity was exhibited by the obese Zucker (*fa/fa*) rats when treated with a soluble TNF-α receptor immunoglobulin. The treated rodents demonstrated a greater response than those left untreated, but remained at least six times more resistant to insulin stimulated glucose uptake than their lean counterparts (Hotamisligil *et al.*, 1993b). However, animal models and human studies show conflicting results as type 2 diabetic patients that were treated with recombinant antibodies to TNF-α did not exhibit any significant changes in fasting glucose, insulin or glucose clearance during insulin sensitivity tests (Ofei *et al.*, 1996; Moller, 2000; Bullo *et al.*, 2002; Grimble, 2002; Muller *et al.*, 2002; Miyazaki *et al.*, 2003).

Resistin

Resistin (FIZZ3) belongs to a family of cysteine-rich C-terminal proteins known as resistin like molecules (RELM; RELMα/FIZZ1 and RELMβ/FIZZ2) of FIZZ (found in inflammatory zone) which are thought to be involved in inflammatory processes (Holcomb *et al.*, 2000; Steppan *et al.*, 2001a, b). This 14-kDa polypeptide is abundantly expressed in the white adipose tissue of rodents and is secreted into the circulation in a dimerized form. Resistin has been proposed as the potential link between obesity, insulin resistance and type 2 diabetes based on observations made on genetically induced (*ob/ob* and *db/db*) and diet-induced (DIO) mouse models of diabetes and obesity (Steppan *et al.*, 2001a).

These studies have shown that in mice, resistin impairs glucose tolerance and insulin action and inhibits adipogenesis in murine 3T3-L1 cell processes (Holcomb *et al.*, 2000; Kim *et al.*, 2001; Lay *et al.*, 2001; Haugen *et al.*, 2001; Levy *et al.*, 2002). The role of resistin in human obesity still remains controversial. Previous resistin mRNA expression have resulted in conflicting reports in respect to the level of expression of this gene in human adipose tissue (Nagaev *et al.*, 2001; Savage *et al.*, 2001; Engeli *et al.*, 2002; McTernan *et al.*, 2002a). However, more recent studies indicate higher levels of expression of both gene and protein in central adipose tissue depots, supporting a role for resistin in linking central obesity to diabetes (McTernan *et al.*, 2002b).

Lazar and co-workers were first to demonstrate that both resistin mRNA and protein were downregulated by TZDs *in vitro* (Holcomb *et al.*, 2000), with the majority of subsequent *in vivo* data supporting these observations (Steppan and Lazar, 2002; Moore *et al*, 2001; Way *et al*, 2001). Furthermore, in their experiments, recombinant resistin induced insulin resistance both *in vivo* and *in vitro* and this effect was blocked by the use of anti-resistin antibodies. These data suggested a potential mechanism for obesity related insulin resistance and also suggested a new mechanism of action for TZDs. These data supported the hypothesis that resistin may be a protein that limits obesity at the expense of glucose tolerance, at least in rodent models.

Although resistin appeared to be a strong candidate protein linking excess adiposity and insulin resistance in rodent models, many early humans studies of resistin mRNA expression concluded that this molecule may not be an important factor linking human obesity to insulin resistance (Nagaev *et al.*, 2001; Savage *et al.*, 2001; Engeli *et al.*, 2002). While subsequent studies have, however, shown that resistin mRNA and protein expression are markedly increased in human central adipose tissue depots (both omental and subcutaneous) compared with thigh and breast adipose tissue (McTernan *et al.*, 2000a, b). Together these data support the potential role for resistin in central obesity. In addition, increased resistin mRNA expression was identified in obese compared with lean subjects (Savage *et al.*, 2001; McTernan *et al.* 2002b). These findings were not related to the contamination of adipose tissue samples by mononuclear blood cells (macrophages), which are known to express resistin (Savage *et al.*, 2001; Nagaev *et al.*, 2001; McTernan *et al.*, 2002b). However the role of resistin in linking obesity-related type 2 diabetes remains controversial as the significance of resistin expression from fat is uncertain (Hotamisligil, 2003; Fain *et al.*, 2003; Patel *et al.*, 2003). It is clear however that macrophages may represent another important site of resistin production although clearly production of resistin from fat may have more significance as fat can represent 30–40 per cent of the total body weight.

JNK-1

A more recently recognized feature of the metabolic syndrome is the association of sub-clinical inflammation (Pick and Crook, 1998). Although, to date, a mechanism linking insulin resistance and inflammation remains unclear, recent studies indicate adipose tissue may have a role in these processes, suggested by c-Jun amino terminal kinase (JNK-1) mice studies. These mice studies suggest that JNK-1 can interfere with insulin action further that JNK-1 can also be activated by pro-inflammatory cytokines such as TNF-α as well as free fatty acids (Aguirre *et al.*, 2000). Studies examining JNK-1 and -2 knock-out mice has strengthened the data providing evidence that obesity is associated with abnormally elevated JNK activity, predominantly provided by JNK-1 present in adipose tissue, liver and muscle. Importantly the absence of JNK-1 in the mice models results in substantial protection from obesity-induced insulin resistance (Hiorsumi *et al.*, 2002). Aberrant production of inflammatory associated cytokines such as TNF-α and FFAs appear important factors in obesity-induced insulin resistance as both factors activate JNK (Boden, 1997; Hiorsumi *et al.*, 2002) which in turn phosphorylates insulin receptor substrate 1 (IRS-1) at serine 307. As such dysregulation of the insulin receptor and reduced tyrosine phosphorylation of the IRS proteins may contribute significantly to peripheral insulin resistance and β-cell failure (Aguirre *et al.*, 2000). Human molecular evidence also indicates that increased JNK activity caused through loss of function-mutations in the JNK closely related protein JIP1 is casual to type 2 diabetes in humans (Waeber *et al.*, 2000). Present studies suggest that JNK1 is an important component of the biochemical pathway responsible for obesity induced insulin resistance *in vivo*, further human genetic mutation of JNK activity is associated with type 2 diabetes development (Waeber *et al.*, 2000). Therefore, analysis of JNK-1 represents a potential therapeutic target for treatment of obesity, insulin resistance and type 2 diabetes.

Adiponectin

Adiponectin expressed in adipose tissue, also known as ACRP30, AdipoQ, and GBP28, is the product of the human apM1 gene and is a 247 amino acid protein consisting of a N-terminal collagenous region and a C-terminal globular domain (Maeda *et al.*, 1996). The protein shares homology with complement factor C1q and other soluble defence collagens as well as the TNF family (Maeda *et al.*, 1996; Shapiro and Scherer, 1998). The importance of the adipocyte-derived hormone known as adiponectin was not immediately recognized when it was first identified in 1993. Several groups have more recently shown that adiponectin plasma concentrations are reduced in patients with type 2 diabetes (Hotta *et al.*, 2000; Lindsay *et al.*, 2002) and cardiovascular disease (Arita *et al.*, 1999; Ouchi *et al.*, 1999; Okamoto *et al.*, 2000) and correlate inversely with both insulin resistance and obesity (Arita *et al.*, 1999). In addition, mouse studies have further shown that administration of adiponectin increases fatty acid oxidation in muscles and decreases hepatic glucose, resulting in enhanced insulin sensitivity and glucose clearance in diabetic mice (Berg *et al.*, 2001; Combs *et al.*, 2001; Fruebis *et al.*, 2001; Yamauchi *et al.*, 2001).

Previous studies have shown that adiponectin appears abundant in the circulating plasma with levels in the range $5-30\,\mu g/ml$ in humans (Scherer et al., 1995; Nakano et al., 1996). Furthermore a depot-specific pattern of mRNA expression of adiponectin in human adipose tissue has been demonstrated, implicating an inverse correlation with adiponectin expression and visceral adiposity (Statnick et al., 2000; Halleux et al., 2001).

Various forms of acrp30 exist within plasma including a truncated form, that consists mainly of the globular domain, as well as homotrimeric and higher order structures. The significance of these different forms of protein remain unclear although studies conducted in mice using both the truncated and full length forms of acrp30 have shown positive effects on the animals' metabolic profile. Administration of acrp30 to mouse models of diabetes results in increased oxidation of fatty acids in muscles, reduced hepatic glucose production and increased insulin sensitivity and glucose clearance. These results indicate that high levels of circulating acrp30 may abate the development of insulin resistance. This theory is further supported by the finding that acrp30 is present in relatively high quantities in non-obese human subjects whilst levels are decreased in both obese and type 2 diabetic subjects.

Other studies have shown that acrp30 accumulates within injured vascular tissue and has the capacity to bind to matrix proteins, indicating a possible role in the repair of these tissues (Okamoto et al., 2000). Some of the functions of acrp30 include the inhibition of phagocytosis by macrophages as well as suppression of TNF-α expression in these same cells (Okamoto et al., 2000). These findings suggest that acrp30 has anti-atherogenic properties, which may help to explain why lower plasma concentrations of acrp30 are associated with increased atherosclerotic risk. Furthermore, circulating plasma levels of acrp30 are higher in females than males, which may partially explain the reduced risk of cardiovascular disease in women.

Acrp30 has been shown to have an inhibitory effect on the nuclear factor (NF)-κB signalling pathway and as NF-κB is involved in the transcription of many pro-inflammatory cytokines, this may be a possible mechanism through which acrp30 ameliorates insulin resistance. However, the acrp30 receptor has, as yet, not been identified and the signalling pathway through which acrp30 produces its effects still remains to be elucidated.

Interleukin-6

IL-6 is another cytokine that has been implicated in the development of insulin resistance and type 2 diabetes in obese individuals. It is produced by a number of different cells including mature adipocytes and the stromal-vascular fraction. Several studies have demonstrated a correlation between circulating levels of IL-6, fat mass and body mass index whilst plasma IL-6 is also elevated in type 2 diabetic patients (Bastard et al., 2000; Kern et al., 2001; Vozarova et al., 2001).

The finding that subcutaneous adipose tissue contributes between 10 and 35 per cent of the body's IL-6 during periods of rest substantiates the importance of subcutaneous adipose tissue as a source of this cytokine (Mohammed-Ali, 1997). In this same study by Mohammed-Ali it was shown that IL-6 release was greater from the abdominal subcutaneous depot of obese subjects. However, studies have also demonstrated that severely obese, non-diabetic subjects produce two to three times more IL-6 from their visceral depot than subcutaneous fat. This suggests that both abdominal subcutaneous and visceral depots are important in IL-6 secretion. IL-6 has strong associations with insulin resistance and provides a possible link between obesity and insulin resistance, although the mechanisms through which it does this remain unclear. IL-6 is known to increase hepatic triglyceride secretion, decrease LPL activity and promote lipolysis, indicating that it may contribute to insulin resistance via an increase in circulating FFAs. In addition TNF-α, which is also strongly associated with insulin resistance, positively modulates IL-6 synthesis (Kern *et al.*, 2001).

Evidence from IL-6 knockout (KO) mice indicates that IL-6 has a central role in regulation of energy expenditure/metabolism. These mice developed mature onset obesity at nine months of age, weighing approximately 20 per cent more than their wild type counterparts (Wallenius *et al.*, 2002). Mature IL-6 KO mice exhibited dyslipidaemia, abnormal carbohydrate metabolism and hyperleptinaemia. Leptin treatment was ineffective in these rodent models whilst administration of recombinant leptin in the wild type mice resulted in a significant reduction in food intake and weight. However, the intracerebroventricular administration of low doses of IL-6 resulted in reduced food intake and decreased body mass in the IL-6 KO mice (Wallenius *et al.*, 2002). Moreover, the presence of IL-6 receptors in the hypothalamic centres of the brain support the possibility that IL-6 may act as an adipostat in much the same way as leptin (Jones *et al.*, 1993).

Summary

Obesity is not a modern problem, although the proportion of the population with obesity is rising and reaching pandemic levels in the current society. This has at present drawn the attention of governments and countries with worries over the socio-economic impact on society today. It may be apparent from our evolutionary background that we were designed to store triglycerides to survive periods of starvation as the original *Homo sapiens* 'hunter–gatherer' might have done. However, today, in the majority of the western world, we find ourselves maintaining a more sedentary lifestyle with increasingly more fat contained within our diets and obesity ensues. As a result, normal metabolic function is altered, ectopic fat deposition occurs altering normal physiological metabolism leading to metabolic diseases and complications. At present, drug therapies are targeting complications of obesity-associated disease as the obvious solution of exercise and reduced calorie intake is not working in the majority. Therefore, as obesity is the source of type 2 diabetes and associated complications, future drug therapies will need to directly target obesity and also adverse fat distribution.

References

Abate N (1996) Insulin resistance and obesity. The role of fat distribution pattern. *Diabetes Care* **19**(3):292–4.

Abate N, Garg A, Pershock RM *et al.* (1995) Relationships of generalised and regional adiposity to insulin sensitivity in men. *J Clin Invest* **96**(1):88–98.

Abate N, Garg A, Pershock RM *et al.* (1996) Relationships of generalised and regional adiposity to insulin sensitivity in men with NIDDM. *Diabetes* **45**(12):1684–93.

Aguirre V, Uchida T, Yenush L *et al.* (2000) The c-Jun NH2-terminal kinase promotes Insulin resistance during association with insulin receptor substrate-1 and phosphorylation of Ser^{307} *J Biol Chem* **275**:9047–54.

Ailhaud G, Fukamizu A, Massiera F *et al.* (2000) Angiotensinogen, angiotensin II, and adipose tissue development. *Int J Obes Relat Metab Disord* **24**(suppl 4):s33–s35.

Ailhaud G and Hauner H (1998) Development of white adipose tissue. In *Handbook of Obesity*, Bray GA, Bouchard C and James WPT (eds). Dekker, New York, pp. 359–78.

Albu JB, Murphy L, Frager DH *et al.* (1997) Visceral fat and race-dependent health risks in obese non-diabetic premenopausal women. *Diabetes* **46**(3):456–62.

Albu JB, Kovera AJ and Johnson JA (2000) Fat distribution and health in obesity. *Ann N Y Acad Sci* **904**:491–501.

Arner P and Eckel RH (1998) Adipose tissue as a storage organ. In *Handbook of Obesity* Bray GA, Bouchard C, James WPT (eds). Dekker, New York, pp. 379–96.

Arita Y, Kihara S, Ouchi N *et al.* (1999) Paradoxical decrease of an adipose-specific protein, adiponectin, in obesity. *Biochem Biophys Res Commun* **257**:79–83.

Armellini F, Zamboni M and Bosello O (2000) Hormones and body composition in humans: clinical studies. *Int J Obes* **24**(Suppl 2):S18–S21.

Banerji MA, Chaiken RL, Gordon D *et al.* (1995) Does intra-abdominal adipose tissue in black men determine whether NIDDM is insulin-resistant or insulin-sensitive? *Diabetes* **44**(2):141–6.

Bastard JP, Jardel C, Bruckert E *et al.* (2000) Elevated levels of interleukin 6 are reduced in serum and subcutaneous adipose tissue of obese women after weight loss. *J Clin Endocrinol Metab* **85**:3338–42.

Bavenholm PN, Kuhl J, Pigon J *et al.* (2003) Insulin resistance in Type 2 diabetes: Association with truncal obesity, impaired fitness and atypical malonyl coenzyme a regulation. *J Clin Endocrinol Metab* **88**:82–7.

Berg AH, Combs TP, Du X *et al.* (2001) The adipocyte-secreted protein Acrp30 enhances hepatic insulin action. *Nat Med* **7**:947–53.

Berger A (2001) Resistin: a new hormone that links obesity with type 2 diabetes. *Br Med J* **322**(7280):193.

Beutler B and Cerami A (1986) Cachectin and tumour necrosis factor as two sides of the same biological coin. *Nature* **320**(6063): 584–8.

Bjorntorp P (1990) 'Portal' adipose tissue as a generator of risk factors for cardiovascular disease and diabetes. *Arteriosclerosis* **10**(4):493–6.

Bjorntorp P, Berchtold P and Tibblin P (1971) Insulin secretion in relation to adipose tissue in men. *Diabetes* **20**(2):65–70.

Boden G (1997) Role of fatty acids in the pathogenesis of insulin resistance and NIDDM. *Diabetes* **46**:3–10.

Bray GA (1990) Obesity: historical development of scientific and cultural ideas. *Int J Obes Relat Metab Disord* **14**:909–26.

Bruun JM, Pederson SB and Richelsen B (2000): Interleukin-8 production in human adipose tissue: inhibitory effects of anti diabetic compounds, the thiazolidinedione ciglitazone and the bigaunide metformin. *Horm Metab Res* **32**(11/12):537–41.

Bullo M, Garcia-Lorda P and Salas-Salvado J (2002) Plasma soluble tumor necrosis factor alpha receptors and leptin levels in normal-weight and obese women: effect of adiposity and diabetes. *Eur J Endocrinol* **146**(3):325–31.

Clausen JO, Borch-Johnsen K, Ibsen H *et al.* (1996) Insulin sensitivity index, acute insulin response, and glucose effectiveness in a population-based sample of 380 young healthy Caucasians: analysis of the impact of gender, body fat, physical fitness, and life-style factors. *J Clin Invest* **98**(5):1195–209.

Campbell PJ and Gerich JE (1990) Impact of obesity on insulin action in volunteers with normal glucose tolerance: demonstration of threshold for the adverse effects of obesity. *J Clin Endocrinol Metab* **70**:1114–8

Considine RV and Caro JF (1997) Leptin and the regulation of body weight. *Int J Biochem Cell Biol* **29**:1255–72.

Considine RV, Sinha MK, Heiman ML *et al.* (1996) Serum immunoreactive-leptin concentrations in normal-weight and obese humans. *N Engl J Med* **334**:292–5.

Combs TP, Berg AH, Obici S *et al.* (2001) Endogenous glucose production is inhibited by the adipose-derived protein Acrp30. *Clin Invest* **108**:1875–81.

Cook KS, Groves DL, Min HY and Spiegelman BM (1985) A developmentally regulated mRNA from 3T3 adipocytes encodes a novel serine protease homologue. *Proc Natl Acad Sci U S A* **82**(19):6480–4.

Czech MP (1976) Cellular basis of insulin insensitivity in large rat adipocytes. *J Clin Invest* **57**(6):1523–32.

Darimont C, Vassaux G, Ailhaud G and Negrel R (1994) Differentiation of preadipose cells: paracrine role of prostacyclin upon stimulation of adipose cells by angiotensin II. *Endocrinology* **135**(5):2030–6.

Despres JP, Lemieux S, Lamarche B *et al.* (1995) The insulin resistance-dyslipidemic syndrome: contribution of visceral obesity and therapeutic implications. *Int J Obes Relat Metab Disord* **19**(Suppl 1)S76–S86.

De Vos P, Saladin R, Auwerx J and Staels B (1995) Induction of the ob gene expression by corticosteroids is accompanied by body weight loss and reduced food intake. *J Biol Chem* **270**:15958–61.

Dobbins RL, Szczepaniak LS, Bentley B *et al.* (2001) Prolonged inhibition of muscle carnitine palmitoyltransferase-1 promotes intramyocellular lipid accumulation and insulin resistance in rats. *Diabetes* **50**(1):123–30.

Durrington PN, Newton RS, Weinstein DB and Steinberg D (1982) Effects of insulin and glucose on VLDL triglyceride secretion by cultured rat hepatocytes. *J Clin Invest* **70**:63–73.

Eckel RH (1989) Alterations in lipoprotein lipase in insulin resistance. *Int J Obes Rel Metab Disord* **320**(16):1060–8.

Engeli JJ, Gorzelniak K, Luft FC, Sharma AM (2002) Resistin gene expression in human adipocytes is not related to insuline resistance. *Obes Res* **10**(1):1–15.

Fain JN, Cheema PS, Bahouth SW, Lloyd Hiler M (2003) Resistin release by human adipose tissue explants in primary culture. *Biochem Biophys Res Commun* **300**(3):674–8.

Farrell GC (2003) Non alcoholic steatohepatitis: what is it, and why is it important in the Asia-Pacific region. *Gastroenterol Hepatol* **18**(2):124–38.

Frayn KN, Coppack SW, Fielding BA and Humphreys SM (1995) Coordinated regulation of hormone sensitive lipase in human adipose tissue invivo: implications for the control of fat storage and fat mobilization. *Adv Enz Regul* **35**:163–78.

Fried SK and Kral JG (1987) Sex differences in regional distribution of fat cell size and lipoprotein lipase activity in morbidly obese patients. *Int J Obes* **11**(2):129–40.

Fried SK, Russel CD, Grauso NL and Brolin RE (1993) Lipoprotein lipase regulation by insulin and glucocorticoids in subcutaneous and omental adipose tissue of obese men and women. *J Clin Invest* **92**:2191–8.

Frübeck G, Gómez-Ambrosi J, Muruzábal FJ and Burrell MA (2001) The adipocyte: a model for integration of endocrine and metabolic signaling in energy metabolism regulation. *Am J Physiol Endocrinol Metab* **280**:E827–E847.

Fruebis J, Tsao TS, Javorschi S *et al.* (2001) Proteolytic cleavage product of 30-kDa adipocyte complement-related protein increases fatty acid oxidation in muscle and causes weight loss in mice. *Proc Natl Acad Sci U S A* **98**:2005–10.

Ganong WF (1997) *Review of Medical Physiology*, eighteenth edition. Appleton & Lange, London.

Gregoire FM, Smas CM and Sul HS (1998) Understanding adipocyte differentiation. *Physiol Rev* **78**(3):783–807.

Greenstein B and Greenstein A (1996) *Medical Biochemistry at a Glance*. Blackwell Science, Oxford.

Grimble RF (2002) Inflammatory status and insulin resistance. *Curr Opin Clin Nutr Metab Care* **5**(5):551–9.

Goodpaster BH Kelley DE (1998) Role of muscle in triglyceride metabolism. *Curr Opin Lipidol* **9**(3):231–6.

Goodpaster BH, Thaete FL, Simoneau JA and Kelley DE (1997) Subcutaneous abdominal fat and thigh muscle composition predict insulin sensitivity independently of visceral fat. *Diabetes* **46**(10):1579–85.

Goodpaster BH, Thaete FL and Kelley DE (2000) Thigh adipose tissue distribution is associated with insulin resistance in obesity and in type 2 diabetes mellitus. *Am J Physiol* **277**(6):E1130–41.

Guan HP, Li Y, Jensen MV, *et al.* (2002) A futile metabolic cycle activated in adipocytes by antidiabetic agents. *Nat Med* **8**(10):1122–8.

Halleux CM, Takahashi M, Delporte ML *et al.* (2001) Brichard SM: Secretion of adiponectin and regulation of apM1 gene expression in human visceral adipose tissue. *Biochem Biophys Res Commun* **288**:1102–7.

Hardardóttir I, Doerrler W, Feingold KR and Grunfeld C (1992) Cytokines stimulate lipolysis and decrease lipoprotein lipase activity in cultured fat cells by a prostaglandin independent mechanism. *Biochem Biophys Res Commun* **186**(1):237–43.

Harris RBS, Ramsay TG, Smith SR and Bruch RC (1996 Early and late stimulation of *ob* mRNA expression in meal-fed and overfed rats. *J Clin Invest* **97**:2020–6.

Haugen F Jorgensen A Drevon CA, Trayhurn P (2001) Inhibition by insulin of resistin gene expression in 3T3-L1 adipocytes. *FEBS letters* **507**:105–8.

Hickman IJ, Clouston AD, Macdonald GA *et al.* (2002) Powell EE: Effect of weight reduction on liver histology and biochemistry in patients with chronic hepatitis C. *Gut* **51**(1): 89–94.

Hill JO and Peters JC (1998) Environmental contributions to obesity. *Science* **282**:1371–3.

Hiorsumi J, Tuncman G, Chang L *et al.* (2002) A central role for JNK in obesity and insulin resistance. *Nature* **420**: 333–6.

Holcomb IN, Kabakoff RC, Chan B, *et al.* (2000) FIZZ1, a novel cysteine-rich secreted protein associated with pulmonary inflammation, defines a new gene family *EMBO J* **19**(15):4046–55.

Hotamisligil GS (2003) The irresistible biology of resistin. *J Clin Invest* **111**(2):173–4.

Hotamisligil GS, Peraldi P and Spiegelman BM (1993a) Adipose expression of tumor necrosis factor-α: direct role in obesity-linked insulin resistance. *Science* **259**:87–91.

Hotamisligil GS, Shargill NS and Spiegelman BM (1993b) Adipose expression of tumour necrosis factor-α: direct role in obesity-linked insulin resistance. *Science* **259**:87–91.

Hotamisligil GS, Arner P, Caro JF *et al.* (1995) Increased adipose tissue expression of tumor necrosis factor-α in human obesity and insulin resistance. *J Clin Invest* **95**: 2409–15.

Hotta K, Funahashi T, Arita Y *et al.* (2000) Plasma concentrations of a novel, adipose-specific protein, adiponectin, in type 2 diabetic patients. *Arterioscler Thromb Vasc Biol* **20**:1595–9.

Hube F and Hauner H (1999) The role of TNF-α in human adipose tissue: prevention of weight gain at the expense of insulin resistance? *Horm Metab Res* **31**:626–1.

IASO/IOTF report (2000) The Asia-Pacific perspective: Redefining obesity and its treatment. WHO (Western Pacific Region).

Iemura A, Douchi T, Yamamoto S *et al.* (2000) Body fat distribution as a risk factor of endometrial cancer. *J Obstet Gynaecol Res* **26**(6):421–5.

Isse N Ogawa Y, Tamura N *et al.* (1999) Structural organisation and chromosomal assignment of the human obese gene. *J Biol Chem* **270**:27728–33.

Jackson TW, Salhanick AI, Elvoson J *et al.* (1990) Insulin regulates apolipoprotein B turnover and phosphorylation in rat hepatocytes. *J Clin Invest* **86**:1746–51.

Jones JH and Kennedy RI (1993) Cytokines and hypothalamic-pituitary function. *Cytokine* **5**:531–8.

Juhan-Vague I and Alessi MC (1997) PAI-1, obesity, insulin resistance and risk of cardiovascular events. *Thromb Haemost* **78**(1):656–60.

Kelley DE and Mandarino LJ (2000) Fuel selection in human skeletal muscle in insulin resistance: a reexamination. *Diabetes* **49**(5):677–83.

Kern PA, Marshall S and Eckel RH (1985) Regulation of lipoprotein lipase in primary cultures of isolated adipocytes. *J Clin Invest* **75**:199–208.

Kern PA, Saghizadeh M Ong JM *et al.* (1995) The expression of tumor necrosis factors in human adipose tissue. *J Clin Invest* **95**:2111–9.

Kern PA, Ranganathan S, Li C *et al.* (2001) Adipose tissue tumor necrosis factor and interleukin-6 expression in human obesity and insulin resistance 2. *Am J Physiol – Endocrinol Metab* **280**:E745–51.

Kim KH, Lee K, Moon YS and Sul HS (2001) A cysteine-rich adipose tissue-specific secretory factor inhibits adipocyte differentiation. *J Biol Chem* **76**(14):11252–6.

Kissebah AH and Krakower GR (1994) Regional adiposity and morbidity. *Physiol Rev* **74**(4): 761–811.

Ko GTC, Chan JCN, Cockram CS and Woo J (1999) Prediction of hypertension, diabetes, dyslipidaemia or albuminuria using simple anthropometric indexes in Hong Kong Chinese. *Int J Obes Relat Metab Disord* **23**(ii):1136–42.

Kolaczynski JW, Nyce MR, Considine RV *et al.* (1996) Acute and chronic effect of insulin on leptin production in humans. *Diabetes* **45**:699–701.

Kopelman PG and Hitman GA (1998) Diabetes: exploding type II. *Lancet* **352**:sIV5–SIV6.

Kruszynska YT (1997) Normal metabolism: the physiology of fuel homeostasis. In Pickup JC, Williams G (eds). *Textbook of Diabetes*. Blackwell Publishers, Oxford.

Kuhn TF (1962) *The structure of Scientific Revolutions*, second edition. University of Chicago Press, Chicago.

Langin D, Holm C and Lafontan M (1996) Adipocyte hormone-sensitive lipase: a major regulator of lipid metabolism. *Proc Nutr Soc* **55**(1B):93–109.

Lay SL, Boucher J, Rey A *et al.* (2001) Decreased resistin expression in mice with different sensitivities to a high-fat diet. *Biochem Biophys Res Commun* **289**: 564–7.

Lefebvre A-M, Laville M, Vega N *et al.* (1998) Depot-specific differences in adipose tissue gene expression in lean and obese subjects. *Diabetes* **47**:98–103.

Leroy P, Dessolin S, Villageois P *et al.* (1996) Expression of the *ob* gene in adipose tissue: regulation by insulin. *J Biol Chem* **101**:2365–8.

Levy JR, Davenport B, Clore JN, Stevens W (2002) Lipid metabolism and resistin gene expression in insulin-resistant Fischer 344 rats. *Am J Physiol Endocorinol Metab* **282**: E626–E633.

Lindsay RS, Funahashi T, Hanson RL *et al.* (2002) Adiponectin and development of type 2 diabetes in the Pima Indian population. *Lancet* **360**:57–8.

Lofgren P, Van Harmelen V, Reynisdottir S *et al.* (2000) Secretion of tumour necrosis factor-alpha shows a strong relationship to insulin-stimulated glucose transport in human adipose tissue. *Diabetes* **49**(5):688–92.

Lönnqvist F, Nordfors L and Schalling M (1999) Leptin and its potential role in human obesity. *J Intern Med* **245**:643–52.

Lonnqvist F, Nordfors L, Jansson M *et al.* (1997 Leptin secretion from adipose tissue in women. Relationship to plasma levels and gene expression. *J Clin Invest* **99**(10):2398–404.

Ludvil B, Nolan JJ, Bolago J *et al.* (1995) Effects of obesity on insulin resistance in normal subjects and patients with NIDDM. *Diabetes* **44**:1121–5

Madej T, Boguski M and Bryant SH (1995) Threading analysis suggests that the obese gene product (leptin) in white adipose tissue and 3T3-L1 adipocytes. *Proc Natl Acad Sci U S A* **373**:13–18.

Maeda K, Okubo K, Shimomura I *et al.* (1996) cDNA cloning and expression of a novel adipose specific collagen-like factor, apM1 (Adipose Most abundant gene Transcript 1). *Biochem Biophys Res Commun* **221**(2):286–9.

Maffei M, Halaas JL, Ravussin E *et al.* (1995) Leptin levels in human and rodent: measurement of plasma leptin and *ob* RNA in obese and weight-reducing subjects. *Nat Med* **1**:1155–60.

Marcus MA, Murphy L, PI-Sunyer FX and Albu JB (1999) Insulin sensitivity and serum triglyceride level in obese white and black women: relationship to visceral and truncal subcutaneous fat. *Metabolism* **48**(2):194–9.

Masuzaki H, Ogawa Y, Isse N *et al.* (1995) Human obese gene expression: adipocyte-specific expression and regional differences in the adipose tissue. *Diabetes* **44**:855–8.

McKeigue PM, Shah B and Marmot MG (1991) Relation of central obesity and insulin resistance with high diabetes prevalence and cardiovascular risk in South Asians. *Lancet* **337**:382–6.

McTernan CL, McTernan PG, Harte AL *et al.* (2002a) Resistin central obesity and type 2 diabetes. *Lancet* **35**:46–7.

McTernan PG, McTernan CL, Chetty R, *et al.* (2002b) Increased resistin gene and protein expression in human abdominal adipose tissue. *J Clin Endocrinol Metab* **87**(5):2407–10.

Miyazaki Y, Pipek R, Mandarino LJ and DeFronzo RA (2003) Tumor necrosis factor alpha and insulin resistance in obese type 2 diabetic patients *Int J Obes Relat Metab Disord* **27**(1):88–94.

Moller DE (2000) Potential role of TNF-alpha in the pathogenesis of insulin resistance and type 2 diabetes. *Trends Endocrinol Metab* **11**(6):212–7.

Mohammed-Ali V, Goodrick S, Rawesh A *et al.* (1997) Subcutaneous adipose tissue releases interleukin-6, but not tumour necrosis factor-α, invivo. *J Clin Endocrinol Metab* **82**: 4196–200.

Mohamed-Ali V, Pinkney JH and Coppack SW (1998) Adipose tissue as an endocrine and paracrine organ. *Int J Obes Relat Metab Dis* **22**(12):1145–58.

Montague CT, Prins JB, Sanders L *et al.* (1997) Depot- and sex-specific differences in human leptin mRNA expression. Implications for the control of regional fat distribution. *Diabetes* **46**:342–7.

Montague CT, Prins JB, Sanders L *et al.* (1998) Depot-related gene expression in human subcutaneous and omental adipocytes. *Diabetes* **47**:1384–91.

Moore GB, Chapman H, Holder JC (2001) Lister CA, Piercy V, Smith SA Clapman JC1: Differential regulation of adipocytokine mRNA by rosiglitazone in *db/db* mice. *Biochem Biophys Res Commun* **286**:735–41.

Mora S and Pessin JE (2002) An adipocentric view of signaling and intracellular trafficking. *Diabetes Metab Res Rev* **18**(5):345–56.

Muller G, Ertl J, Gerl M and Preibisch G (1997) Leptin impairs metabolic actions of insulin in isolated rat adipocytes. *J Biol Chem* **272**(16):10585–93.

Muller S, Martin S, Koenig W *et al.* (2002) Impaired glucose tolerance is associated with increased serum concentrations of interleukin 6 and co-regulated acute-phase proteins but not TNF-alpha or its receptors. *Diabetologia* **45**(6):805–12.

Nadler ST and Attie AD (2001) Please pass the chips: genomic insights into obesity and diabetes. *J Nutr* **131**(8):2078–81.

Nagaev I and Smith U (2001) Insulin resistance and type 2 diabetes are not related to resistin expression in human fat cells or skeletal muscle. *Biochem Biophys Res Commun* **285**:561–4.

Nakao K, Nakata K, Ohtsubo N *et al.* (2002) Association between nonalcholic fatty liver, markers of obesity, and serum leptin level in young adults. *Am J Gastroenterol* **97**(7):1796–1801.

Nakano Y, Tobe T, Choi-Miura NH *et al.* (1996) Isolation and characterisation of GBP28, a novel gelatain-binding protein purified from human plasma. *J Biochem* **120**:803–12.

Nolan JJ, Olefsky JM, Nyce MR *et al.* (1996) Effect of troglitazone on leptin production. Studies *in vitro* and in human subjects. *Diabetes* **45**:1276–8.

Odeleeye OE, de Courten M and Ravussin E (1995) Insulin resistance as a predictor of body weight gain in 5–10 year old Pima Indians. *Diabetes* **44**(suppl 1):7a.

Obici S, Feng Z, Morgan K *et al.* (2002) Central administration of Oleic acid inhibits glucose production and food intake. *Diabetes* **51**:271–5.

Ofei F, Hurel S, Newkirk J, Sopwith M and Taylor R (1996) Effects of an engineered human anti-TNF-α-antibody (CDP571) on insulin sensitivity and glycemic control in patients with NIDDM. *Diabetes* **45**:881–5.

Okamoto Y, Artia Y, Nishida M *et al.* (2000) An adipocyte-derived plasma protein, adiponectin, adheres to injured vascular walls. *Horm Metab Res* **32**:47–50.

Ouchi N, Kihara S, Arita Y *et al.* (1999) Novel modulator for endothelial adhesion molecules: adipocyte-derived plasma protein adiponectin. *Circulation* **100**:2473–6

Paolisso G, Tataranni PA, Foley JE *et al.* (1995) A high concentration of fasting plasma non-esterified fatty acids is a risk factor for the development of NIDDM. *Diabetologica* **38**(10):1213–17.

Patel L, Buckels AC, Kinghorn IJ *et al.* (2003) Resistin is expressed in human macrophages and directly regulated by PPAR gamma activators. *Biochem Biophys Res Commun* **300**(2): 472–6.

Pelleymounter MA, Cullen MJ, Baker MB *et al.* (1995) Effects of the obese gene product on body weight regulation in ob/ob mice. *Science* **269**:543–6.

Pick JC and Crokk MA (1998) Is type II diabetes mellitus a disease of the innate immune system? *Diabetologia* **41**:1241–8.

Pittenger MF, Mackay AM, Beck SC *et al.* (1999) Multilineage potential of adult human mesenchymal stem cells. *Science* **284**(5411):143–7.

Ramirez ME, McMurray MP, Wiebke GA *et al.* (1997) Evidence for sex steroid inhibition of lipoprotein lipase in men: comparison of abdominal and femoral adipose tissue. *Metabolism* **46**(2):179–85.

Ramsay TG, White ME and Wolverton CK (1989) Insulin like growth factor 1 induction of differentiation of porcine preadipocytes. *J Anim Sci* **67**(9):2452–9.

Rangwala SM and Lazar MA (2000) Transcriptional control of adipogenesis [in process citation]. *Annu Rev Nutr* **20**:535–59.

Ravussin E and Smith SR (2002) Increased fat intake, impaired fat oxidation, and failure of fat cell proliferation result in ectopic fat storage, insulin resistance and type 2 diabetes mellitus. *Ann N Y Acad Sci* **967**:363–78.

Reaven GM (1988) Role of insulin resistance in human disease. Banting Lecture. *Diabetes* **37**:1595–1607.

Reaven GM (1995) The fourth Musketeer–from Alexandre Dumas to Claude Bernard. *Diabetologia* **38**:3–13.

Richelsen B, Pederson SB, Moller-Pederson T and Bak JF (1991) Regional differences in triglyceride breakdown in human adipose tissue: effects of catecholamines, insulin and prostaglandin E2. *Metabolism* **40**(9):990–6.

Robbins DC, Danforth E, Horton ES *et al.* (1979) The effect of diet on thermogenesis in acquired lipodystrophy. *Metabolism* **28**(9):908–16.

Robbins DC, Hortin ES, Tulp O and Sims EA (1982) Familial partial lipodystrophy: complications of obesity in the non-obese? *Metabolism* **31**(5):445–52.

Rosell S and Belfrage E (1979) Blood circulation in adipose tissue. *Physiol Rev* **59**(4): 1078–104.

Ryysy L, Hakkinen AM, Goto *et al.* (2000) Hepatic fat content and insulin action on free fatty acids and glucose metabolism rather than insulin absorption are associated with insulin requirements during insulin therapy in type 2 diabetic patients. *Diabetes* **49**(5):749–58.

Saladin R, De Vos P, Guerre-Millo M *et al.* (1995) Transient increases in obese gene expression after food intake or insulin administration. *Nature* **377**:527–9.

Samad F and Loskuttof DJ (1996) Tissue distribution and regulation and regulation of plasminogen activator inhibitor-1 in obese mice. *Mol Med* **2**(5):568–82.

Savage DB, Sewter CP, Klenk ES (2001) Resistin/FIZZ3 expression in relation to obesity and peroxisome proliferator-activated receptor-γ action in humans. *Diabetes* **50**:2199–202.

Scheen AJ and Luyckx FH (2003) Nonalcoholic steatohepatitis and insulin resistance: interface between gastroenterologists and endocrinologists. *Acta Clin Belg* **58**(2):81–91.

Scherer PE, Williams S, Fogliano M *et al.* (1995) A novel serum protein similar to Clq, produced exclusively in adipocytes. *J Biol Chem* **270**:26746–5749.

Schwartz MW, Selley RJ, Campfield LA *et al.* (1996) Identification of leptin action in rat hypothalamus. *J Clin Invest* **98**:1101–6.

Seidell JC, Muller DC, Sorkin JD and Andres R (1992) Fasting respiratory exchange ration and resting metabolic rate as predictors of weight gain: the Baltimore Longitudinal Study on Aging. *Int J Obes Relat Metab Disord* **16**(9):667–74.

Serrero G and Lepak N (1996) Endocrine and paracrine negative regulators of adipose differentiation. *Int J Obes Relat Metab Disord* **20**(5):58–64.

Shapiro L and Scherer PE (1998) The crystal structure of a complement-1q family protein suggests an evolutionary link to tumor necrosis factor. *Curr Biol* **8**:335–8

Shimomura I, Hammer RE, Ikemoto S *et al.* (1999) Leptin reverses insulin resistance and diabetes mellitus in mice with congenital lipodystrophy. *Nature* **401**(6748):73–6.

Shulman GI (2000) Cellular mechanism of insulin resistance. *J Clin Invest* **106**(2):171–6.

Slieker LJ, Sloop KW, Surface PL *et al.* (1996) Regulation of expression of *ob* mRNA and protein by glucocorticoids and cAMP. *J Biol Chem* **271**:5301–4.

Smith SR, Lovejoy JC, Greenway F *et al.* (2001) Contributions of total body fat, abdominal subcutaneous adipose tissue compartments, and visceral adipose tissue to the metabolic complications of obesity. *Metabolism* **50**(4):425–35.

Spaulding L, Trainer T and Janiec D (2003) Prevalence of non-alcoholic steatohepatitis in morbidly obese subjects undergoing gastric bypass. *Obes Surg* **13**(3):347–9.

Spranger J, Kroke A, Mohlig M *et al.* (2003) Inflammatory cytokines and the risk to develop type 2 diabetes: results of the prospective population-based European Prospective Investigation into Cancer and Nutrition (EPIC)-Potsdam Study. *Diabetes* **52**(3):812–7.

Statnick MA, Beavers LS, Conner LJ *et al.* (2000) Decreased expression of apM1 in omental and subcutaneous adipose tissue of humans with type 2 diabetes. *Int J Exp Diabetes Res* **1**:81–8.

Steppan CM, Bailey ST, Bhat S *et al.* (2001a) The hormone resistin links obesity to diabetes. *Nature* **409**:307–12.

Steppan CM, Brown EJ, Wright CM *et al.* (2001b) A family of tissue-specific resistin like molecules. *Proc Natl Acad Sci U S A* **98**:505–6.

Steppan CM, Lazar MA (2002) Resistin and obesity-associated insulin resistance. *TRENDS Endocrinol Metab* **13**:18–23.

Swinburn BA, Nyomba BL, Saad MF *et al.* (1991) Insulin resistances associated with lower rates of weight gain in Pima Indians. *J Clin Invest* **88**:168–73.

Tartaglia LA, Dembski M, Weng X *et al.* (1995) Identification and expression cloning of a leptin receptor, OB-R. *Cell* **83**:1263–71.

Ukkola O (2002) Resistin–a mediator of obesity-associated insulin resistance or an innocent bystander? *Eur J Endocrinol* **147**:571–4.

Vague J (1956) The degree of masculine differentiation of obesity: a factor determining predisposition to diabetes. Atherosclerosis, gout and uric calculus disease. *Am J Clin Nutr* **4**:20–34.

Valtuena S, Salas-Salvado J and Lorda PG (1997) The respiratory quotient as a prognostic factor in weight loss rebound. *Int J Obes Relat Metab Disord* **21**(9):811–17.

Van Gaal, LF, Wauters MA, Mertens IL *et al.* (1999) Clinical endocrinology of human leptin. *Int J Obes Relat Metab Disord* **23**(Suppl 1):29–36.

Van Harmelen V, Ariapart P, Hoffstedt J *et al.* (2000) Increased adipose angiotensinogen gene expression in human obesity. *Obes Res* **8**(4):337–41.

Vaughan M, Steinberg D, Liberman F and Stanley S (1965) Activation and inactivation of lipase in homogenates of adipose tissue. *Life Sci* **4**(10):1077–83.

Vozarova B, Weyer C, Hanson K *et al.* (2001) Circulating interleukin-6 in relation to adiposity, insulin action and insulin secretion. *Obes Res* **9**:414–7.

Waeber G. Delplanque J, Bonny C *et al.* (2000) The gene MAPK8IPI, encoding islet brain-1, is a candidate for type 2 diabetes. *Nat Genet* **24**:291–5.

Walker BR (2001) Steroid metabolism in metabolic syndrome X. Ballières Best *Pract Res Clin Endocrinol Metab* **15**(1):111–22.

Wallenius V, Wallenius K, Ahrén B *et al.* (2002) Jansson JO: Interleukin-6-deficient mice develop mature-onset obesity. *Nat Med* **8**:75.

Way JM, Gorgun CZ, Tong Q *et al.* (2001) Adipose tissue resistin expression is severely suppressed in obesity and stimulated by PPARγ agonists. *J Biol Chem* **276**:25651–3.

Weyer C, Foley JE, Bogardus C *et al.* (2000) Enlarged subcutaneous abdominal adipocyte size, but not obesity itself, predicts type II diabetes independent of insulin resistance. *Diabetologica* **43**:1498–1506.

WHO (1998) Obesity–preventing and managing the global epidemic. Report of a WHO consultation on obesity 1998. World Health Organization, Geneva.

Wion KL, Kirchgessner TG, Lusis AJ *et al.* (1987) Human lipoprotein lipase complementary DNA sequence. *Science* **235**:1638–41.

Woods SC, Seeley RJ, Porte D and Schwartz (1998) Signals that regulate food intake and energy homeostasis. *Science* **280**:1378–80.

Yamauchi T, Kamon J, Waki H *et al.* (2001) The fat-derived hormone adiponectin reverses insulin resistance associated with both lipotrophy and obesity. *Nat Med* **7**:941–6.

Yaspelkis BB 3rd, Ansari L, Ramey EL *et al.* (1999) Chronic leptin administration increases insulin-stimulated skeletal muscle glucose uptake and transport. *Metabolism* **48**(5):671–6.

Yki-Jarvinem H (2002) Ectopic fat accumulation: an important cause of insulin resistance in humans. *J Roy Soc Med* **95**(suppl 42):39–45.

Zhang B, Graziano MP, Doebber TW *et al.* (1996) The down regulation of the expression of the obese gene by antidiabetic thiazolidinedione in Zucker diabetic fatty rats and *db/db* mice. *J Biol Chem* **271**(16):9455–9459.

Zhang Y, Proenca R, Maffei M *et al.* (1994) Positional cloning of the mouse obese gene and its human homologue. *Nature* **372**:425–32.

Zurlo F, Lillioja A, Esposito-Del Puente *et al.* (1990) Low ration of fat carbohydrate oxidation as predictor of weight gain: study of 24-h RQ. *Am J Physiol* **259**(5 part 1):E650–E657.

5
Obesity and Prevention of Type 2 Diabetes

Jaakko Tuomilehto, Jaana Lindström and
Karri Silventoinen

Obesity and the risk of type 2 diabetes

Several prospective studies have documented that obesity is probably the most powerful predictor of the development type 2 diabetes (Knowler *et al.*, 1981; Colditz *et al.*, 1990; Manson *et al.*, 1992). However, not every obese subject develops diabetes, i.e. obesity alone is not sufficient to cause type 2 diabetes; there are other factors that considerably modify the effect of obesity on diabetes risk. For instance, it is likely that genetic susceptibility to diabetes is a necessary prerequisite for diabetes. This was demonstrated in the Pima Indians in whom the incidence increases more steeply with body mass index (BMI) in those whose parents have diabetes than in those who do not (Knowler *et al.*, 1981). Vice versa, in non-obese people the incidence of type 2 diabetes is low in the middle-aged even in populations such as the Pima Indians where the overall risk of the disease is very high. However, a large proportion of the human populations possess genes that permit type 2 diabetes to develop, well documented by a high prevalence of diabetes and impaired glucose regulation among the elderly (DECODE Study Group, 2003; Qiao *et al.*, 2003). Age-specific incidence rates of diabetes were also shown to vary according to BMI (kg/m^2) in the Pima Indians (Knowler *et al.*, 1981): in younger age groups subjects with a high BMI have higher incidence rates than those with lower BMI. It is, however, possible that many genetically predisposed subjects will develop type 2 diabetes or milder forms of impaired glucose regulation in the

Obesity and Diabetes.   Edited by Anthony H. Barnett and Sudhesh Kumar
© 2004 John Wiley & Sons, Ltd   ISBN: 0-470-84898-7

elderly in absence of gross obesity, particularly with decreasing physical activity and other conditions increasing with ageing.

Several studies indicate that other anthropometric indicators such as waist circumference or waist–hip ratio are strong risk factors for type 2 diabetes, independent of BMI, and may be better risk indicators than BMI alone (Chan et al., 1994; Boyko et al., 2000; Despres, 2001). Such data suggest that the distribution of body fat is an important determinant of risk as these measures reflect abdominal or visceral obesity. In Japanese American men, for example, the intra-abdominal fat, as measured from computed tomography scans, was the best anthropometric predictor of diabetes incidence (Boyko et al., 2000). More recent data indicate that intra-abdominal fat is more active than subcutaneous fat in secreting inflammatory cytokines that are associated with the development of type 2 diabetes (Spranger et al., 2003).

Obesity has increased rapidly in most populations in recent years. As expected, this increase has been accompanied by increasing prevalence of type 2 diabetes. Since obesity is such a strong predictor of diabetes incidence, it appears that the rapid increases in the prevalence of type 2 diabetes seen in many populations in recent decades are almost certainly related to increasing obesity. Furthermore, interventions directed to reducing obesity reduce the incidence of type 2 diabetes in obese individuals with impaired glucose tolerance (Tuomilehto and Lindström, 2003).

Obesity is the outcome of a positive energy balance in which energy intake has exceeded energy expenditure over time. Although this implies that obese individuals constantly eat more than they need, there is increasing evidence to support the idea that there are genetically determined metabolic difference between individuals who gain excessive weight and those that do not (Bergstrom and Hernell, 2001). However, endogenous factors alone do not sufficiently explain the massive increase in the prevalence of obesity worldwide in both developed and developing countries. The cause of this increasing prevalence can be ascribed largely to the increasing urbanization and its consequences. Some of the consequences have been the availability of 'affluent foods' (energy-dense foods that are high in fats and simple sugars and also low in dietary fibre) and an overall decrease in peoples' physical activity (Grundy, 1998). Decreased physical activity over a long period results in an imbalance of energy with excess energy being stored as fat in adipose tissue (Grundy, 1998; World Health Organization, 1998). In the presence of excess energy intake, the adaptive range is extremely small (<5 per cent) and the body energy reserve as adipose tissue increases rapidly (World Health Organization, 1998).

Many dietary studies show an inverse relation between reported energy intakes and body weight. This could be due to several reasons: first, obese people tend to under-report their energy intakes (Ravussin and Swinburn, 1992). Second, increased obesity prevalence could be the result of a gradual reduction in physical activity over many years (Schoeller, 2001), and third, it could also be the result of metabolic differences between lean and obese individuals (World Health Organization, 1998).

There is a tendency for weight gain with age (Martikainen and Marmot, 1999; Lahmann *et al.*, 2000). Most of this increment in weight occurs in adipose tissue. Grundy (1998) has estimated that a relatively small energy imbalance underlies most relative obesity in the general population. About 1255 kJ (300 kcal) maintains about 10 kg (22 lb) of excess weight. Theoretically therefore small weight losses should not be difficult to attain.

There has been a great deal of controversy regarding which macronutrients are responsible for causing a high prevalence of obesity in populations. Many investigators have favored the causative effects of a high fat diet in this regard (Flatt, 1988; Sclafani, 1992; Shah and Grag, 1996). However, several studies have indicated that despite decreasing fat intakes, average body weight is increasing in the US (Shah *et al.*, 1991; Kuczmarski *et al.*, 1994). In contrast many countries in Europe, which have higher per capita consumption of fat than the US, have lower prevalence's of obesity (Grundy, 1998). Data from the Third National Health and Nutrition Examination Survey (NHANES III) have shown a significant decrease in the mean percentage of total food intake from fat since the 1960s (Troiano *et al.*, 2000), but still the prevalence of obesity and NIDDM have continued to rise (Flegal *et al.*, 1998). However, other studies have showed increasing trends in energy consumption in the USA, and thus it is possible that the results about decreased food intake may be due to, for example, recall bias, and actually energy consumption has increased in the USA (Harnack *et al.*, 2000; Nielsen *et al.*, 2002). A recent meta-analysis in this regard by Swinburn *et al.* (2001) showed that relatively simple messages regarding fat restriction could however lead to weight loss. A meta-analysis based on 19 controlled, *ad libitum*, low-fat 2–12-month intervention studies, showed that *ad libitum*, low fat diets cause weight loss. The effect is more pronounced in subjects with a higher initial body weight (Astrup *et al.*, 2000). Ultimately, however, the overall energy intake will determine whether weight is lost, regardless of the source (Grundy, 1998).

Nutritional goals and guidelines are necessary to prevent the pathological consequences of an excessive energy intake. Recommendations, based on the energy density of foods with emphasis being on the consumption of nutrient-dense foods versus energy-dense foods, have been made by an Expert Consultation Group (1985). Nutrient-dense foods are foods, which are low in energy per unit volume, yet are high in micronutrients and dietary fibre. An example of such a food group would be green and yellow vegetables. Lower consumption of energy-dense foods is possible by restricting foods high in fats and simple sugars. Consideration should be given to rural populations in developing countries who have a high fibre intake. Recommended nutrient intakes may need to be increased between 5–15 per cent depending on the extent of fibre consumption (Expert Consultation Group, 1985).

With respect to ideal adult weight a BMI of less than 25 has been proposed, based on the evidence that up to two-thirds of type 2 diabetes could be prevented by maintaining BMI at less than this (Tuomilehto and Lindström, 2003). However more recently a population mean BMI of 21 has been promoted based on the fact that Oriental populations have a much lower BMI normal range (James *et al.*, 2001).

Even though primary prevention of type 2 diabetes was first proposed 80 years ago (Joslin, 1921) and more recently stressed by the WHO (WHO Study Group, 1994) only a limited number of studies have attempted to assess the value of measures aimed at controlling its modifiable risk factors. To be able to prevent a chronic disease such as type 2 diabetes, certain requirements have to be met. Knowledge about its natural history with a pre-clinical phase, modifiable risk factors, effective and simple screening tool to identify high-risk subjects and effective intervention that is affordable and acceptable are necessary. In addition, the efficacy of the intervention has to be proven under a clinical trial setting. It is well known that obesity and physical inactivity are the major risk factors and in people genetically predisposed to the disease the probability to develop type 2 diabetes is very high once exposed to 'unhealthy' lifestyles. Type 2 diabetes results from a dual process: a deficit in early insulin secretion and insulin resistance of liver, muscle and adipose tissue. During this process early prandial insulin secretion is blunted already in people with impaired glucose tolerance (IGT) (Sartor *et al.*, 1980; Bruce *et al.*, 1988; Eriksson and Lindgarde, 1991), and it worsens with a longer duration of diabetes. Post-prandial hyperglycaemia *per se* may contribute to the progressive deterioration of β-cells with early insulin secretion deficiency in type 2 diabetes as a vicious cycle. Thus, a detectable pre-clinical stage suitable for an intervention exists prior to the development of type 2 diabetes.

In testing the potential for prevention of type 2 diabetes, important questions must be answered: (1) Is lifestyle intervention efficacious to prevent type 2 diabetes? (2) What is the magnitude of the preventive intervention? (3) Does lifestyle intervention work in different ethnic groups and cultural settings? Observational cross-sectional and prospective studies have provided a large body of data that leanness and physically active lifestyles are associated with a low prevalence of type 2 diabetes and vice versa communities where obesity and sedentary lifestyle are common have a high risk of diabetes (Sartor *et al.*, 1980; Bruce *et al.*, 1988; Eriksson and Lindgarde, 1991). A very high prevalence of type 2 diabetes in some communities was previously attributed to special genetic constellation in these populations, and also the 'thrifty genotype' hypothesis was formed (Neel, 1962; Kahn *et al.*, 1996). Currently, however, type 2 diabetes has become common all over the world and is increasing in most countries (King *et al.*, 1998); the obvious inference is that there is no ethnic group with a particular genetic protection against the disease.

While observational data are important to identify risk factors for a disease and their possible independent role in the natural history of a disease, trials where risk factor exposures are modified are needed to determine their value in the prevention of the disease. Also, pharmacologic agents may be used to prevent hyperglycaemia or to halt the progressive increase in glucose levels in people with impaired glucose regulation. In the modern evidence-based medicine era the strongest evidence is considered to be coming from controlled clinical trials. Until recently, proper evidence regarding the prevention of type 2 diabetes tested and confirmed under a randomized clinical trial setting was virtually missing. Nevertheless, several attempts to intervene upon people who had various types and degrees of impaired glucose regulation have been carried out during the last decades. Most of them had major problems with design, sample size or conduct. These studies are summarized with comments recently by Hamman (2002). Today, there is evidence to suggest that the vicious circle in the natural history of type 2 diabetes can be stopped and the worsening from impaired glucose regulation to frank diabetes can be halted or delayed by influencing the causal environmental risk factors. In this paper we review the results from the major intervention studies for the prevention of diabetes and discuss their implications for public health applications and for the further research needs.

Lifestyle intervention studies

The main lifestyle issues that have been intervention targets in the prevention of type 2 diabetes are body weight, diet and physical activity. The intervention methods used to modify lifestyle have varied between the studies, since it is obvious that socio-cultural issues and the available facilities and personnel have dictated the application of the intervention. Also study designs have varied: both randomized and non-randomized studies have been conducted. The type of intervention, its duration and intensity has been very different in earlier preventive studies of type 2 diabetes (Hamman, 2002). One of the largest early intervention studies was the Malmöhus study in Sweden (Sartor *et al.*, 1980), comprising 267 men. A significant difference in the rates of development of type 2 diabetes was found between IGT subjects randomized to treatment and those randomized to no therapy. In an early intervention study in 10 years, the incidence of overt diabetes was 13 per cent in treated subjects (diet alone, tolbutamide or combined) compared with 29 per cent in the untreated subjects; the difference was statistically significant. The adherence with the treatment regimens was poor; for instance less than half of the people randomized to tolbutamide continued to take the drug throughout the study. It is also unclear as to what kind of dietary advice was actually given and how well the men randomized to diet groups actually followed these. Nevertheless, this trial suggested that the worsening from IGT to diabetes could be prevented or delayed. More recently, a few trials have tested this hypothesis: we may call them as the 'major lifestyle trials in prevention of type 2 diabetes'. These are described below.

The Malmö feasibility study (Eriksson and Lindgarde, 1991)

The feasibility of diet and exercise intervention in 217 men with IGT was assessed in the Malmö feasibility study. The effect of exercise and diet was compared to a reference group with no intervention. The reference group consisted of men who themselves decided not to join the intervention programme. Thus, the groups were not assigned at random. By the end of the 5-year study period 10.6 per cent of the intervention group and 28.6 per cent of the reference group had developed diabetes. Thus, the relative risk reduction in the incidence in the intervention group was 59 per cent and the absolute risk reduction was 17 per cent. This study was important in demonstrating the feasibility of carrying out a diet–exercise programme for 5-years among the volunteers, and furthermore it suggested that the incidence of type 2 diabetes might be halved with diet and exercise intervention. Overall, the progression to diabetes in these Swedish men was relatively low even in the reference group compared with the data from the observational studies. Even though the men who did not want to join the intervention programme, some of them may have changed their lifestyle as a result of the screening programme. Thus, these results based on intention-to-treat analysis may underestimate the true effect of lifestyle changes.

In this study, no difference was found between groups assigned to either diet alone, exercise alone or combined diet-exercise programs. The intervention actually resulted in significant changes in lifestyle and physiological parameters. The estimated maximal oxygen uptake increased by 10 per cent while it decreased by 5 per cent in control men. BMI decreased by 2.5 per cent in the intervention group but increased by 0.5 per cent in the control group. While the results on diabetes risk in the Malmö feasibility study are likely to be due to the effects on diet and exercise, it is not possible to generalize these results since the men in the study were not assigned to the treatment groups randomly.

The Da-Qing Study (Pan *et al.*, 1997)

Another important study was carried out in Da-Qing, China based on a large population-based screening programme to identify people with IGT. The 33 participating clinics were randomized to carry out the intervention according to one of the four specified intervention protocols (diet alone, exercise alone, diet-exercise combined or none). Data on the preventive effect of a diet and exercise intervention have been reported from this cluster-randomized clinical trial on 577 subjects with IGT in 1986. The cumulative 6-year incidence of type 2 diabetes was lower in the three (diet alone, exercise alone, diet-exercise combined) intervention groups (41–46 per cent) compared with the control group (68 per cent). Because no *individual* allocation of study subjects to the intervention and control groups was done, but the participating clinics were allocated, the results based on individual data analysis must be interpreted with caution. Furthermore, the study subjects were relatively lean, the mean BMI 25.8 kg/m^2 making inferences for other ethnic groups, where IGT subjects are usually obese, difficult. The mean BMI was 25.8 kg/m^2. Also, the progression from IGT to diabetes was high, more than 10 per cent per year in the control group, which is more than usually reported by observational studies. In this study the relative risk reduction was approximately 40 per cent while the absolute risk reduction was 22–26 per cent during the 6-year period.

In clinics assigned to dietary intervention, the participants were encouraged to reduce weight if BMI was >25 kg/m^2, aiming at <24 kg/m^2, otherwise a high-carbohydrate and low-fat diet was recommended. Counselling was done by physicians and also group sessions were organized weekly for the first month, monthly for 3 months and every 3 months thereafter. In clinics assigned to physical exercise, counselling sessions were arranged at a similar frequency. In addition, the participants were encouraged to increase their level of leisure-time physical activity by at least 1–2 'units' per day. One unit would correspond, for instance, to 30 min slow walking, 10 min slow running or 5 min swimming.

The overall changes in risk factor patterns were relatively small. Body weight did not change in lean subjects, and there was a modest, less than 1 kg reduction in subjects with baseline BMI > 25 kg/m^2. Also, the estimated changes in habitual dietary nutrient intakes were small and non-significant between groups. Exercise intervention seemed to produce best effects. Thus, it is not easy to determine the factors responsible for the beneficial effects on the risk of type 2 diabetes. It is nevertheless obvious that weight control was not the key issue. Thus, physical activity and qualitative changes in diet that are difficult to measure on individual level probably played a key role.

The Finnish Diabetes Prevention Study (DPS) (Eriksson *et al.*, 1999; Uusitupa *et al.*, 2000; Tuomilehto *et al.*, 2001)

The Finnish Diabetes Prevention Study is the first proper controlled trial on prevention of type 2 diabetes where the study subjects were individually randomly allocated into the intervention and control groups. The first part of the DPS was carried out during 1992 to 2000 in five clinics in Finland, aiming at preventing type 2 diabetes with lifestyle modification alone. A total of 522 individuals at high risk to develop diabetes were recruited into the study, mainly by opportunistic screening for IGT in middle-aged (age 40–64 years), overweight (BMI > 25 kg/m^2) subjects. The presence of IGT before randomization was confirmed in two successive 75-g oral glucose tolerance tests; the mean of the two values had to be within the IGT range. From previous studies it was estimated that the cumulative diabetes incidence in such a high-risk group would be 35 per cent in 6 years. The study subjects were randomly allocated either into the control group or the intensive intervention group. The subjects in the intervention group had frequent consultation visits with a nutritionist (seven times during the first year and every 3 months thereafter). They received individual advice about how to achieve the intervention goals: reduction in weight of 5 per cent or more, total fat intake less than 30 per cent of energy consumed, saturated fat intake less than 10 per cent of energy consumed, fibre intake of at least 15 g/1000 kcal, and moderate exercise for 30 min per day or more. Frequent ingestion of whole-meal products, vegetables, berries and fruit, low-fat milk and meat products, soft margarines, and vegetable oils rich in monounsaturated fatty acids were recommended. The dietary advice was based on 3-day food records completed four times per year. The subjects had seven sessions with a nutritionist during the first year of the study and every 3 months thereafter. They were also individually guided to increase their level of physical activity. Endurance exercise (walking, jogging, swimming, aerobic ball games, skiing) was recommended to increase aerobic capacity and cardiorespiratory fitness. Supervised, progressive, individually tailored circuit-type resistance training sessions to improve the functional capacity and strength of the large muscle groups were also offered.

The control group subjects were also given general advice about healthy lifestyle at their annual visits to the study clinic. An oral glucose tolerance test was done annually and if either fasting or 2-h glucose values reached diabetic levels a confirmatory oral glucose tolerance test was performed. The study end-point, type 2 diabetes, was only recorded if the second test also reached diabetic levels; otherwise the subjects continued with their randomized treatment. The subjects in the control group were given general verbal and written diet and exercise information at baseline and at subsequent annual visits, but no specific individually tailored information.

During the first year of the study body weight decreased on average 4.2 kg in the intervention group and 0.8 kg in the control group subjects ($P = 0.0001$). Most of the weight reduction was maintained during the second year. Also indicators of central adiposity and fasting glucose and insulin, 2-h post-challenge glucose and insulin, and HbA1c reduced significantly more in the intervention group than in the control group at both 1-year and 2-year follow-up examinations. At the 1-year and 2-year examinations intervention group subjects reported significantly more beneficial changes in their dietary and exercise habits, based on dietary and exercise diaries.

According to the study plan an interim analysis of the trial was carried out when approximately half of the 160 endpoints expected during the 6-year study period had occurred. In March 2000, a total of 86 incident cases of diabetes had been diagnosed among the 522 subjects with IGT randomized into the DPS trial when the median follow-up duration of the study was 3 years. Of them, 27 occurred in the intervention group and 59 in the control group. The absolute risk of diabetes was 32/1000 person-years in the intervention group and 78/1000 person-years in the control group. The effect of the intervention was rapid: the difference in incidence of diabetes between the groups was statistically significant already after two years: 6 per cent in the intervention group and 14 per cent in the control group. The cumulative incidence of diabetes was 11 per cent (95 per cent CI 6 to 15 per cent) in the intervention group and 23 per cent (95 per cent CI 17 to 29 per cent) in the control group after 4 years. Based on life-table analysis the risk of diabetes was reduced by 58 per cent ($P < 0.001$) during the trial in the intervention group compared with the control group. The absolute risk of diabetes was 32/1000 person-years in the intervention group and 78/1000 person-years in the control group. Thus the absolute risk reduction was 12 per cent at that point. From this it is possible to calculate the numbers needed to treat to prevent one case of diabetes: 22 subjects with IGT need to be treated for 1 year or 5 people for five years with such a lifestyle intervention to prevent one case of diabetes. Both men and women benefited from lifestyle intervention: the incidence of diabetes was reduced by 63 per cent and in women by 54 per cent in the intervention group compared with the control group. Interestingly, none of the people (either in the intervention or control group) who had reached all five lifestyle targets developed diabetes, while approximately one-third of the people who did not reach a single one of the targets developed type 2 diabetes. This is direct empirical proof that the reduction of the diabetes risk was indeed mediated through the lifestyle changes.

The Diabetes Prevention Program (DPP) (The Diabetes Prevention Program Research Group, 1999; Knowler *et al.*, 2002; The Diabetes Prevention Program Research Group, 2002)

The Diabetes Prevention Program was a multicentre randomized clinical trial carried out in the United States. It compared the efficacy and safety of three interventions: an intensive lifestyle intervention, or standard lifestyle recommendations combined with metformin or placebo. The study focused on high-risk individuals ($n = 3234$) with IGT who also had slightly elevated fasting plasma glucose (>5.5 mmol/l). The original closing date of the study was planned to be in year 2002. However, the study was terminated prematurely soon after the publication of the Finnish DPS results (Tuomilehto *et al.*, 2001) leading to an unscheduled interim data analysis of the DPP. The data safety and monitoring board then advised the closure the DPP trial because the results had unequivocally answered the main research questions regarding the reduction in incidence of diabetes. In DPP, intensive lifestyle intervention with a 58 per cent reduction in type 2 diabetes risk compared with the placebo group was also superior to the metformin group where type 2 diabetes risk was reduced by 31 per cent compared with placebo.

The lifestyle intervention in DPP was primarily done by special educators, 'case managers', not regular health personnel, and was quite intense (The Diabetes Prevention Program Research Group, 2002). Thus, the translation of such intervention to a routine primary health care may not be easy. The lifestyle intervention commenced with a 16-session structured core curriculum within

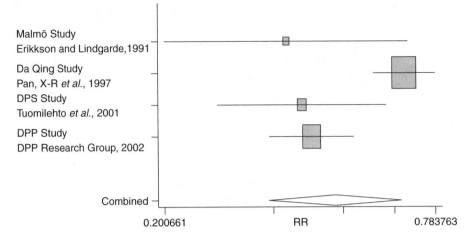

Figure 5.1   Relative risks (RR) with 95 per cent confidence intervals (control versus intervention group) in diabetes incidence in diabetes prevention studies.

the first 24 weeks after randomization was carried out in each. The focus of the dietary intervention was first on reducing total fat intake. Later on the concept of calorie balance was introduced and fat and calorie goals set as means to achieve weight loss goal rather than as a goal in and of itself. The weight loss goal for all participants was a 7 per cent weight reduction and to maintain it throughout the trial. The physical activity goal was approximately 700 kcal per week expenditure from physical activities, which was translated to correspond 150 min of moderate physical activity such as brisk walking. Clinical centres also offered supervised activity sessions where attendance was voluntary. Of the DPP participants assigned to intensive lifestyle intervention 74 per cent achieved the study goal of ≥150 min of activity per week at 24 weeks. At 1-year follow-up the mean weight loss was 7 kg (about 7 per cent).

Figure 5.1 displays relative risks between the control and the intervention groups in the above diabetes intervention studies. The risk reduction was very similar in the Malmö, the DPS, and the DPP studies (more than 50 per cent) but clearly less in the Da-Qing Study (less than 40 per cent). It is too early to argue whether this smaller effect in China is due to factors related to study protocol or other technical questions or whether it reflects real differences between ethnic groups and cultures. The Da-Qing Study differed from the three Western studies also because incidence of type 2 diabetes was much higher in this study, which may also have affected the found differences in relative risk.

Other intervention studies

There are also other interventions that are relevant to the prevention of type 2 diabetes. Promising results on the treatment of obesity come from the Swedish

SOS Intervention Study where gastric surgery was used in very obese subjects (Sjöström *et al.*, 1999). The 2-year incidence of diabetes was 30 times lower in surgically treated grossly obese subjects compared to control subjects receiving regular care. The corresponding weight losses were 28 kg versus 0.5 kg ($P < 0.0001$). These results suggest that severe obesity can and should be treated and that the reduction of obesity results in a marked reduction in the incidence of hypertension, diabetes and some lipid disturbances.

In the SLIM (Study on Lifestyle Intervention and Impaired Tolerance Maastricht) Study in the Netherlands 102 men and women were randomized into two groups (Mensink *et al.*, 2003). Inclusion criteria for all participants were that they are over 40 years old, have a family history of diabetes or BMI 25 kg/m^2 or more, and have impaired glucose tolerance but are not diabetics. In the intervention group, participant received detailed instructions how to regulate diet and increase physical activity. Participants took part in individual follow-up visits every third month. In the control group, participants received only brief information about recommended diet and physical activity. After 1-year follow-up the participants in the intervention group had lost averagely 2.7 kg of their weight whereas in the control group the average weight loss was only 0.3 kg ($P < 0.01$). A difference was also found in glucose tolerance (-0.8 in the intervention group and $+0.2$ in the control group, $P < 0.05$) but in fasting glucose statistically significant differences were not found between the groups. These 1-year preliminary results of this 3-year intervention study confirm the previous results that it is possibly to affect BMI and diabetes risk by lifestyle counselling. The participants in this study were leaner (average BMI 29.5 kg/m^2) than in the Finnish DPS (31.2 kg/m^2) or in the DPP (33.9 kg/m^2) studies and show that lifestyle interventions have beneficial effect also in a population where the risk level of type 2 diabetes is lower than in these two previous interventions.

In a single blind intervention study in Italy 120 menopausal (20–46 years old) obese women (BMI $\geq$ 30 kg/m^2) were randomly divided into two groups (Esposito *et al.*, 2003). Women with impaired glucose tolerance or diabetes were excluded. In the intervention group the participants received detailed instructions how to reduce weight by 10 per cent by regulating diet and increasing physical activity. The methods to use included food diaries, personal goal setting, monthly small group sessions, and access to behavioural and psychological counselling. In the control group, women received general information about healthy dieting and physical exercise at baseline and in subsequent monthly visits but not specific individualized programme. The intervention had a beneficial effect on weight, fat distribution, and fasting plasma glucose; after 2-year follow-up these indicators had decreased more in the intervention group (14 kg for weight, 0.08 for waist–hip ratio, and 9 mg/dl for plasma glucose) than in the control group (3 kg, 0.04, and 2 mg/dl, respectively). All these differences between these two groups were statistically significant.

In another Italian intervention study 122 non-insulin-treated type 2 diabetes patients, half of them women, were randomized into two groups (Trento *et al.*, 2002). In the intervention group, patients were divided into small groups including nine or ten patients. Educational sessions were held every 3 months including topics about meal planning, burden of overweight, smoking cessation, and physical exercise. In the control group, patients continued individual consultation. After 4-year follow-up, statistically significant decrease in body weight was found in the intervention group (2.5 kg, $P < 0.001$) but not in the control group (weight decrease 0.9 kg, NS). Also, fasting blood glucose was measured, but it did not show statistically significant change in either of these groups. Weight reduction in the control and the intervention groups in the above three obesity intervention studies are given in Figure 5.2.

Additional evidence for the importance of weight reduction was recently derived from a placebo-controlled multicentre trial called Xendos (Xenical in the Prevention of Diabetes in Obese Subjects; Sjöström *et al.*, 2002). It used a weight loss agent, orlistat (Xenical®) compared with weight reduction with diet alone for the prevention of type 2 diabetes over a period of 4 years. Overweight (BMI $\geq 30 \, \text{kg/m}^2$) subjects aged 30–60 years of whom 21 per cent had IGT at baseline received lifestyle counselling every 2 weeks for the first 6 months of the study and monthly thereafter. They were prescribed a calorie-reduced diet and encouraged to take part in moderate daily physical exercise. At four years mean weight reduction was 4.1 kg in the lifestyle+placebo group and 6.9 kg in

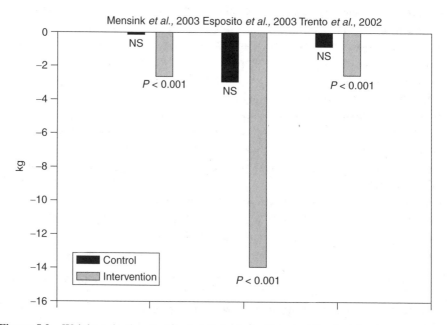

Figure 5.2 Weight reduction (kg) and statistical significance (P-value) in the control and intervention groups in obesity intervention studies.

the lifestyle+orlistat group. Cumulative incidence of type 2 diabetes was 9.0 per cent in the lifestyle+placebo group and 6.2 per cent in the lifestyle+orlistat group, with a 37 per cent risk reduction in the orlistat group compared with the placebo group. The major problem with this study like with most of other drug intervention studies in type 2 diabetes prevention was a high drop-out rate: only 52 per cent of the lifestyle+orlistat group subjects and 34 per cent of the lifestyle+placebo group subjects completed the 4-year treatment phase. Nevertheless, there is no doubt that weight control in obese subjects is an efficient way to prevent the development of type 2 diabetes and there are many ways to reach effective weight reduction in addition to dietary means which obviously is the basis for any weight management in obesity.

In the Fasting Hyperglycaemia Study (FHS) II (Dyson *et al.*, 1997) 227 subjects with fasting plasma glucose in the range of 5.5 to 7.7 mmol/l on two consecutive tests were randomized to reinforced or basic healthy-living advice and sulphonylurea treatment or control group in a two-by-two factorial design. Two hundred and one subjects completed the 1-year follow-up study. Reinforced advice recommending dietary modification and increased exercise was given every 3 months, and basic advice was given once at the initial visit. Both the reinforced and basic advice groups had a significant mean reduction in body weight (1.5 kg) at 3 months, although the weight subsequently returned to baseline. After 1 year, subjects allocated to reinforced advice versus basic advice showed no change in fasting plasma glucose, glucose tolerance, or haemoglobin A1c (HbA1c). Thus, this study was unable to show any effect on the risk of type 2 diabetes of 'healthy-living advice', but it seems that the intervention was not particularly successful since no significant weight change was achieved. Also, compared with other recent trials on type 2 diabetes prevention in high-risk subjects with IGT, this study differed regarding the glucose inclusion criteria that were based on fasting values only. Therefore, while it is clearly shown that type 2 diabetes can be prevented in subjects with IGT, we are still lacking the data on the risk on the reduction of the risk of type 2 diabetes in people screened for high fasting glucose. Prospective studies show that people with high fasting glucose (impaired fasting glycaemia) also have an increased risk of developing type 2 diabetes, even though the risk is lower than that for IGT (Shaw *et al.*, 1999). Nevertheless, thus far there is no evidence that screening for fasting glucose is a justified strategy for the prevention of type 2 diabetes.

Conclusions

The results from the recent major type 2 diabetes prevention trials have now provided unequivocal evidence that type 2 diabetes can be prevented, at least in high-risk individuals. It is striking that the two individually randomized trials yielded similar results when the DPP confirmed the 58 per cent relative risk reduction (Knowler *et al.*, 2002) obtained in the Finnish DPS study only a year earlier (Tuomilehto *et al.*, 2001). Even more striking is that the previous non-randomized Malmö feasibility study had almost identical result, 59 per cent risk reduction (Eriksson and Lindgarde, 1991), and also in 1980 the Malmöhus study showed a 56 per cent risk reduction between the intervention and the control groups (Sartor *et al.*, 1980). Also, the absolute risk reductions were very similar among these studies: a 16–18 per cent reduction in the incidence during the 3–6 year period. The data from the Chinese Da Qing study (Pan *et al.*, 1997) were slightly different: while the relative risk reduction was somewhat less, about 40 per cent, the absolute risk reduction was higher, 27 per cent, due to the fact that the overall incidence in the Chinese was higher.

The public health implications of these results are very wide. The primary prevention of type 2 diabetes is possible by a non-pharmacological intervention that can be implemented in the primary health care setting. It has been speculated that there might be differences in the acceptance and compliance with lifestyle modification between different ethnic groups, especially in the United States (Tataranni and Bogardus, 2001). The reasoning for this has probably been based on the findings from observational studies suggesting that certain ethnic or socio-economic groups have an increased risk of type 2 diabetes. It may, however, be misleading to imply that an observed disease risk differential between subgroups would also lead to a similar differential in the effect of interventions. On the contrary, one should assume that whenever and wherever unhealthy lifestyles are corrected the individual disease risk should reduce regardless the demographic background. The recent trials have now confirmed that lifestyle intervention, once carried out properly, is an efficient way to prevent type 2 diabetes. It is worth noting that the metformin arm of the DPP and other trials (Chiasson *et al.*, 2002) have shown that antidiabetic drugs may also prevent worsening of IGT to frank type 2 diabetes, but the pharmacologic intervention compared with lifestyle intervention seems inferior. This is not surprising since in the lifestyle intervention causal factors influencing the natural history of type 2 diabetes are modified while antidiabetic drugs have specific and limited modes of action leading to a relative lowering of blood glucose concentration.

In order to prevent the emerging epidemic of type 2 diabetes worldwide it is necessary that the primary prevention of type 2 diabetes will receive more serious attention than it has got in the past. Unfavourable lifestyle patterns are no longer an issue only among adults but also in children and adolescents. As a consequence, the age-at-onset of type 2 diabetes has become younger, not only in special small ethnic groups like Pima Indians, but also in many societies in both developed and developing countries (Dabelea *et al.*, 1998; Ehtisham *et al.*, 2000; Sinha *et al.*, 2002). The effect of these lifestyle patterns is particularly deleterious in those who have born small and thin and who subsequently become heavy already in childhood and adolescence (Dabelea *et al.*, 1999). It is however important to note that in the DPP people aged over 60 years at baseline benefited more from lifestyle intervention than younger ones (Knowler *et al.*, 2002).

Similar results have been observed from the DPS (Tuomilehto, unpublished data). Thus, it is not too late to prevent diabetes in older people with IGT, but the immediate benefits are likely to be even greater than in younger subjects since the absolute risk of type 2 diabetes in the short term is higher in older than in younger people.

While it is useful to accumulate more information from interventions in other populations and cultural environments, the evidence to initiate intensive actions to prevent type 2 diabetes is clearly sufficient. The identification of high-risk subjects for type 2 diabetes is relatively easy; no biochemical or other costly tests are required. It is now recognized that from the prevention point of view, screening for type 2 diabetes is not the same as measuring blood glucose, but one can determine the risk of developing type 2 diabetes using non-invasive data before testing for blood glucose. Recently, such a Diabetes Prediction Risk Score has been developed based on the prospective study in Finland (Lindström and Tuomilehto, 2003). It is also important to note that most of the high-risk subjects for type 2 diabetes are already regular customers of primary health care services for various reasons. What is needed in the health care system is to determine the future risk of type 2 diabetes using a diabetes risk score in clients that seem to be potential candidates for type 2 diabetes, and to target a systematic lifestyle intervention to these individuals regardless their current glucose levels. It is necessary that such an intervention will become a part of routine preventive care in order to reduce the burden of type 2 diabetes that is reaching epidemic proportions in many countries. At the same time, it is also necessary to develop national programmes for the primary prevention of type 2 diabetes that include not only the high-risk strategy but also the population strategy, i.e. to reduce the risk factors for type 2 diabetes such as obesity and physical inactivity in the entire population. The trials on prevention of type 2 diabetes have included high-risk subjects only since this is the most efficient way to test the efficacy of preventive measures. The efficacy of lifestyle intervention is now confirmed.

According to the estimates derived from the US third National Health and Nutrition Examination Survey 11 per cent of the US adults aged 40–74 years meet the DPP eligibility criteria (Benjamin *et al.*, 2003). This illustrates well the magnitude of the problem: the number of subjects at high risk of type 2 diabetes who would benefit from lifestyle intervention is large. It will be a major challenge for the health care systems to implement the necessary action to prevent or postpone type 2 diabetes in these people (Saydah *et al.*, 2002). The interventions on high-risk subjects alone will, however, not be sufficient for the successful prevention of type 2 diabetes in the community. It is also necessary to initiate actions based on the population approach. These include actions that will assure the shift of the risk factor distribution in the entire population to a lower level without screening for high-risk subjects (Uusitupa *et al.*, 2000). Such efforts are likely to be even more important than individual interventions alone, as seen from the prevention of cardiovascular disease in the recent past. The coordinated combination of the high-risk approach together with systematic population approach programmes simultaneously will be the most efficient, and also necessary, strategy to reverse the current increasing trend in the incidence of type 2 diabetes. Such actions are overdue and are only now starting in some countries. For instance, the national consensus conference on diabetes control in Finland in 2000 listed the primary prevention of type 2 diabetes as the primary issue among all activities in diabetes care. A national programme is being developed currently in Finland. Other countries are likely to develop similar activities in the near future. In such programmes it is necessary to realize that the primary prevention of type 2 diabetes must have a long-term plan and it has to include a range of activities targeted to different age groups from fetal life to the elderly (Eriksson *et al.*, 2001).

References

Astrup A, Grunwald GK, Melanson E *et al.* (2000) The role of low-fat diets in body weight control: a meta-analysis of ad libitum intervention studies. *Int J Obes* **24**: 1545–52.

Benjamin SM, Valdez R, Geiss LS *et al.* (2003) Estimated number of adults with prediabetes in the US in 2000: opportunities for prevention. *Diabetes Care* **26**: 645–9.

Bergstrom R and Hernell O (2001) Obesity and insulin resistance in childhood and adolescence. In *Primary and Secondary Preventive Nutrition*, Bendich A and Deckelbaum RJ (eds). Humana Press Inc., Totowa, NJ, pp. 165–83.

Boyko EJ, Fujimoto WY, Leonetti DL and Newell-Morris L (2000) Visceral adiposity and risk of type 2 diabetes: a prospective study among Japanese Americans. *Diabetes Care* **23**: 465–71.

Bruce DG, Chisholm DJ, Storlien LH and Kraegen EW (1988) Physiological importance of deficiency in early prandial insulin secretion in non-insulin-dependent diabetes. *Diabetes* **37**: 736–44.

Chan JM, Rimm EB, Colditz CA *et al.* (1994) Obesity, fat distribution, and weight gain as risk factors for clinical diabetes in men. *Diabetes Care* **17**: 961–9.

Chiasson JL, Josse RG, Gomis R *et al.* and the STOP-NIDDM Trial Research Group (2002) Acarbose for prevention of type 2 diabetes mellitus: the STOP-NIDDM randomised trial. *Lancet* **369**: 2072–7.

Colditz GA, Willett WC, Stampfer MJ *et al.* (1990) Weight as a risk factor for clinical diabetes in women. *Am J Epidemiol* **132**: 501–13.

Dabelea D, Hanson RL, Bennett PH *et al.* (1998) Increasing prevalence of type II diabetes in American Indian children. *Diabetologia* **41**: 904–10.

Dabelea D, Pettitt DJ, Hanson RL *et al.* (1999) Birth weight, type 2 diabetes, and insulin resistance in Pima Indian children and young adults. *Diabetes Care* **22**: 944–50.

DECODE Study Group (2003) Age- and sex-specific prevalences of diabetes and impaired glucose regulation in 13 European cohorts. *Diabetes Care* **26**: 61–9.

Despres JP (2001) Health consequences of visceral obesity. *Ann Med* **33**: 534–41.

Dyson PA, Hammersley MS, Morris RJ *et al.* (1997) The Fasting Hyperglycaemia Study: II randomized controlled trial of reinforced healthy-living advice in subjects with increased but not diabetic fasting plasma glucose. *Metabolism* **46** (suppl. 1): 50–5.

Ehtisham S, Barrett TG and Shaw NJ (2000) Type 2 diabetes in UK children – an emerging problem. *Diabetes Med* **17**: 867–71.

Eriksson J, Lindström J and Tuomilehto J (2001) Potential for the prevention of type 2 diabetes. *Br Med Bull* **60**: 183–99.

Eriksson J, Lindström J, Valle T *et al.* (1999) Prevention of Type II diabetes in subjects with impaired glucose tolerance: the Diabetes Prevention Study (DPS) in Finland – Study design and 1-year interim report on the feasibility of the lifestyle intervention programme. *Diabetologia* **42**: 793–801.

Eriksson KF and Lindgarde F (1991) Prevention of type 2 (non-insulin-dependent) diabetes mellitus by diet and physical exercise. The 6-year Malmö feasibility study. *Diabetologia* **34**: 891–8.

Esposito K, Pontillo A, Di Palo C *et al.* (2003) Effect of weight loss and lifestyle changes on vascular inflammatory markers in obese women: a randomized trial. *JAMA* **289**: 1799–1804.

Expert Consultation Group (1985) *Energy and protein requirements. Report of a Joint FAO/UNU/WHO Expert Consultation.* World Health Organization, Geneva (WHO Technical Report Series No. 724).

Flatt JP (1988) Importance of nutrient balance in body weight regulation. *Diabet Metab Rev* **4**: 571–81.

Flegal KM, Carroll MD, Kuczmarski RJ and Johnson CL (1998) Overweight and obesity in the United States: prevalence and trends, 1960–1994. *Int J Obes* **22**: 39–47.

Grundy SM (1998) Multifactorial causation of obesity: implications for prevention. *Am J Clin Nutr* **67** (Suppl. 3): 563S–572S.

Hamman RF (2002) Prevention of type 2 diabetes. In *The Evidence Base for Diabetes Care*, R. Williams *et al.* (eds). John Wiley & Sons, Ltd, Chichester, pp. 75–176.

Harnack LJ, Jeffery RW and Boutelle KN (2000) Temporal trends in energy intake in the United States: an ecologic perspective. *Am J Clin Nutr* **71**: 1478–84.

James PT, Leach R, Kalamara E and Shayeghi M (2001) The worldwide obesity epidemic. *Obes Res* **9** (Suppl. 4): 228S–233S.

Joslin E (1921) The prevention of diabetes mellitus. *JAMA* **76**: 79–84.

Kahn CR, Vicent D and Doria A (1996) Genetics of non-insulin-dependent (type-II) diabetes mellitus. *Annu Rev Med* **47**: 509–31.

King H, Aubert RE and Herman WH (1998) Global burden of diabetes, 1995–2025: prevalence, numerical estimates, and projections. *Diabetes Care* **21**: 1414–31.

Knowler WC, Pettitt DJ, Savage PJ and Bennett PH (1981) Diabetes incidence in Pima Indians: contributions of obesity and parental diabetes. *Am J Epidemiol* **113**: 144–56.

Knowler WC, Barrett-Connor E, Fowler SE *et al.* and Diabetes Prevention Program Research Group (2002) Reduction in the incidence of type 2 diabetes with lifestyle intervention or metformin. *N Engl J Med* **346**: 393–403.

Kuczmarski RJ, Flegal KM, Campbell SM and Johnson CL (1994) Increasing prevalence of overweight among US adults. The National Health and Nutrition Examination Surveys, 1960 to 1991. *JAMA* **273**: 205–11.

Lahmann PH, Lissner L, Gullberg B and Berglund G (2000) Sociodemographic factors associated with long-term weight gain, current body fatness and central adiposity in Swedish women. *Int J Obes* **24**: 685–94.

Lindström J and Tuomilehto J (2003) The Diabetes Risk Score: a practical tool to predict type 2 diabetes risk. *Diabetes Care* **26**: 725–31.

Manson JE, Nathan DM, Krolewski AS *et al.* (1992) A prospective study of exercise and incidence of diabetes among US male physicians. *JAMA* **268**: 63–7.

Martikainen PT and Marmot MG (1999) Socioeconomic differences in weight gain and determinants and consequences of coronary risk factors. *Am J Clin Nutr* **69**: 719–26.

Mensink M, Feskens EJM, Saris WHM *et al.* (2003) Study on Lifestyle Intervention and Impaired Glucose Tolerance Maastricht (SLIM): preliminary results after one year. *Int J Obes* **27**: 377–84.

Neel JV (1962) Diabetes mellitus: a 'thrifty' genotype rendered detrimental by progress? *Am J Hum Genet* **14**: 353–62.

Nielsen SJ, Siega-Riz AM and Popkin BM (2002) Trends in energy intake in US between 1977 and 1999: similar shift seen across age groups. *Obes Res* **10**: 370–8.

Pan XR, Li GW, Hu YH *et al.* (1997) Effects of diet and exercise in preventing NIDDM in people with impaired glucose tolerance. The Da Qing IGT and Diabetes Study. *Diabetes Care* **20**: 537–44.

Qiao Q, Hu G, Tuomilehto J *et al.* (2003) Age- and sex-specific prevalence of diabetes and impaired glucose regulation in 11 Asian cohorts. *Diabetes Care* **26**: 1770–80.

Ravussin E and Swinburn BA (1992) Pathophysiology of obesity. *Lancet* **340**: 404–8.

Sartor G, Schersten B, Carlstrom S *et al.* (1980) Ten-year follow-up of subjects with impaired glucose tolerance: prevention of diabetes by tolbutamide and diet regulation. *Diabetes* **29**: 41–9.

Saydah SH, Byrd-Holt D and Harris MI (2002) Projected impact of implementing the results of the diabetes prevention program in the US population. *Diabetes Care* **25**: 1940–45.

Schoeller DA (2001) The importance of clinical research: the role of thermogenesis in human obesity. *Am J Clin Nutr* **73**: 511–16.

Sclafani A (1992) Dietary obesity models. In *Obesity* Bjorntorp P and Brodoff BN (eds). JB Lippincott, Philadelphia, pp. 241–8.

Shah M and Grag A (1996) High-fat and high-carbohydrate diets and energy balance. *Diabetes Care* **19**: 1142–52.

Shah M, Hannan PJ and Jeffery RW (1991) Secular trend in body mass index in adult population of three communities from the upper mid-western part of the USA: the Minnesota Heart Health Program. *Int J Obes* **15**: 499–503.

Shaw JE, Zimmet PZ, de Courten M *et al.* (1999) Impaired fasting glucose or impaired glucose tolerance. What best predicts future diabetes in Mauritius? *Diabetes Care* **22**: 399–402.

Sinha R, Fisch G, Teague B *et al.* (2002) Prevalence of impaired glucose tolerance among children and adolescents with marked obesity. *N Engl J Medi* **346**: 802–10.

Sjöström CD, Lissner L, Wedel H and Sjöström L (1999) Reduction in incidence of diabetes, hypertension and lipid disturbances after intentional weight loss induced by bariatric surgery: the SOS Intervention Study. *Obes Res* **7**: 477–84.

Sjöström L, Torgerson JS, Hauptman J and Boldrin M (2002) XENDOS (Xenical in the prevention of Diabetes in Obese Subjects): a landmark study. Sao Paulo, Brazil.

Spranger J, Kroke A, Möhlig M *et al.* (2003) Inflammatory cytokines and the risk to develop type 2 diabetes. Results of the prospective population-based European Prospective Investigation into cancer and nutrition (EPIC) Potsdam Study. *Diabetes* **52**: 812–17.

Swinburn B, Metcalf PA and Ley SJ (2001) Long-term (5-year) effects of a reduced fat diet in individuals with glucose intolerance. *Diabetes Care* **24**: 619–24.

Tataranni PA and Bogardus C (2001) Changing habits to delay diabetes. *N Engl J Med* **344**: 1390–2.

The Diabetes Prevention Program Research Group (1999) The Diabetes Prevention Program: design and methods for a clinical trial in the prevention of type 2 diabetes. *Diabetes Care* **22**: 623–34.

The Diabetes Prevention Program Research Group (2002) The Diabetes Prevention Program (DPP): description of lifestyle intervention. *Diabetes Care* **25**: 2165–72.

Trento M, Passera P, Bajardi M *et al.* (2002) Lifestyle intervention by group care prevents deterioration of Type II diabetes: a 4-year randomized controlled clinical trial. *Diabetologia* **45**: 1231–9.

Troiano RP, Briefel RR, Carroll MD and Bialostosky K (2000) Energy and fat intakes of children and adolescents in the United States: data from the National Health and Nutrition Examination Surveys. *Am J Clin Nutr* **72**: 1343S–1353S.

Tuomilehto J and Lindström J (2003) The major diabetes prevention trials. *Curr Diab Rep* **3**: 115–22.

Tuomilehto J, Lindström J, Eriksson J *et al.* (2001) Prevention of type 2 diabetes mellitus by changes in lifestyle among subjects with impaired glucose tolerance. *N Engl J Med* **344**: 1343–50.

Uusitupa M, Louheranta A, Lindström J *et al.* (2000) The Finnish Diabetes Prevention Study. *Br J Nutr* **83** (Suppl. 1): S137–S142.

WHO Study Group (1994) *Primary Prevention of Diabetes Mellitus*. World Health Organization, Geneva (Technical Report Series No. 844).

World Health Organization (1998) *Preparation and use of food-based dietary guidelines, report of a joint FAO/WHO consultation*. World Health Organization, Geneva (WHO Technical Report Series No. 880).

6

Diet and Food-based Therapies for Obesity in Diabetic Patients

Iain Broom

Introduction

The strategies for delivering diet-based therapies for the management of obesity may differ in type 1 (insulin-dependent) and type 2 (insulin-independent) diabetes mellitus. The role of diet, however, in the management of type 1 diabetes mellitus is primarily in minimizing the short-term fluctuations in plasma glucose, specifically hypoglycaemia and to reduce the risks of long-term complications (micro- and macrovascular).

Despite approaches in the past where emphasis was placed on eating less carbohydrate in type 1 diabetes mellitus, this possibly leading to increased atherogenesis in this group, the general nutritional requirements of the diabetic patient are now deemed to be no different from that of the non-diabetic population. Thus dietary recommendations are no different from the general population (Table 6.1). The same is also true for type 2 diabetes mellitus but other approaches may be adopted in treating obesity associated with type 2 diabetes mellitus, which is resistant to standard dietary approaches (see below).

Type 2 diabetes

Obesity is the main aetiological factor in the development of type 2 diabetes mellitus with 70–80 per cent of type 2 diabetes patients presenting with obesity (body mass index; BMI $> 30 \text{kg/m}^2$). This obese phenotype is associated with insulin-resistance and thus differs metabolically from type 1 diabetes, which is an insulin-deficient state. Thus, in general, obesity management in diabetes is

Obesity and Diabetes. Edited by Anthony H. Barnett and Sudhesh Kumar
© 2004 John Wiley & Sons, Ltd ISBN: 0-470-84898-7

Table 6.1   General principles for the management of diabetic patients

* Energy intake	Recommendations for diabetes mellitus to approach and maintain BMI of 25
Carbohydrate	>55% of total energy
Fat:	<30–35% of total energy[†] (Saturated fat ≤ 10%)
Protein:	10–15% of total energy
Salt:	<6 g daily (<3 g if hypertensive)
Sucrose (added)	<25 g per day
Dietary fibre	>30 g per day
'Diabetic foods' (as labelled)	None

BMI, body mass index ([Weight in kg] × [height in m]$^{-2}$).
*Dependent on sex, age and activity.
[†]A higher total fat intake is allowed if monosaturated fatty acids form a major component of the diet, e.g. olive oil.

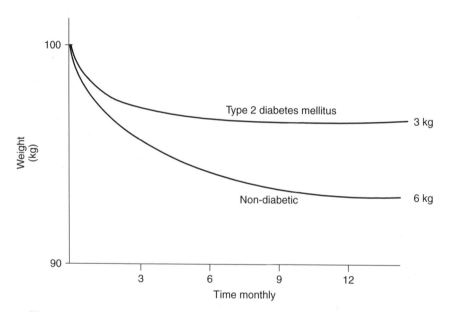

Figure 6.1   Weight loss in type 2 diabetes mellitus compared to non-diabetics.

primarily a problem of type 2 diabetes and further discussion will be centred around management of the type 2 diabetic patient.

Patterns of weight loss in diabetes

The obese diabetic patient provides a particular challenge in terms of achieving sustainable weight loss. In all studies, when compared to the non-diabetic patient, weight loss achieved at 1 year is approximately 50 per cent (Hollander *et al.*, 1998; Avenell *et al.*, 2004) when the best diet and lifestyle advice and support is given (Figure 6.1) Thus, the presence of type 2 diabetes gives the patient increased problems in achieving clinically significant weight loss. As an added confounder the natural history of weight alteration in the diabetic patient is for this to slowly increase, the rate of increase being dependent on drug therapy used (UK Prospective Diabetes Study Group, 1998), both insulin and sulphonylurea increasing the rate of weight gain.

On achieving sustainable weight loss and maintenance, it is important to recognize the above and to relay this information to the parent to allow his/her better understanding of energy metabolism. Clear and frank discussion with patients in respect of difficulties in achieving and maintaining weight loss are essential. The approach to the patient by the whole healthcare delivery team as to the role of diet and lifestyle alteration needs to send the same message. It is also important that non-verbal communication to patients from the diabetic management team reinforces the verbal statements. Contradictory messages will lead to patient confusion, lack of confidence, and ultimate failure in achieving weight reduction and hence failure to achieve improved glycaemic control, blood pressure and/or lipid parameters.

Target setting

Goal-setting is a pre-requisite prior to the initialization of diet therapy. It is essential to set a realistic target of weight loss in a fixed period of time, e.g. 5–10 per cent of body weight in 6 months. Patients should be advised that achieving an 'ideal weight' for height, i.e. to give a BMI of $<25\,\mathrm{kg/m^2}$ may not be an achievable target, and that not achieving such an ideal weight should not be seen as failure. Other targets to discuss with the patient are achievable changes in food intake, increased activity and decreased inactivity. It is not appropriate in attempting to alter diet and lifestyle to institute absolute negative attitudes towards certain foodstuffs or current lifestyle but to slowly change attitudes to both with positive as opposed to negative reinforcement. Such target setting may allow small but sustainable weight losses that are clinically significant and allow patients to stabilize at a new lower weight, with consequent improvement in glycaemic control and other outcomes, prior to attempting further weight reduction measures at a later date (Figure 6.2).

Dietary and lifestyle alterations

It is important to address alterations in diet and lifestyle simultaneously and diet alone should not be targeted in an attempt to achieve sustainable weight loss (Usitupa, 1996; Torjesen *et al.*, 1997; Eriksson *et al.*, 1999; Avenell *et al.*, 2003). In addition, the use of cognitive behaviour therapy has clearly shown to add benefits to sustainable weight loss when used in conjunction with diet and lifestyle changes. It is therefore appropriate to use an holistic approach when dealing with weight loss and maintenance in obese individuals be they diabetic or non-diabetic (Avenell *et al.*, 2003).

It is important to understand, however, dietary intake cannot be reliably estimated in the overweight patient as they consistently understate their food

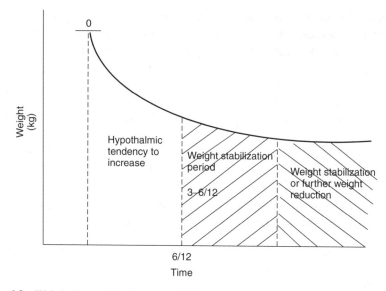

Figure 6.2   Weight loss and maintenance including the influence of hypothalamic control. Weight loss programmes should be carried out in 6-monthly stages with periods of weight stabilization.

intake by the order of 20 per cent. (Prentice *et al.*, 1986). The energy intake required to maintain body weight is best estimated by using standard formulae derived from metabolic rate measurements and appropriate reductions in intake advised by altering proportions of foodstuffs in the diet.

Currently Diabetes UK recommends energy intake prescriptions for diabetes patients to be that required to maintain a BMI of 25 kg/m² (Diabetes UK, 2003). In the obese diabetes patient this may be too strict an energy deficit to allow longer-term adherence with consequent patient and treatment failure. It is more appropriate to induce small changes in energy intake to allow an approximate deficit of 500–600 kcal per day (Lean and James, 1986). This standard approach to BMI of 25 kg/m² is reasonable for Caucasian populations, although rarely attainable in practice. In Asian populations the susceptibility to type 2 diabetes and metabolic syndrome increases dramatically at a lower BMI (23 kg/m²). Certainly in disease prevention such targets should be considered as maximal desirable within the relevant populations.

The subsequent discussion will be restricted to diet and food-based treatment only. The independent effects of exercise on weight loss and maintenance, improved insulin sensitivity and well-being will be discussed elsewhere, as will the effects of CBT.

Dietary nutrient composition in type 2 diabetes

There is considerable evidence in support of high fat, relatively low-carbohydrate (but high sugar), low-fibre diets of Western societies being a major

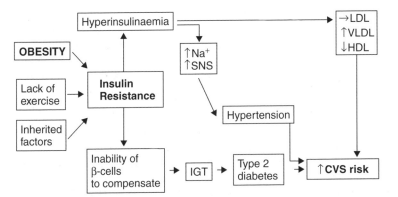

Figure 6.3 Metabolic syndrome. LDL, low-density lipoprotein; VLDL, very low density lipoprotein; HDL, high-density lipoprotein; SNS, sympathetic nervous system; IGT, impaired glucose tolerance; CVS, cardiovascular system.

aetiological factor in susceptible individuals. Excess dietary fat is more easily converted to adipose tissue lipid stores than carbohydrate (Flatt, 1985); diet-induced thermogenesis is less with fat than carbohydrates or protein thus inducing lower metabolic rates with high fat diets (Lean and James, 1988; Lean *et al.*, 1989); dietary fat has minimal effects on both appetite and satiety (Caterson and Broom, 2001); hyperinsulinaemia has been associated with high fat intakes possibly through components of the hormonal enteroinsular axis (Grey and Kipnes, 1971). The associated hyperinsulinaemia will favour further fat deposition and aggravate the insulin resistance of type 2 diabetes, increasing the associated metabolic dysregulation, e.g. dyslipidaemia (Figure 6.3).

In addition, in the obese individual dietary-induced thermogenesis is lower than in the non-obese, and hence further weight increase is more likely with energy-dense diets (Bruce *et al.*, 1990).

For the vast majority of type 2 diabetes patients therefore, diets based on reduced fat intake and higher unrefined carbohydrates are recommended (Table 6.2). Such approaches in association with mild energy restriction should lead to weight reduction and maintenance of this reduced weight.

Changing to such a diet is frequently sufficient to induce weight loss without this energy restriction especially in males.

It is clear, therefore, that specific dietary recommendations in type 2 diabetes do *not* differ from dietary recommendations in the non-diabetic population (DHSS-COMA, 1984; European Association for the Study of Diabetes, 1988; Diabetes UK, 2003). If, however, in the overweight (90 per cent) or obese (60–70 per cent) type 2 diabetes patients there is no reduction in weight, or indeed an increase in weight, then additional dietary energy restriction has to be instituted. Overweight type 2 diabetes patients will need reassurance from the *whole* diabetes management team that such alterations in diet are effective both in controlling their disease but also in achieving small but sustainable weight

Table 6.2   Advantages of high carbohydrate versus high fat intake in achieving and maintaining weight loss in type 2 diabetes

High carbohydrate	High fat
Low energy density	High energy density
Appetite suppression (inclusive of bulk effect of fibre)	Low appetite suppression
Increased satiety	No satiety effects
Reduced food intake	Increased food intake
Reduced hyperinsulinaemia	Tendency to hyperinsulinaemia
Increased diet-induced thermogenesis	Decreased diet-induced thermogenesis
Increased intake: reduced tendency to fat deposition	Increased intake: tendency to fat deposition
Reduction in metabolic dysregulation	Increased metabolic dysregulation

↓ Atherogenic effects ↑

loss. It is also important that consistent messages are given to these patients that diet (and lifestyle) are the major factors involved in achieving adequate diabetes control and that weight loss in the overweight/obese is a prerequisite to this improved control.

The approach to dietary prescription

The initial approach to the patient and the initial emphasis on diet and dietary alterations are of extreme importance. This may be the only advice the patient remembers, and first approaches to dietary intervention are liable to provide the best outcomes relative to both improved control and weight loss in the overweight/obese diabetic. The restriction of single nutrients such as sugar, is not advised but dietary habits in general should be discussed, as well as the modification and reduction or increase in specific food groups, e.g. reduction in overall fat and increase in complex carbohydrate.

Simple guidelines for dietary manipulation, suitable for the primary care health team to provide at the time of diagnosis, are preferable until, and if, fuller advice is given by the community and hospital dietitian. It is well recognized, however, that weight loss and maintenance in the overweight/obese diabetic is more difficult than in the non-diabetic, generally speaking about half that expected in the non-diabetic (Hollander *et al.*, 1998; Broom *et al.*, 2002; Avenell *et al.*, 2004). This will therefore require the re-emphasis of diet and weight loss in achieving optimum control and the setting of achievable targets for patients in both the short and the longer term. It is better and easier to bring weight down in stages with intervening periods of weight stabilization than to attempt more major weight reductions in the obese type 2 diabetic.

Failure of therapy

Because of the reduced rate of weight loss seen in Type 2 diabetes when compared with the non-diabetic population and indeed the general failure with lifestyle advice to achieve sustainable weight loss over the longer term (most individuals returning to initial weight by 5 years) (Lean, 1998), 'failure' is seen as inevitable. Failure is, however, a relative term and the explanation to patients of patterns of weight loss and gain are essential. The importance of small amounts of weight lost relative to improvements in disease outcomes should be emphasized and the importance of maintaining good control by dietary means alone without the need for pharmacotherapy also stressed (UK PDS, 1998). It is equally important for the clinician and the healthcare workers to understand patterns of weight loss and gain and for such individuals to provide continual encouragement. It is particularly unhelpful to continually castigate the patient about his/her 'failure to comply' with diet adherence. Indeed such attitudes often have the opposite effect and increase the rate of weight gain, and alienate the patient towards further therapeutic approaches based on lifestyle modification.

Again, in the 'failing patient', it is important to emphasize the positive effects of achieving further modest reductions in weight without dwelling on the negative. Here, patient motivation is important and changing his/her attitudes towards weight loss paramount. Lastly, failure in patients is frequently *not* that, but one of treatment withdrawal after short-term 3–6 months' intensive support. Weight loss and maintenance require long-term input and support by both healthcare workers and the family unit.

Fat or carbohydrate

For the majority of patients (diabetic and non-diabetic) who have a problem with weight maintenance, targeting fat in the diet is appropriate for the reasons outlined above. This is also the sensible option for Government to adopt as far as population targets are concerned. It must be realized, however, that high carbohydrate intakes can also lead to marked obesity and consequently increase the likelihood of the development of type 2 diabetes. Individual patient therapy may therefore differ from that applied to population or generally applied to achieve weight reduction. Where increased carbohydrate is identified as the main dietary energy substrate involved in the aetiology of obesity in an individual, strategies to reduce weight based on increased carbohydrate intake are likely to fail. Cognizance must therefore be taken of other approaches to reduce weight and optimize metabolic control.

There is considerable controversy over the use of low-carbohydrate, high-protein diets especially in type 2 diabetes. The most common of these is the Atkins diet (Atkins, 1998), although there are a number of such diet treatments based on switching energy substrate metabolism from a carbohydrate base to a

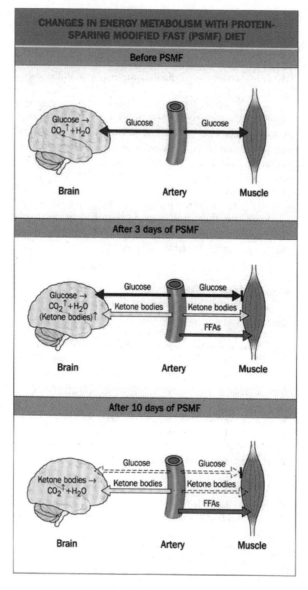

Figure 6.4 Patterns of fat and ketone body utilization with time in patients on reduced carbohydrate intake.

fat base, involving ketogenesis and ketone body utilization by brain and peripheral tissues. The appropriate utilization of fat as an energy substrate by the brain takes time to develop (Figure 6.4), but once this occurs there is marked appetite suppression. It is interesting that William Banting described the first low-carbohydrate diet to achieve popular success in the 1860s and claimed that on this diet he was never hungry (Banting, 1863).

Numerous professional bodies have, however, at the least cautioned against the use of low-carbohydrate diets. They have suggested that such diets have serious medical consequences particularly for patients with known cardiovascular disease, type 2 diabetes, dyslipidaemia or hypertension. It should be said that such statements have been made without good evidence. A recent meta-analysis and systematic review of such dietary treatment by Bravata *et al.* (2003) have stated that there is insufficient evidence to make such recommendations against the use of such dietary therapy. In addition there was no evidence to suggest adverse effects on glycaemia, blood pressure or serum lipids. This is also substantiated by two recent papers in the *New England Journal of Medicine* (Foster *et al.*, 2003; Samaha *et al.*, 2003).

The jury is therefore out as to the efficacy and longer-term safety of such approaches. It is clear, however, that patients in general do not adopt this dietary approach for longer than 6 months with both weight loss and fall in HbA$_1$c being maximal at this time period (Robertson *et al.*, 2002) (Figure 6.5).

This study also demonstrated no adverse effects on renal function with time, although there were insignificant increases in serum creatinine secondary to increase creatine intake in meat. With the associated high protein intake there is also a rise in serum area concentration as would be expected.

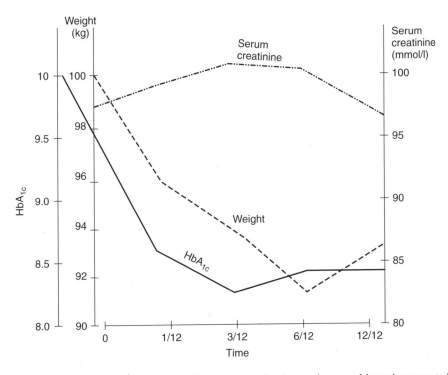

Figure 6.5 Patterns of weight loss and improvement in glycaemic control in patients treated with low-carbohydrate, high-protein diets.

Table 6.3 Nutrient content of high protein low-carbohydrate diets (1000 kcal intake)

Nutrient	Weight (g)	%Energy	Absolute energy (kcal)
Protein	120	41	408
Carbohydrate	40	16	160
* Fat	43	43	432

*Absolute amount of fat in standard healthy eating −600 kcal (Diabetes UK) is 51–59 g based on 1600 kcal intake, i.e. 30–35% total energy.

In general these diets are classified as high in fat (Table 6.3). This is the case when fat is expressed as percentage of energy consumed but in absolute terms the amount of fat consumed is low and the tendency to overeat suppressed by the action of such diets on control mechanisms affecting appetite and satiety.

Such diets can use standard food components with protein comprising at least 120 g per day or may be constituted in powder format. These latter act as meal replacement therapy.

Approaches based on low-carbohydrate intake are usually supplemented with additional vitamins or trace elements. Calcium is also frequently added as loss of bone mineral mass has been suggested to accompany such high protein intakes although again evidence for this is lacking (Bravata *et al.*, 2003).

Meal replacement therapy

Many companies offer meal replacement techniques in an effort to reduce weight. Such therapies can be based on standard low energy intakes but are nutrient complete (e.g. Slimfast) or are based on low-carbohydrate intakes (e.g. Modifast, Cambridge Diet, etc.). The success of such treatments remains to be confirmed and appropriate trials in this area are sadly lacking, especially in the management of type 2 diabetes. Recently 'Diet Trials' on BBC television examined in detail meal replacement therapies and found these to be as good as but no better than other weight loss strategies when compared to no therapeutic approach. (Truby, personal communication.)

Very low calorie diets (VLCD)

A variety of synthetic and food based formula diets are available which give energy intakes of 300–400 kcal/day. These are complete with appropriate vitamin and trace element supplements as part of the formulation. Such diets appear to be safe in the short-to-medium term although a number of side effects have been reported (Hanefield and Weck, 1989). Certainly in the short term VLCD produce excellent weight loss but this appears not to be sustained at 1 year when they confer no advantage over standard approaches (Avenell *et al.*, 2004).

Such diets were used to good effect in drug-associated weight loss and maintenance studies to effect rapid and large weight loss in the first three months of treatment (James *et al.*, 2000).

Modern VLCDs must be distinguished from those used in the 1960s and 1970s to effect weight reduction. These latter dietary approaches were associated with sudden death syndrome, thought to be due to electrolyte and micronutrient deficiencies. Modern VLCDs do not induce such deficiencies. It is clear that short-term use of VLCDs produces improvements in glycaemic control, blood pressure and lipids. Longer-term effects both on weight and other outcomes remains to be investigated.

Conclusions

Dietary modification remains the cornerstone in the management of the obese type 2 diabetic, and the best long-term outcomes are achieved when optimal control is achieved by this means. There remains considerable research to determine the best way of delivering such therapy to achieve long-term weight reduction and optimum metabolic control. Identification of patient-specific dietary therapy remains the ideal goal. It is clear that no one approach to diet and food-based therapies is applicable to all patients. Further work is therefore needed to identify patient-matched diet treatment for long-term sustained weight loss possibly in association with drug-based therapies.

References

Atkins RC (1998) *Dr Atkins New Diet Revolutions*. Avon Books, New York.

Avenell A, Broom J, Brown TJ *et al.* (2004) Systematic review of the long-term outcomes of the treatments for obesity and implications for health improvement and the economic consequences for the National Health Service. *Health Technology Assessment*.

Banting W (1863) *Letter on corpulence, addressed to the public*, 2nd edn. Harrison and Sons, London.

Bravata DM, Sanders L, Huang J *et al.* (2003) Efficacy and safety of low-carbohydrate diets. *JAMA* **289**:1837–49.

Broom J, Wilding J, Stott P and Myers N (2002) Randomised trial of the effect of orlistat on body weight and cardiovascular risk profile in obese patients; the UK. Multimorbidity study. *Int J Clin Pract* **56**: 494–9.

Bruce AC, McNurlan MA, McHardy KC *et al.* (1990) Protein synthesis in human tumour and muscle is enhanced more by TPN than by solutions enriched with branched-chain amino acids. *Clin Nutr* **9**(Suppl):21–2.

Caterson ID and Broom J (eds) (2001) *In Pocket Picture Guide Obesity*. Harcount Health Communications.

DHSS-COMA (1984) Diet and cardiovascular disease. Report on Health and Social Subjects Vol. 28 HMSO, London.

Diabetes UK, Nutrition Subcommittee of the Diabetes Care Advisory Committee (2003) The implementation of nutritional advice for people with diabetes. *Diabet Med* **20**:786–807.

Eriksson J, Lindstrom J, Valle T *et al.* (1999) Prevention of type 2 diabetes in subjects with impaired glucose tolerance: the Diabetes Prevention Study (DPS) in Finland. Study design and 1 year interim report on the feasibility of the lifestyle intervention programme. *Diabetologica* **42**:793–801.

European Association for the Study of Diabetes, Nutrition and Diabetes Study Group (1988) Nutritional recommendations and principles for individuals with diabetes mellitus. *Diabet Nutr Metab* **1**:145–9.

Flatt JP (1985) Energetics of intermediary metabolism. In *Substrate and Energy Metabolism*. Farrow JS and Halliday D (eds). J Libbey, London, pp. 58–69.

Foster GD, Wyatt HR, Hill JO *et al.* (2003) A randomised trial of low-carbohydrate diet for obesity. *N Engl J Med* **348**:2082–90.

Grey N and Kipnes DM (1971) Effect of diet composition on the hyperinsulinaemia of obesity. *N Engl J Med* **285**:827–31.

Hanefield M and Weck M (1989) Very low calorie diet therapy in obese non-insulin dependent diabetes patients. *Int J Obes* **13** (Suppl 2):33–7.

Hollander PA, Elbein SC, Hirsch IB *et al.* (1998) Role of orlistat in the treatment of obese patients with type 2 diabetes. A 1-year randomised double-blind study. *Diabetes Care* **21**:1288–94.

James WPT, Astrup A, Finer N *et al.* (2000) Effect of sibutramine on weight maintenance after weight loss: A randomised trial. *Lancet* **356**:2119–25.

Lean MJ and James WPT (1986) Prescription of diabetic diets in the 1985. *Lancet* **I**:723–5.

Lean MJ and James WPT (1988) Metabolic effects of isoenergetic nutrient exchange over 24 hours in relation to obesity in women. *Int J Obes* **12**:15–28.

Lean MJ, James WPT and Garthwaite PH (1989) Obesity without overeating? In *Obesity in Europe 88*. Bjorntrop P and Rössner S (eds). J Libbey, London, pp. 281–6.

Lean MJ (1998) *Clinical Handbook, of Weight Management*. Dunitz IV, London.

Prentice AM, Black AE and Loward WA (1986) High levels of energy expenditure in obesity. *Br Med J* **242**:83–7.

Robertson AM, Broom J, McRobbie LJ and MacLennan GS (2002) Low carbohydrate diets in overweight patients with type 2 diabetes. *Proceedings of 9th International Congress on Obesity, Brazil. International Journal of Obesity*.

Samaha FF, Iqbal N, Seshadri P *et al.* (2003) A low carbohydrate as compared with a low-fat diet in severe obesity. *N Engl J Med* **348**: 2074–81.

Torjesen PA, Hjermann I, Birkeland KI *et al.* (1997) Lifestyle changes may reverse development of the insulin resistance syndrome–The Oslo Diet and Exercise Study: a randomised trial. *Diabetes Care* **20**:26–31.

UK Prospective Diabetes Study Group (1998) Effect of intensive blood glucose control with metformin on complications in overweight patients with type 2 diabetes (UKPDS 34). *Lancet* **352**:854–6.

Uusitupa MI (1996) Early lifestyle intervention in patients with non-insulin-dependent diabetes mellitus and impaired glucose tolerance. *Ann Med* **28**:445–9.

7

Behavioural Modification in the Treatment of Obesity

Brent Van Dorsten

Introduction

The alarming global increase in the prevalence of overweight and obesity is now a worldwide health epidemic (Hill *et al.*, 1995; Popkin and Doak, 1998; Wadden *et al.*, 2002). Obesity appears closely associated with several major health risks including hypertension, diabetes, high cholesterol, cardiovascular disease, and certain cancers (Must *et al.*, 1999), and may shorten life expectancy in even young adults (Fontaine *et al.*, 2003). A persistent increase in obesity prevalence has been observed in the United States over the past three decades despite increased awareness. Mokdad *et al.* (1999) reported an increase in the prevalence of obesity (body mass index (BMI) $\geq 30\,\mathrm{kg/m^2}$) from 12 per cent (1991) to 17.9 per cent (1998), and a recent review of National Health and Nutrition Examination Survey (NHANES) data report that 64.5 per cent of the US population is currently overweight (BMI $\geq 25\,\mathrm{kg/m^2}$), with the prevalence of obesity now reaching 30.5 per cent (Flegal *et al.*, 2002). Most recently, Mokdad and colleagues (2003) reported a 5.6 per cent one-year increase (2000–2001) in the prevalence of obesity, accompanied by an 8.2 per cent increase in the prevalence of diabetes from 7.35 to 7.9 per cent in this same year. These data confirm increases in the prevalence of these disorders across both genders, all age ranges, educational levels, and ethnicities. As the rate of obesity and its associated health disorders rapidly reaches crisis proportions, there are many proposed explanations to account for these increases including genetics, and the influence of an environment which promotes unhealthy lifestyle practices.

Obesity and Diabetes. Edited by Anthony H. Barnett and Sudhesh Kumar
© 2004 John Wiley & Sons, Ltd ISBN: 0-470-84898-7

Genetics

Many years of data support a relationship between genetics, other biological factors, and body mass regulation (Bouchard, 1994; Price, 2002). While the matrix of potential gene defects, and factors influencing their expression on body weight remains unknown, promising insights such as identification of the OB mouse obese or 'leptin' gene have been obtained (Zhang *et al.*, 1994). Severely obese ob/ob mice were found to be deficient in leptin production, prompting hope of a similar, and assumably correctable, deficit in obese humans. However, to date, this finding has not been reliably replicated in humans, spurring, investigations into leptin insensitivity (Campfield *et al.*, 1995). While promising work in genetics remains ahead, it follows that certain individuals possess a greater genetic predisposition to obesity which may be readily activated by the environment (Wadden *et al.* 2002).

The 'toxic environment'

The rapid escalation of overweight and obesity across genders, ages, ethnicities and countries, strongly suggests etiological factors that supercede genetics alone (Hill and Peters, 1998; Popkin and Doak, 1998). The term 'toxic environment'(Battle-Horgen and Brownell, 2002; Wadden *et al.*, 2002) is now commonly used to denote the rapid global changes shared by developed and developing countries. Unwarranted personal attributions regarding body size have allowed environmental factors to escape professional scrutiny until the recent past. Perceptions that obesity signifies personal weakness or failure, and a public proclivity to blame or hold individuals with emotional or physical problems responsible for their circumstance (Wortman and Silver, 1985, cited in Brownell and Rodin, 1993) have been difficult to overcome. In fact, a recent published survey of clinicians and researchers specialising in obesity similarly identified a significant perpetuation of anti-fat biases and stereotypes even among informed professionals (Schwartz *et al.*, 2003) given the current population demographics, the 'average' person in the population is now overweight, and gaining quickly. It is beyond debate that prevalent environmental obstacles to weight loss exist. Multiple dietary challenges exist including ready access to inexpensive, nutrient-rich foods, drive-through and meal delivery, popularity of buffet dining, television advertising of unhealthy products, school contracts with soft drink companies and availability of fast food outlets on school properties. An increase in the sedentary nature of the population reflects the 'double-edged sword' of technological advances that require less energy expenditure via physical labour, available transportation, increased leisure time, computers, internet, videogames, increased television viewing, decreased availability and emphasis on physical education in schools, and ever-increasing safety concerns which restrict access to walking, playgrounds, and other outdoor pursuits. While the health benefits of consistent, moderate intensity exercise are well known, the significant challenge to motivate and sustain behaviour change efforts against these factors is apparent (Dubbert, 2002).

Components of obesity treatment

Behavioural lifestyle modification

Persons with BMI of 25.0–29.9 kg/m^2 who have two or more health risk factors are encouraged to consume a low-calorie diet and increase physical activity consistent with the US Surgeon General's recommendation for 30 min or more per day most days of the week (NHLBI and NAASO, 2000; US Department of Health and Human Services, 1996). Behavioural lifestyle modification has comprised the cornerstone of weight loss treatment for decades, and typically involves group-led weekly meetings focusing on dietary change, activity increase and instruction in behaviour change techniques. Programme lengths have doubled from an average of 20 weeks in the 1980s to 40 or more weeks at present (Perri et al., 1989; Wing, 2002), with the active instructional phases most commonly lasting 16–26 weeks, and follow-ups typically extended to one or more years. Dietary recommendations include limiting calories to 1000–1800 kcal/day, with no more than 20–30 per cent of calories from fat. Behaviour change strategies include improving food choices and decreasing portion sizes, as well as modifying the environments, cognitions, or emotions associated with maladaptive health patterns. Exercise prescriptions typically entail brisk walking some 30–40 min per day most days per week. In a recent study by Manson et al. (2002), moderate intensity walking produced similar cardioprotective benefits as vigorous exercise for post-menopausal women while controlling for baseline age, race, and BMI. Further, cumulative short bouts of exercise (i.e. 10 min) throughout day have been associated with improved adherence and health benefits, and availability of home exercise equipment may also enhance outcomes (DeBusk et al., 1990; Jakicic et al., 1999). While of limited value in producing initial weight losses, exercise appears to strongly contribute to improving weight maintenance (Grilo, 1995; Jeffrey et al., 1998b; Pronk and Wing, 1994; Wing, 1999).

Medication

Published guidelines from a National Institutes of Health (NIH) expert panel on obesity recommend that pharmacological interventions are appropriate for persons with BMI $\geq$ 30.0 kg/m^2, BMI $\geq$ 27 kg/m^2 with additional co-morbid health conditions, or for those who have not achieved weight reduction with repeated conservative efforts (NHLBI & NAASO, 2000). A history of adverse events has plagued pharmacological attempts at weight management (Bray, 1998, 2002), and there are currently only two Federal Drug Administration (FDA) approved medications for obesity treatment. Sibutramine (Meridia) is a central nervous system agent that inhibits the reuptake of norepinephrine and serotonin, and functions by reducing appetite and energy intake (Rolls *et al.*, 1998). This medication has been shown to produce both initial and sustained weight loss with and without the addition of behavioural therapy (Lean, 1997; Rolls *et al.*, 1998).

In contrast, orlistat (Xenical) does not act on the central nervous system, but rather functions as a lipase inhibitor blocking the absorption of about one-third of consumed fat. Orlistat may also modify food preference via aversive conditioning and the unpleasant gastrointestinal symptoms commonly experienced after high fat intake. Both medications are typically prescribed as an adjunct to diet, exercise and behaviour modification to produce greater initial losses, while receiving the reduction in health risks associated with healthy lifestyle.

Surgery

Bariatric surgeries for weight loss are typically reserved for persons with BMI $\geq 40\,\text{kg/m}^2$, or for individuals with BMI $\geq 35\,\text{kg/m}^2$ and other significant co-morbid health conditions. Available data suggests that medical weight reduction programmes are unsuccessful for extreme obesity patients (BMI $\geq 40\,\text{kg/m}^2$), and that most regain all weight lost, and more, within two years (Latifi *et al.*, 2002). The two most common surgical procedures are gastric bypass (GB) and vertical banded gastroplasty (VBG) in which a small pouch is either surgically created or silicone banded at the base of the oesophagus to limit volume and absorption. While cost and surgical risk (e.g. gastric perforation, postoperative gallstone formation) may pose an obstacle for some, surgical interventions are capable of producing losses of two-thirds of excess weight within two years, superior long-term maintenance of large weight losses (Latifi *et al.*, 2002; Sjostrom *et al.*, 1999), and extensive health benefits including improved control of type 2 diabetes (Pories *et al.*, 1995).

Features of behavioural lifestyle change

While often considered a specific treatment, behaviour modification is better conceptualized as the application of a set of behaviour change strategies derived from the experimental analysis of human behaviour (Miltenberger, 1997). These strategies can be applied in a variety of combinations to create adaptive desirable behaviours, strengthen and sustain their performance, and promote long-term durability of these behaviours. Brownell *et al.* (1986) proposed three phases of behaviour change including exacting the commitment and motivation for change, initial change, and maintenance of change. Behaviour change techniques can be applied to observable behaviours, cognitions or thoughts, and affect or mood. They are ubiquitously applied in weight management to modify environmental stimuli, behaviours, and thoughts influencing food intake and physical activity. A fundamental assumption in applying behavioural strategies to weight loss is that the balance between behaviours controlling food intake and energy expenditure is tipped in the direction of excessive intake, and that these behaviours are learned and thus can be modified to produce a shift in this balance towards energy expenditure (Jeffery *et al.*, 2000).

Behavioural lifestyle modification strategies can be applied in weight management *before* a person begins walking, or makes their first intentional dietary change. Determining readiness to attempt behavioural change has been suggested as a useful factor in predicting participation with health behaviour change efforts (Prochaska *et al.*, 1992, 1994), and has been specifically applied to readiness for behaviour change associated with weight loss (Clark *et al.*, 1992, 1996; Greene *et al.*, 1999).

In assessing readiness for change, obesity treatment providers are increasingly utilizing motivational interviewing techniques (Miller and Rollnick, 2002) to assist patients in clarifying their personal reasons for attempting weight loss, and to acknowledge and validate the feelings of ambivalence an individual may feel about starting weight change efforts. Motivational interviewing is designed to anticipate specific obstacles one might encounter during change efforts, and identify available personal resources to address these barriers. These techniques have been successfully applied to adherence with adult behavioural weight control and dietary change efforts in children (Smith *et al.*, 1997; Berg-Smith, 1999).

A 5–10 per cent reduction in body weight is considered successful given the associated improvement in health risk factors and potential for reasonable weight maintenance. However, previous research has obviated the need to explicitly identify patient goals for weight reduction. Foster *et al.* (1997) assessed the 'dream weight', 'happy weight', 'goal weight', 'acceptable weight', and 'disappointing weight' of 60 obese women prior to beginning a 48-week behavioural weight loss treatment programme. Surprisingly, this group identified a 32 per cent reduction as their average weight loss goal. Nearly half of the 45 women who completed the 48-week treatment did not achieve even the 'disappointing' weight loss goal, despite an average 16-kg weight loss during the programme. This 16-kg loss – a 16 per cent total body weight reduction in this study – was only approximately one-third of the desired loss, and none of the participants reached their 'dream' weight. Foster *et al.* (2001) reported similarly unreasonable weight loss goals for patients seeking weight loss via either behavioural interventions or surgery, with the heaviest of participants desiring the greatest absolute weight losses to meet their satisfaction. Unrealistic weight loss expectations were also identified in persons seeking pharmacological treatment for obesity as pre-treatment goals for weight loss desires were nearly 25 per cent of total body weight (Wadden *et al.* 2001). Of significant clinical interest, Wadden *et al.* (2003) recently reported that explicit provision of both verbal and written information regarding what participants might reasonably expect for weight loss with one year of Sibutramine use (5–15 per cent of total body weight) had little impact on the unreasonable expectations of participants throughout weight loss treatment.

Behavioural modification strategies in obesity treatment

There are multiple published articles describing the commonly employed behavioural modification strategies for dietary change, exercise adoption, and relapse prevention (Brownell, 2000; Foreyt and Poston, 1998; Poston and Foreyt; 2000; Wing, 1998). Establishing reasonable, specific short- and long-term goals, daily self-monitoring of dietary intake and exercise behaviours, using stimulus control techniques to modify environmental and intrapersonal factors that precede and cue food intake, cognitive restructuring to address maladaptive thoughts impacting behaviour change, problem-solving environmental, emotional, or motivational challenges to change efforts, enlisting social support resources, and relapse prevention training are useful techniques in modifying behaviours associated with weight loss. Several examples of how the primary behavioural modification strategies might be incorporated throughout the weight loss process are provided in Table 7.1.

Goal setting

Considering the important potential divergence of treatment goals between providers and treatment seekers, the development of realistic, attainable goals prior to beginning weight loss is critical to facilitating personal acceptance and maintenance of losses actually achieved. Various behaviour change goals in obesity treatment may include targeting a specific number of grams to lose (as opposed to a more obscure goal of 'losing some weight'), specific metabolic or psychosocial improvements, or potential changes in medication intake or insulin requirements for co-morbid conditions. Potential decreases in oral medication requirements for co-morbid health conditions are often a salient motivation for individuals to begin and maintain behavioural lifestyle changes. Behavioural weight loss goals of 10 per cent total body weight are attainable and can produce important health risk reductions. Further, establishing a modest weight loss goal may be associated with more successful achievement and long-term maintenance of this goal (Jeffrey et al., 1998a). Any overall weight loss goal can be sub-divided into weekly goals for 500–750-g losses, with precise identification of the incremental behaviour changes necessary to produce this outcome. Typically these incremental changes include restricting calorie and fat intake, and gradually increasing minutes of physical activity. Explicit behavioural commitments or contracts between an individual and a counsellor or group can assist in clarifying the frequency, intensity and duration of activities the person will perform to attain these weekly or monthly goals. These behaviour change contracts, often publicly signed by others witnessing the commitment, can be important strategies in motivating patients to maintaining efforts over time (Ureda, 1980; Zandee and

Table 7.1 Potential applications of five primary behavioural modification strategies in weight loss and diabetes management

Behavioural technique	General purpose(s)	Potential targets/examples

Goal setting	Specify realistic, measurable, obtainable incremental goals for target behaviours	Gradual weight loss
		  0.5–1 kg per week weight loss
		  daily calorie range goal
		  daily fat gram intake goal
		Activity increase
		  minutes per day/week
		  number of steps on pedometer
		  number of days per week

Self-monitoring	Increase awareness of behaviour patterns Increase accuracy of behaviour estimates Reinforce changes in target behaviours	Dietary intake (fat, calories) Eating pattern (time, portions) Activity minutes Factors influencing food intake mood, social events Medication adherence Self-monitoring blood glucose

Stimulus control/cues	Prompt occurrence of target behaviours	Keep walking shoes in sight
		Colour dots to prompt behaviours
		  blood glucose checks
		  medication intake
		  exercise initiation
		  reminder of calorie goals

Problem-solving	Provide step-wise structure to modify challenges to consistent efforts at behaviour change	Obstacles to exercise adherence
		  adverse weather
		  minor injury
		  social pressure to limit
		Obstacles to healthy food intake
		  holidays/social parties
		  eating in restaurants
		  skipping meals
		  social pressure to eat

Cognitive restructuring	Identify and modify self-defeating thoughts and increase self-rewarding thoughts to motivate change efforts	Inaccurate self-perceptions
		  'slow metabolism' problem
		  lazy, weak, failure
		  lack will-power
		Encouraging thoughts
		  can do it this time
		  will succeed in the long run
		  little changes will help
		  lapse is not a crisis
		  proud of myself for trying

Oermann, 1996). Behavioural contracts should clearly specify the contingencies under which the person will reward themselves for the efforts they have made to change behaviour. Since weight itself is not a behaviour, but rather an artifact of several behaviours, rewards must be contingent upon behavioural effort (i.e.

number of times walked or number of minutes accumulated) and not outcome (i.e. number of grams lost).

Self-monitoring

Self-monitoring describes the systematic recording of a behaviour that is targeted for change. In behavioural weight loss, calories or fat grams consumed, minutes of daily walking, number of steps taken, and even emotional factors influencing food intake, can be either objectively or subjectively quantified via self-monitoring. Self-recording may serve many purposes including establishing baseline values of a behaviour, increasing awareness of personal patterns, improving accuracy of unstructured behaviour estimates, and providing feedback and reinforcement for changes in a target behaviour. Ensuring accurate base rates of targeted behaviours is critical, as the published error in unstructured estimates of caloric intake and energy expenditure may reach 50 per cent (Bandini et al., 1990; Irwin et al., 2001; Lichtman et al., 1992). Consistent and accurate self-monitoring has been identified as an important component in maintaining long-term weight loss (Klem et al., 1997), and successfully maintaining weight during shorter 'high-risk for regain' periods such as the holidays (Boutelle and Kirschenbaum, 1998; Boutelle et al., 1999).

Stimulus control

Stimulus control is the term applied to the behaviour change strategy designed to identify and modify environmental cues associated with food intake or activity patterns. Environmental cues which prompt overeating or sedentary behaviours may be modified to those which more adaptively prompt and support improved eating habits or physical activity (Foreyt and Goodrick, 1993). For example, cues (e.g. colour dots) may be intentionally *placed* in a person's home to prompt medication adherence, walking shoes can be placed in visible sight to cue increased walking, and snack foods may be removed from the home to *remove* a cue for eating undesirable foods. Considering the media bombardment of cues that promote food intake and inactivity, the utilization of personal environmental cues can be immensely helpful in 'reminding' patients of behaviour change goals and agreements in the interim between group or counsellor visits. While a 167:1 ratio may be considered weak in mathematical terms, this ratio represents the 'best case scenario' in weight loss treatment. Specifically, if a counsellor meets with a weight loss client weekly for 1 hour, 167 hours remain in this week for the person to independently attempt implement changes, and any available prompts to motivate and prompt their daily efforts need be utilized.

Problem solving

In prolonged obesity treatment, few patients might accurately anticipate the number and intensity of obstacles they might encounter as they strive to initiate and sustain diet and activity changes across time and settings. As such, a valuable component of behavioural skill instruction is providing individuals with a framework for identifying, defining and problem solving physical, environmental, or psychosocial challenges to sustained performance. Problem-solving strategies compose five steps including: (1) identification and detailed definition of a specific challenge; (2) brainstorming potential alternatives; (3) weighing the relative benefits and disadvantages of each option; (4) selecting and implementing the option that holds the highest probability for rectifying the circumstance; and (5) evaluating efficacy after implementation. These strategies can be flexibly applied to any number of challenges including time management or schedule conflicts, employment or transportation issues, adverse weather, minor physical injuries, holidays or restaurant eating, or mood or negative self-talk challenges. As most active treatment programs are time-limited, problem-solving training can provide individuals with a systematic framework to define and solve unforeseen challenges to attaining their weight loss goals. Perri *et al.* (2001) reported that the inclusion of problem-solving significantly improved weight loss maintenance.

Cognitive restructuring

Emotional factors may have considerable impact on a person's dedication to weight change and may be a strong antecedent to overeating or abandoning activity. Negative affect and self-defeating cognitions regarding one's ability to succeed in making behavioural changes may hamper future efforts. Most obese persons have endured many unsuccessful weight loss attempts and this history can fuel maladaptive expectations of future failure if not addressed as a part of comprehensive behavioural treatment. Negative self-attributions associated with failure to lose weight (e.g. 'can't do it', 'weak', or 'don't have the willpower'), or inaccurate physical attributions such as having a resistant or 'slow metabolism' are frequently encountered in weight treatment. While the latter may seem desirable as a potential explanation for failure to achieve weight loss despite repeated efforts, one recent study rejected this phenomenon as a primary explanation for failure to lose weight (Lichtman *et al.*, 1992).

Based upon the work of Beck and colleagues, cognitive-behavioural theory suggests that cognition and behaviour are in part determined by perceptions of self and the factors believed to control one's world. Tailored cognitive restructuring involves teaching individuals to become aware of maladaptive cognitive perceptions or "distortions" (Beck and Weishar, 1989), and to explicitly describe and actively challenge maladaptive self-perceptions. A variety of behavioural change strategies may be combined to increase awareness (e.g. self-monitoring of cognitions), devise a change plan (e.g. problem-solving alternatives to negative self-talk), and reinforcing efforts to challenge the validity of these perceptions.

Social support

Existing data suggests that people with greater perceived social support, attending weight loss groups, or involving family or friends in weight loss efforts may produce better outcomes (Foreyt and Goodrick, 1991, 1994; Renjilian *et al.*, 2001; Wing and Jeffrey, 1999). Behavioural weight loss is typically conducted in closed groups as peer familiarity, validation of struggles, modelling coping and incremental success, encouragement, and group accountability to meet goals all add important dimensions to the weight loss process. In order to promote real-world adoption of behavioural changes, primary social support may be transitioned from weight loss counsellors or the weight loss group to resources in the person's social circle. The frequency of group meetings is typically faded over time and participants are taught to engender personal social support resources to maintain their efforts. These personal social supports may include family, friends, physicians, community support groups or electronic contacts (e.g. diet-related websites, chat rooms).

Relapse prevention

The most commonly identified problem in obesity treatment is long-term maintenance of weight loss (DePue *et al.*, 1995; Foreyt and Goodrick, 1991; Perri, 1998). A primary factor known to contribute to adherence with behaviour change strategies and maintenance of weight loss is maintaining episodic long-term contact with treatment providers and/or peers (Perri *et al.*, 1984, 1986, 1987). These follow-up contacts can be accomplished with face-to-face meetings, by telephone (Lindstrom *et al.*, 1976), or via electronic e-mail. The optimal frequency of maintenance contacts is largely unknown, but should be devised in response to attendance and weight maintenance data. Restart programmes which give patients the opportunity to re-engage in an active intervention strategy for a short period of time (e.g. exercise groups or meal replacements for 6 weeks) may be offered to re-establish the benefits and behavioural patterns of the active intervention. It should be noted however that Smith and Wing (1991) found that repeated diets produced lower levels of programme adherence and less weight loss than was achieved during an original intervention period. Alternatively, provision of personal trainers and monetary incentives (Jeffrey *et al.*, 1984, 1998b), and group-contingent work site competitions (Brownell *et al.*, 1984; Zandee and Oermann, 1996) have been successfully used to achieve ongoing participation with weight-loss programmes.

Many unique insights regarding successful maintenance of weight loss have been gained from the members of the National Weight Control Registry (NWCR), a roster of several thousand people who have lost at least 13 kg and maintained this loss for at least 1 year (Klem *et al.*, 1997). In fact, the average weight loss of registry members is 30 kg with an average successful maintenance period of over 5 years. While registry members endorsed using several dietary strategies to lose weight, three primary strategies have been utilized in their efforts to maintain losses. Consistent self-monitoring of intake, frequent weighing, and increasing physical activity beyond that required to produce initial weight loss appear as strong recommendations. The need to increase energy expenditure for successful weight maintenance has also been emphasized by other studies (Kayman *et al.*, 1990, Jakicic *et al.*, 1999, Jeffrey *et al.*, 1998b). On a positive note, NWCR members have reported that as time since original weight loss increases, maintenance requires fewer strategies and becomes more pleasurable (Klem *et al.*, 2000). Considering the importance of sustained physical exercise to weight maintenance, it is somewhat encouraging that two recent studies have reported that participants who exercised in the convenience of their homes, as compared to exercising at a weight loss clinic or health club, demonstrated increased adherence, weight maintenance, and in some cases continued weight reduction (King *et al.*, 1997; Perri *et al.*, 1997; Leermarkers *et al.*, 1998). This finding, coupled with the evidence supporting the benefits of accumulating short bouts of activity, provides promise for achieving the increased activity levels necessary for maintenance.

Efficacy of combination treatments

It is difficult to succinctly evaluate the efficacy of 'behavioural management' of obesity because the term generally encompasses all facets of treatment apart from surgery. Considering the multiple variations of diet, physical activity and behavioural modification strategies and adding adherence techniques, relapse prevention, meal replacements, and medication use to this matrix – an exponential number of combinations exist against which to assess the success of treatment packages. A brief review of the relative contribution of these components to obesity treatment follows.

Behavioural treatments

Behavioural treatments for weight loss are designed to produce a 0.5–1.0 kg average weekly weight reduction, or an approximate 8.5–9.0 kg decrease (8–10 per cent of total body weight) from pre- to post-treatment, with attrition rates generally under 20 per cent (Poston *et al.*, 1998; Perri, 2002; Wing, 2002).

In an early report of the efficacy of behavioural-based treatment, Bjorvell and Rossner (1985) assigned 107 severely obese subjects (basal BMI women 40.5, men 42.9) to receive a 6-week clinic-based intervention consisting of twice weekly group behavioural therapy, a supervised 600 kcal/day clinic diet plus nutritional advice on low-fat cooking, and therapist-led exercise three times per week. This programme also provided a remarkable 4-year maintenance programme with optional weekly weighing and nutritional 'booster sessions'.

Those who did not attend boosters were frequently contacted via telephone or letter, and those who relapsed were provided short-term 'refresher courses'. Mean weight losses for women and men at 6 weeks, 1 year, and 4 years were 10.0/12.2 kg, 15.0/30.9 kg, and 11.5/18.4 kg, respectively. Study attrition at 4 years was 31 per cent. A follow-up of this study indicated average weight losses maintained at 10–12 year follow-up equaled 9.5 kg for women, and 17.5 kg for men (Bjorvell and Rossner, 1992). While the authors concluded that a comprehensive behavioural modification programme could produce positive long-term weight loss results, the findings are difficult to compare with current studies given the comprehensiveness and duration of the intervention.

Few recent studies have specifically compared different combinations of diet and exercise versus diet alone, and some recent reports surprisingly fail to support the benefits of combining strategies. Skender and colleagues (1996) reported marginal but non-significant differences in diet plus exercise versus diet alone, in a study whose conclusions were limited by attrition. Wadden *et al.* (1998) reported the 1-year follow-up of a clinical trial which compared four conditions: including diet alone, diet plus either aerobic or strength training, or combination of all. All participants received similar diets and a 48-week group behavioural programme. At week 48, participants across all groups averaged a 15.1 kg weight loss, and no significant difference was noted between groups. Weight losses were well maintained, but no group differences were found at one-year follow-up. Wing (2002) suggests that these study results may fail to support combining strategies as each reported that participants struggled to maintain sufficient long-term exercise adherence to adequately assess the potential effect.

Both the provision of food products and structured meal plans have been reported to improve weight loss results. Jeffrey *et al.* (1993) found that patients who were prescribed standard reduced calorie diets, and were provided most of the food for this diet, lost significantly more weight after six and 18 months of treatment than did patients who were randomized to a self-selected decreased calorie diet. Wing *et al.* (1996) expanded these results by reporting that the provision of structured meal plans (i.e. what to eat for specific meals) produced similar results without providing the foods.

Two recent national studies have provided further evidence that standard behavioural recommendations for weight loss including reduced calorie diet and increased physical activity can produce moderate sustained weight loss, decreased health risks, and prevention or delayed development of type 2 diabetes in those at high risk for up to 3 years (Diabetes Prevention Program Research Group, 2002; Tuomilehto *et al.*, 2001).

Very low calorie diets (VLCD)

Very-low-calorie diets typically provide less than 800 kcal/day (as compared with low-calorie-diets (LCD) 800–1500 kcal/day), but include sufficient amounts of protein (i.e. lean meat, fowl, or liquid formula) to minimize loss of lean muscle mass during weight loss. Several studies in the past two decades have confirmed the capacity of VLCD to produce superior weight loss and maintenance (Wadden *et al.*, 1988, 1989; Wing *et al.*, 1994). The common features of these studies include stringent dietary intake restrictions, with or without provision of behavioural counselling, and follow up of 1–8 years (Kirschner *et al.*, 1988; Wadden *et al.*, 1988, 1989). Aggregate results of these investigations suggest that VLCD typically produces weight reductions of 15–25 per cent of baseline body weight with 8–16 weeks of treatment (Wadden and Osei, 2002). While this weight loss is significant in comparison to the low calorie self-selected food diets, rapid regain is common with VLCD diets and non-significant differences in weight loss are common between the two dietary approaches at even 1-year post treatment (Wadden *et al.*, 1994; Wing *et al.*, 1994). The addition of behaviour therapy in addition to VLCD alone appears to marginally improve weight loss maintenance.

As before, the efficacy of behavioural weight loss approaches is diminished by the disappointing durability of changes. Problems with weight regain are well known, with most patients regaining at least 30–40 per cent of initial weight loss at one year, and more than half regaining all weight lost within 3–5 years (Institute of Medicine [IOM], 1995). These results must be viewed however, in light of epidemiological observations that without treatment most obese individuals naturalistically gain 0.5–1 kg per year (Williamson, 1993; Rothacker, 2000).

Liquid meal replacements

Despite their historical public popularity, liquid meal replacements have received little empirical attention until the recent past. Ditschuneit *et al.* (1999) conducted a study in which 100 patients received nutrition consultation and random assignment for three months to either a 1200–1500 kcal/day self-selected diet or an isoenergetic diet in which two meals and two snacks per day were replaced by SlimFast products. After the initial 3-month treatment period, both groups were prescribed a similar energy-restricted 1200–1500 kcal/day diet with one meal and one snack replacement for an additional 2 years. Three month results indicated mean weight losses of 1.5 kg and 7.8 kg for the respective groups, with increased weight losses to 3.2 kg and 8.4 kg per respective group approximately 4 years after treatment initiation (Flechtner-Mors *et al.*, 2000).

In an interesting minimal contact, community-based intervention, Rothacker (2000) provided further support for the efficacy of meal replacements in producing weight loss. In this study, 141 participants replaced two meals per day with liquid meal replacements for 3 months, then one to two per day until reaching an unspecified weight goal. If regain of more than 1–2 kg occurred over the following 5 years, patients were encouraged to return to the twice a day replacements. After weekly weighing at a local facility for the first 12 weeks, patients were then seen twice yearly for maintenance with no other treatment provided. Data for this treatment group was compared against age and weight-matched no treatment controls who simply provided weights in 1992 and 1997. In the initial 3-month treatment phase, weight loss for treatment males and females were 7.4 kg and 6.4 kg, with losses of 5.9 kg and 4.2 kg maintained at 5 years. Control males and females *gained* 6.7 kg and 6.5 kg, respectively, over the 5-year period. This investigation suggests that meal replacements, with even minimal additional contact, may be capable of producing modest weight losses. Taken together, these investigations suggest that meal replacement strategies may produce larger initial weight losses and improved maintenance of losses versus standard dietary changes alone. Continued investigation of the strategic use of these products in weight loss programmes appears warranted.

Pharmacotherapy

Phelan and Wadden (2002) proposed several reasons that medications are most commonly prescribed adjunctively to behavioural treatments including a preference to implement the least intrusive treatment first, receiving the health improvements associated with physical exercise, and pursuing larger weight losses with combined therapy. Combined pharmacological and behavioural interventions for weight loss are hypothesized to produce a synergistic effect acting on both internal cues that influence hunger and/or nutrient absorption, and external environmental cues which influence diet and exercise patterns (Wadden and Osei, 2002). Phelan and Wadden (2002) provide a comprehensive review of published double-blind, placebo controlled trials of both orlistat and sibutramine and lifestyle modification for obesity. Similar to results of behavioural treatment, obesity medications typically produce losses of 8–10 per cent of initial weight for up to 2 years with continued use (Bray, 2002; Wadden and Osei, 2002), and the combination of strategies appears to enhance both initial weight losses and maintenance.

Bray *et al.* (1999) reported a clear dose-response relationship for sibutramine between 5 and 30 mg with losses of 3–12 per cent of initial weight. James *et al.* (2000) reported significantly greater losses for sibutramine versus placebo treatment, and 90% maintenance of initial weight loss between years one and two. Wadden *et al.* (2001) reported significantly greater weight losses and patient satisfaction at 1 year when behavioural care was added to sibutramine treatment alone.

Similarly, two recent studies reported significantly greater losses and one-year maintenance with orlistat and behavioural care versus placebo and behavioural care (Lindgarde, 2000; Miles *et al.*, 2002). Orlistat has been shown to produce losses of 5–13 per cent of initial weight, with 2-year maintenance of the majority of weight lost (Phelan and Wadden 2002). Hoping to combine mechanisms of action, Wadden *et al.* (2000) found no additional benefit of adding orlistat to patients who had lost weight during 1 year of treatment with sibutramine plus lifestyle. Nonetheless, continued investigation of the optimal combinations of medications, doses, and behavioural packages appears strongly indicated.

Conclusions and future work

Despite the advances in the treatment of obesity observed in the past 20 years, practitioners have clearly not been successful in stemming the tide of the obesity epidemic. Significant environmental challenges to behaviour change will continue, and substantiate the need to continue to refine and improve treatments. Based upon existing data, obesity treatment programmes must necessarily be designed to provide extended provider contact, and flexibly combine behavioural, meal replacement and pharmacological treatment strategies. Combination treatment packages appear more promising in achieving long-term weight loss than single treatments, and multidisciplinary provider teams may improve adherence, initial losses and maintenance. Treatment programmes should include both community-based and in-home resources for increasing physical activity whenever possible. Obesity must be conceptualized as a chronic health condition similar to diabetes or hypertension, and physicians using pharmacotherapy must be prepared to provide long-term management (Hill *et al.*, 1999). Additionally, non-behavioural community providers need be increasingly trained to competently utilize behavioural modification strategies with their patients on a daily basis, because until more treatment resources are obtained, the bulk of the responsibility for weight change may continue to reside with the individual and their primary care providers.

References

Bandini LG, Schoeller DA, Cyr HN and Dietz WH (1990) Validity of reported energy intake in obese and non-obese adolescents. *Am J Clin Nutr* **52**:421–5.

Battle-Horgen K and Brownell KD (2002) Confronting the toxic environment: Environmental and public health actions in a world crisis. In Wadden TA and Stunkard AJ (eds), *Handbook of Obesity Treatment* Guilford Press, New York, pp. 95–107.

Beck AT and Weishar M (1989) Cognitive therapy. In Freeman A, Simon KM, Beutler LE and Arkowitz H (eds), *Comprehensive Handbook of Cognitive Therapy* Plenum Publishing Company, New York.

Berg-Smith SM, Stevens JJ, Brown KM, *et al.* (1999) A brief motivational intervention to improve dietary adherence in adolescents. *Health Educ Res* **14**:399–410.

Bjorvell H and Rossner S (1985) Long-term treatment of severe obesity: Four year follow-up of results of combined behavioral modification programme. *Br Med J* **291**:379–82.

Bjorvell H and Rossner S (1992) A ten year follow-up of weight change in severely obese subjects treated in a behavior modification programme. *Int J Obes* **16**:623–5.

Bouchard CB (1994) Genetics of obesity: Overview and research direction. In Bouchard CB (ed.); *The Genetics of Obesity* CRC Press, Boca Raton, FL, pp. 223–33.

Boutelle KN and Kirschenbaum DS (1998) Further support for consistent self-monitoring as a vital component of successful weight control. *Obes Res* **6**:219–24.

Boutelle KN, Kirschenbaum DS, Baker RC and Mitchell EM (1999) How can obese weight controllers minimize weight gain during the high risk holiday season? By self-monitoring very consistently. *Health Psychol* **18**:364–8.

Bray GA (1998). Drug treatment of obesity: Don't throw the baby out with the bath water. *Am J Clin Nutr* **67**:1–2.

Bray GA (2002) Drug treatment of obesity. In Wadden TA and Stunkard AJ (eds), *Handbook of Obesity Treatment*. Guilford Press, New York, pp. 317–38.

Bray GA, Blackburn GL, Ferguson JM *et al.* (1999) Sibutramine produces dose-related weight loss. *Obes Res* **7**:189–98.

Brownell KD (2000) The LEARN program for weight management 2000. Dallas, TX, American Health.

Brownell KD and Cohen LR (1995) Adherence to dietary regimens 2: Components of effective interventions. *Behav Med* **20**:155–64.

Brownell KD and Rodin J (1993) The dieting maelstrom: Is it possible and advisable to lose weight. *Am Psychol* **49**:781–91.

Brownell KD, Yopp-Cohen R, Stunkard AJ *et al.* (1984) Weight loss competitions at the work site: Impact on weight, morale, and cost-effectiveness. *Am J Public Health* **74**:1283–5.

Brownell KD, Marlatt GA, Lichtenstein E and Wilson GT (1986) Understanding and preventing relapse. *Am Psychol* **41**:765–82.

Campfield LA, Smith FJ, Guisez Y *et al.* (1995) Recombinant mouse OB protein: Evidence for a peripheral signal linking adiposity and central neural networks. *Science* **269**:546–9.

Clark MM, Pera V, Goldstein MG *et al.* (1996) Counseling strategies for obese patients. *Am J Prevent Med* **12**:266–70.

Curry SJ, Kristal AR and Bowen DJ (1992) An application of the stage model of behavior change to dietary fat reduction. *Health Educ Res* **7**:97–105.

DeBusk RF, Stenestrand U, Sheehan M and Haskell WL (1990) Training effects of long versus short bouts of exercise in healthy subjects. *Am J Cardiol* **65**:1010–13.

DePue JD, Clark MM, Ruggiero L *et al.* (1995) Maintenance of weight loss: A needs assessment. *Obes Res* **3**:241–7.

Diabetes Prevention Program Research Group (2002) Reduction in the incidence of type 2 diabetes with lifestyle intervention and metformin. *N Engl J Med* **346**:393–403.

Ditschuneit HH, Flechtner-Mors M, Johnson TD and Adler G (1999) Metabolic and weight loss effects of long-term dietary intervention in obese patients. *Am J Clin Nutr* **69**:198–204.

Dubbert PM (2002) Physical activity and exercise: Recent advances and current challenges. *J Consult Clin Psychol* **70**:526–36.

Flechtner-Mors M, Ditschuneit HH, Johnson TD *et al.* (2000) Metabolic and weight loss effects of long-term dietary intervention in obese patients: Four-year results. *Obes Res* **8**:399–402.

Flegal KM, Carroll MD, Ogden CL and Johnson CL (2002) Prevalence and trends in obesity among US adults, 1999–2000. *JAMA* **288**:1723–7.

Fontaine KR, Redden DT, Wang C *et al.* (2003) Years of life lost due to obesity. *JAMA* **289**:187–93.

Foreyt JP and Goodrick GK (1991) Factors common to successful therapy for the obese patient. *Med Sci Sports Exerc* **23**:292–7.

Foreyt JP and Goodrick GK (1993) Evidence for success of behavioral modification in weight loss and control. *Ann Intern Med* **119**:698–701.

Foreyt JP and Goodrick GK (1994) Attributes of successful approaches to weight loss and control. *Appl Prevent Psychol* **3**:20–215.

Foreyt JP and Poston WSC (1998) What is the role of cognitive-behavioral therapy in patient management? *Obes Res* **6** (Suppl.):18S–22S.

Foster GD, Wadden TA, Vogt RA and Brewer G (1997) What is reasonable weight loss? Patient's expectations and evaluations of obesity treatment outcomes. *J Consult Clin Psychol* **65**:79–85.

Foster GD, Wadden TA, Phelan S *et al.* (2001) Obese patient's perceptions of treatment outcomes and the factors that influence them. *Arch Intern Med* **161**:2133–9.

Greene GW, Rossi SR, Rossi JS *et al.* (1999) Dietary applications of the stages of change model. *J Am Diet Assoc* **99**:673–678.

Grilo CM (1995) The role of physical activity in weight loss and weight loss management. *Med Exerc Nutr Health* **4**:60–76.

Hill JA, Rogers PJ and Blundell JE (1995) Techniques for the experimental measurement of human eating behaviour and food intake: A practical guide. *Int J Obes* **19**:361–75.

Hill JO and Peters JR (1998) Environmental contributions to the obesity epidemic. *Science* **280**:1371–4.

Hill JO, Hauptman J, Anderson JW *et al.* (1999) Orlistat, a lipase inhibitor, for weight maintenance after conventional dieting: A 1-year study. *Am J Clin Nutr* **69**:1108–16.

Institute of Medicine (1995) *Weighing the options: Criteria for evaluating weight management programs*. National Academy Press, Washington DC.

Irwin ML, Ainsworth BE and Conway JM (2001) Estimation of energy expenditure from physical activity measures: determinants of accuracy. *Obes Res* **9**:517–25.

Irwin ML, Yasui Y, Ulrich CM *et al.* (2003) Effect of exercise on total and intra-abdominal body fat in postmenopausal women. *JAMA* **289**:323–30.

Jakicic J, Winters C, Lang W and Wing RR (1999) Effects of intermittent exercise and use of home exercise equipment on adherence, weight loss, and fitness in overweight women. *JAMA* **282**:1554–60.

James WP, Astrup A and Finer N (2000) Effect of sibutramine on weight maintenance after weight loss: a randomized trial. STORM Study Group. *Lancet* **356**:19–25.

Jeffrey RW, Bjornson-Benson WM, Rosenthal BS *et al.* (1984) Effectiveness of monetary contracts with two repayment schedules on weight reduction in men and women from self-referred and population samples. *Behav Ther* **15**:273–9.

Jeffrey RW, Wing RR, Thorson C *et al.* (1993) Strengthening behavioral interventions for weight loss: A randomized trial of food provision and monetary incentives. *J Consult Clin Psychol* **61**:1038–45.

Jeffrey RW, Wing RR and Mayer RR (1998a) Are smaller weight losses or more achievable weight loss goals better in the long term for obese patients? *J Consult Clin Psychol* **66**:641–5.

Jeffrey RW, Wing RR, Thorson C and Burton LR (1998b) Use of personal trainers and financial incentives to increase exercise in a behavioral weight loss program. *J Consult Clin Psychol* **66**:777–83.

Jeffery RW, Epstein LH, Wilson GT *et al.* (2000) Long-term maintenance of weight loss: Current status. *Health Psychol* **19** (Suppl.):5S–16S.

Kayman S, Bruvold W and Stern JS (1990) Maintenance and relapse after weight loss in women: Behavioral aspects. *Am J Clin Nutr* **52**:800–7.

King AC, Keirnan M, Oman RF *et al.* (1997) Can we identify who will adhere to long-term physical activity? Signal detection methodology as a potential aid to clinical decision making. *Health Psychol* **16**:380–9.

Kirschner MA, Schneider G, Ertel NH and Gorman J (1988) An eight year experience with a very-low-calorie formula diet for control of major obesity. *Int J Obes* **12**:69–80.

Klem ML, Wing RR, McGuire MT *et al.* (1997) A descriptive study of individuals successful at long-term maintenance of substantial weight loss. *Am J Clin Nutr* **66**:239–46.

Klem ML, Wing RR, Lang W *et al.* (2000) Does weight loss maintenance become easier over time? *Obes Res* **8**:438–44.

Latifi R, Kellum JM, DeMaria EJ and Sugarman HJ (2002) Surgical treatment of obesity. In Wadden TA and Stunkard AJ (eds), *Handbook of Obesity Treatment* Guilford Press, New York, pp. 339–56.

Lean MEJ (1997) Sibutramine – a review of clinical efficacy. *Int J Obes* **21** (Suppl.):30–6.

Leermarkers EA, Jakicic JM, Viteri J and Wing RR (1998) Clinic-based vs. home-based interventions for preventing weight gain in men. *Obes Res* **6**:346–52.

Lichtman SW, Pisarska K, Berman ER *et al.* (1992) Discrepancy between self-reported and actual caloric intake and exercise in obese subjects. *N Engl J Med* **327**:1893–8.

Lindgarde F (2000) The effect of orlistat on body weight and coronary heart disease risk profile in obese patients: The Swedish Multimorbidity Study. *J Intern Med* **248**:245–54.

Lindstrom LL, Balch P and Reese S (1976) In person versus telephone treatment for obesity. *J Behav Ther Exp Psychiatry* **7**:367–9.

Lowe MR, Miller-Kovach K and Phelan S (2001) Weight loss maintenance in overweight individuals one to five years following successful completion of a commercial weight loss program. *Int J Obes* **25**:325–31.

Manson JE, Greenland P, LaCroix AZ *et al.* (2002) Walking compared with vigorous exercise for the prevention of cardiovascular events in women. *N Engl J Med* **347**:716–25.

Miles JM, Leiter L, Hollander P *et al.* (2002) Effect of orlistat in overweight and obese patients with type 2 diabetes treated with metformin. *Diabetes Care* **25**:1123–8.

Miller WR and Rollnick S (2002) *Motivational Interviewing: Preparing People for Change.* Guilford Press, New York.

Miltenberger RG (1997) *Behavior Modification: Principles and Procedures.* Brooks/Cole Publishing Company, Pacific Grove, CA.

Mokdad AH, Serdula MK, Dietz WH *et al.* (1999) The spread of the obesity epidemic in the United States, 1991–98. *JAMA* **282**:1519–22.

Mokdad AH, Ford ES, Bowman BA *et al.* (2003) Prevalence of obesity, diabetes, and obesity-related health risk factors, 2001. *JAMA* **289**:76–9.

Must A, Spadano J, Coakley EH *et al.* (1999) The disease burden associated with overweight and obesity. *JAMA* **282**:1523–9.

National Heart, Lung, and Blood Institute (NHLBI) & North American Association for the Study of Obesity (NAASO) (2000) *Practical Guide to the Identification, Evaluation, and Treatment of Overweight and Obesity in Adults.* National Institutes of Health, Bethesda, MD.

Perri MG (1998) The maintenance of treatment effects in the long-term management of obesity. *Clin Psychol Sci Pract* **5**:526–43.

Perri MG and Corsica JA (2002) Improving the maintenance of weight lost in behavioral treatment of obesity. In Wadden TA and Stunkard AJ (eds), *Handbook of Obesity Treatment* Guilford Press, New York, pp. 357–79.

Perri MG, McAdoo WG, Spevak PA and Newlin DB (1984) Effect of a multicomponent maintenance program on long-term weight loss. *J Consult Clin Psychol* **52**:480–1.

Perri MG, McAdoo WG, McAllister DA *et al.* (1986) Enhancing the efficacy of behavior therapy for obesity: Effects of aerobic exercise and a multicomponent maintenance program. *J Consult Clin Psychol* **54**:670–5.

Perri MG, McAdoo WG, McAllister DA *et al.* (1987) Effects of peer support and therapist contact on long term weight loss. *J Consult Clin Psychol* **55**:615–17.

Perri MG, Nezu AM, Patti ET and McCann KL (1989) Effect of length of treatment on weight loss. *J Consult Clin Psychol* **57**:450–2.

Perri MG, Martin AD, Leermarkers EA *et al.* (1997). Effects of group versus home-based exercise in the treatment of obesity. *J Consult Clin Psychol* **65**:278–85.

Perri MG, Nezu AM, McKelvey WF *et al.* (2001) Relapse prevention training and problem-solving therapy in the long-term management of obesity. *J Consult Clin Psychol* **69**:722–6.

Phelan S and Wadden TA (2002) Combining behavioral and pharmacological treatments for obesity. *Obes Res* **10**: 560–74.

Popkin BM and Doak CM (1998) The obesity epidemic is a worldwide phenomenon. *Nutr Rev* **56**:106–14.

Poston WSC and Foreyt JP (2000) Successful management of the obese patient. *Am Fam Phys* **61**:3615–22.

Poston WSC, Foreyt JP, Borrell L and Haddock CK (1998) Challenges in obesity management. *South Med J* **91**:710–20.

Pories WJ, Swanson MS, MacDonald KG *et al.* (1995) Who would have thought it? An operation proves to be the most effective therapy for adult-onset diabetes mellitus. *Ann Surg* **222**:339–52.

Price RA (2002) Genetics and common obesities: Background, current status, strategies, and future prospects. In Wadden TA and Stunkard AJ (eds), *Handbook of Obesity Treatment* Guilford Press, New York, pp. 73–94.

Prochaska JL, DiClemente CC and Norcross JC (1992) In search of how people change: Applications to addictive behaviors. *Am Psychol* **47**:1102–14.

Prochaska JL, Redding C and Evers K (1994) The transtheoretical model of behavioral change. In Glanz K, Lewis FM and Rimer BK (eds), *Health Behavior and Health Education: Theory, Research and Practice*, 2nd edn. Jossey Bass, San Francisco, pp. 60–84.

Pronk NP and Wing RR (1994) Physical activity and long-term maintenance of weight loss. *Obes Res* **2**:587–99.

Renjilian DA, Perri MG, Nezu AM *et al.* (2001) Effects of matching participants to their treatment preference. *J Consult Clin Psychol* **69**:717–21.

Rolls BJ, Shide DJ, Thorwart ML and Ulbrecht JS (1998) Sibutramine reduces food intake in non-dieting women with obesity. *Obes Res* **6**:1–11.

Rothacker DQ (2000) Five-year self-management of weight using meal replacements: comparison with matched controls in rural Wisconsin. *Nutrition* **16**:344–8.

Schwartz MB, O'Neal Chambliss H, Brownell KD *et al.* (2003) Weight bias among health professionals specializing in obesity. *Obes Res* **11**: 1033–9.

Sjostrom CD, Lissner L, Wedel H and Sjostrom L (1999) Reduction in incidence of diabetes, hypertension, and lipid disturbance after intentional weight loss induced by bariatric surgery: the SOS intervention study. *Obes Res* **7**:477–84.

Skender MS, Goodrick GK, Del Jungo DJ *et al.* (1996) Comparison of 2-year weight loss trends in behavioral treatments of obesity: Diet, exercise and combination interventions. *J Am Diet Assoc* **96**:342–6.

Smith DE and Wing RR (1991) Diminished weight loss and behavioral compliance during repeated diets in obese patients with type II diabetes. *Health Psychol* **10**: 378–83.

Smith D, Heckemeyer C, Kratt P and Mason D (1997) Motivational interviewing to improve adherence to a behavioral weight-control program for older obese women with NIDDM. *Diabetes Care* **20**:52–8.

Tuomilheto J, Lindstrom J, Eriksson JG *et al.* (2001) Prevention of type 2 diabetes mellitus by changes in lifestyle among subjects with impaired glucose tolerance. *N Engl J Med* **344**:1343–9.

United States Department of Health and Human Services (1996) *Physical Activity and Health: A Report of the Surgeon General.* Centers for Disease Control, Atlanta, GA.

Ureda JR (1980) The effect of contract witnessing on motivation and weight loss in a weight control program. *Health Educ Q* **7**:163–84.

Wadden TA and Osei S (2002) The treatment of obesity: an overview. In Wadden TA and Stunkard AJ (eds), *Handbook of Obesity Treatment*. Guilford Press, New York, pp. 229–48.

Wadden TA, Stunkard AJ and Liebschutz J (1988) Three-year follow-up of the treatment of obesity by very low calorie diet, behavior therapy, and their combination. *J Consult Clin Psychol* **56**:925–8.

Wadden TA, Sternberg JA, Letizia KA *et al.* (1989) Treatment of obesity by very low calorie diet:, behavior therapy, and their combination: A five year perspective. *Int J Obes* **13**:39–46.

Wadden TA, Foster GD and Letizia KA (1994) One-year behavioral treatment of obesity: Comparison of moderate and severe caloric restriction and the effects of maintenance therapy. *J Consult Clin Psychol* **62**:165–71.

Wadden TA, Vogt RA, Foster GD and Anderson DA (1998) Exercise and maintenance of weight loss: 1-year follow-up of a controlled clinic trial. *J Consult Clin Psychol* **66**:429–33.

Wadden TA, Berkowitz RI, Womble LG *et al.* (2000) Effects of sibutramine plus orlistat in obese women following 1 year of treatment by sibutramine alone: A placebo-controlled trial. *Obes Res* **8**:431–7.

Wadden TA, Berkowitz RI, Sarwer DB *et al.* (2001) Benefits of lifestyle modification in the pharmacological treatment of obesity. *Arch Intern Med* **161**:218–27.

Wadden TA, Brownell KD and Foster GD (2002) Obesity: Responding to the Global Epidemic. *J Consult Clin Psychol* **70**:510–25.

Wadden TA, Womble LG, Sarwer DB *et al.* (2003) Great expectations: 'I'm losing 25% of my weight no matter what you say.' *J Consult Clin Psychol* **71**:1084–9.

Williamson DF (1993) Descriptive epidemiology of body weight and weight changes in US adults. *Ann Intern Med* **119**:646–9.

Wing RR (1998) Behavioral approaches to the treatment of obesity. In Bray G, Bouchard C and James WPT (eds), *Handbook of Obesity*. Marcel Dekker, New York, pp. 855–73.

Wing RR (1999) Physical activity in the treatment of adulthood overweight and obesity: Current evidence and research issues. *Med Sci Sports Exerc* **31**:S547–S552.

Wing RR (2002) Behavioral weight control. In Wadden TA and Stunkard AJ (eds), *Handbook of Obesity Treatment* Guilford Press, New York, pp. 301–16.

Wing RR and Jeffrey RM (1999) Benefits of recruiting participants with friends and increasing social support for weight loss maintenance. *J Consult Clin Psychol* **67**:132–8.

Wing RR, Blair EH, Marcus MD *et al.* (1994) Year-long weight loss treatment for obese patients with type 2 diabetes: Does including an intermittent very-low-calorie diet improve outcome? *Am J Med* **97**:354–62.

Wing RR, Jeffrey RM, Burton LR *et al.* (1996) Food provisions vs. structured meal plans in the behavioral treatment of obesity. *Int J Obes* **20**:56–62.

Zandee GL and Oermann MH (1996) Effectiveness of contingency contracting. *AAOHN J* **44**:183–8.

Zhang Y, Proenca R, Maffei M *et al.* (1994) Positional cloning of the mouse obese gene and its human homologue. *Nature* **372**:425–2.

8
Physical Activity, Obesity and Type 2 Diabetes

Carlton B. Cooke and Paul J. Gately

Introduction

Overweight and obesity are increasing around the globe (WHO, 1997). Throughout most of human existence, the accessibility and availability of food has been limited. The ability to conserve energy has always been an advantage to the survival of humans. It is likely that genetic influences have promoted the intake of energy dense foods, the ability to efficiently store energy and the ability to minimize energy expenditure (Rosenbaum and Leibel, 1998). However, industrialization, modernization and globalization have affected dramatic decreases in daily energy expenditure and increases in food accessibility and availability in many parts of the world. It is these changes in the environment, coupled with a genetic predisposition to weight gain in some individuals, that has led to the dramatic increase in overweight and obesity around the globe. The environmental influences on physical activity and eating behaviour are most likely to have had the greatest impact on the increasing prevalence of this disease (NIH, 1998). The 'obesegenic environment' is influenced by a variety of factors, these include: a reduction in daily energy expenditure and physical activity, due to sedentary behaviours during work and leisure time; an increase in availability of highly palatable energy-dense foods; and intensive marketing of these foods to individuals, particularly children, using innovative campaigns.

In parallel with the dramatic and continued increase in the prevalence of overweight and obesity (Joint Health Surveys Unit, 1998) is the associated increase in the prevalence of type 2 diabetes. Risk factors for type 2 diabetes include:

Obesity and Diabetes.   Edited by Anthony H. Barnett and Sudhesh Kumar
© 2004 John Wiley & Sons, Ltd   ISBN: 0-470-84898-7

older age, obesity, minority ethnicity, fat distribution, family history of diabetes and inactivity (Albright *et al.*, 2000). Of these risk factors only obesity, fat distribution and physical inactivity are modifiable. Overweight and obesity strongly predict risk of developing type 2 diabetes, it is estimated that just under two-thirds of cases of type 2 diabetes in men and three-quarters in women could be prevented if everyone had a body mass index (BMI) below $25\,kg/m^2$ (Sargeant *et al.*, 2000).

Until recently it was believed that children and adolescents that were sedentary and had a poor diet were storing up problems for later life. They needed to be exposed to unhealthy behaviours for years before the consequences became manifest in the form of cardiovascular disease, chronic obesity and type 2 diabetes. However, Drake *et al.* (2002) in the UK have produced cases of white obese adolescents who have been diagnosed as type 2 diabetic and Freedman *et al.* (1999) in the US have shown that overweight (greater than the 85th percentile for BMI) adolescents are exceeding risk factor thresholds for hyperinsulinaemia, hypertension, hypercholesterolaemia and hypertriglyceridaemia.

As a consequence of obesity many people experience reduced glucose tolerance from an increase in insulin resistance, which causes excessive insulin output (hyperinsulinaemia). For such individuals, many of whom will develop type 2 diabetes, regular physical activity or exercise can reduce resting plasma insulin levels and lower insulin output during fasted oral glucose tolerance tests, thereby indicating improved insulin sensitivity. There is no doubt that regular physical activity and exercise can provide an important contribution to the prevention and treatment of both obesity and type 2 diabetes. This chapter evaluates the research evidence regarding the role that physical activity can play in the prevention and treatment of obesity and type 2 diabetes. It also offers guidance on how physical activity can be increased in the lives of those who are obese and/or type 2 diabetic.

Physical activity and exercise, what is the difference?

Physical activity is defined as any bodily movement produced by skeletal muscles that results in energy expenditure, whereas exercise is planned, and repetitive bodily movement done to improve or maintain one or more of the components of fitness (Casperson *et al.*, 1985; American College of Sports Medicine, 1998). Exercise may include training, sports participation or going to some form of regular exercise class. Physical activity is therefore the umbrella term with types of exercise, sport and physical recreation forming subsets of physical activity. Physical activity can therefore take many forms, as a means of transport, occupational requirements, daily living activity and leisure time activity. Although there are differences in definitions of exercise, sport and physical activity it is important to realize that most individuals do not discriminate between them in this way. If you ask people how active they are, evidence suggests that they will probably interpret the question as to how much sport or exercise they do. According to the Allied Dunbar National Fitness Survey (Activity and Health Research, 1992) 75 per cent of the participants knew that exercise is good for your health, but many people do not recognize that they can look to their everyday life to find ways to be more active without the need to engage in formal exercise if they do not wish to. Working from an understanding of the perspective and lifestyle of the obese or type 2 diabetic individual is therefore important in supporting their efforts to increase their physical activity. This is especially important since they will commonly view exercise and sport participation as unattainable and not desirable, as they may have had bad previous experiences of exercise and sport.

Current physical activity behaviour and guidelines

The results of the Allied Dunbar National Fitness Survey (Activity and Health Research, 1992) showed that in terms of physical activity 7 out of 10 men and 8 out of 10 women fell below their age-appropriate activity level necessary to achieve a health benefit.

Current guidelines in the UK recommend that adults build up gently towards participating in 30 min of moderate physical activity on at least 5 days per week (Physical Activity Task Force, 1995). It is suggested that each 30 min session would ideally be completed in one go, but this could be achieved by shorter periods of 10 minutes or so, accumulating a total of 30 min over the day. Moderate physical activities are defined as those that raise the heart rate sufficiently to leave you warm and slightly out of breath and include brisk walking, climbing stairs, swimming, social dancing and heavy DIY, gardening and housework.

Increasing heart rate to between 60 and 90 per cent of its estimated maximum (220 beats per minute minus age in years) during regular sustained physical activity (three times per week for at least 30 min) will improve cardiorespiratory fitness and decrease the risk of heart disease, stroke and metabolic disorders (ACSM, 1995). There is also increasing evidence to support the health benefits of shorter periods of physical activity accumulated throughout the day, which is how sedentary obese and type 2 diabetics should start to engage in a more active lifestyle (ACSM, 1995). For most adults who are not regularly active but are able to walk comfortably, walking can become a good way to establish an active lifestyle. It is important to build up activity and fitness gradually and for most inactive adults taking longer walks more often and more briskly is an excellent way to improve activity and health.

Adults can also make the most of other opportunities to be active in their everyday life by walking up stairs instead of taking the lift, walking to the shops or work rather than taking the car or bus (or getting off to walk part of the way if public transport is necessary because of the distance of the journey), spending more time in heavy gardening or DIY jobs around the house, playing with the children or being active as a family. Adults should consider taking up a sport or physical recreation activity as exercising with others is more sociable and you do not need to be a 'sporty person' to have fun and enjoyment in the many different indoor and outdoor activities available. The emphasis on fun and enjoyment in physical activity, be it play or sport, is also crucial to keep young people participating in an active lifestyle.

For most inactive people starting off gradually and working towards the recommendations is very safe, but any person who has any concerns or questions regarding specific health issues should be encouraged to consult their GP before they begin their more active lifestyle. Any person who has been diagnosed as a type 2 diabetic or is chronically obese should consult their GP or consultant before starting regular physical activity.

In terms of health benefits three main rationales were identified by the Health Education Authority for encouraging young people to take part in regular physical activity:

- to optimize physical fitness, current health and well-being, and growth and development;

- to develop active lifestyles that can be maintained throughout adult life;

- to reduce the risk of chronic diseases of adulthood (Biddle *et al.*, 1998).

In terms of tracking physical activity through childhood and into adulthood there is a moderate relationship between the amount and type of physical activity in childhood with that in youth, but low levels of tracking from youth into adulthood. However, in specific groups such as overweight and obese children the persistence of obesity is high, as shown by Freedman *et al.* (2001), where 77 per cent of obese children remained obese at 17 years follow up. Given the physical, psychological and social changes that occur across the life span that profoundly influence and shape our lives, it is perhaps not surprising that the amount and type of activity does not track well from childhood through to adulthood. Individuals alter their priorities in life and their motivation towards different types of physical activity change.

The Health Education Authority recommended that all young people (5–18 years) should participate in physical activity of at least moderate intensity for 1 hour per day. Moderate physical activities again include brisk walking, cycling, swimming dance and most sports. Again it is recognized that this activity could be accumulated intermittently throughout the day, which, given the intermittent nature of young children's activity and play, seems practical. Those who currently do very little should aim for half an hour per day. A secondary recommendation was that at least twice a week, some of these activities should help to enhance and maintain muscular strength, flexibility and bone health (Biddle *et al.*, 1998).

It is important to note that most individuals who are obese and/or type 2 diabetic will have most probably led a very sedentary existence for a number of years. Such individuals will have impaired exercise tolerance and may have a number of co-morbidities that require clinical treatment or monitoring in order that physical activity may be undertaken safely. However, any individual that has been previously sedentary for some considerable time must always start with very gradual increases towards the achievement of the general physical activity recommendations for adults and children.

In the case of obese individuals weight-bearing exercise may be difficult and painful to sustain for any period of time that will have a significant impact on calorific expenditure. In such cases individuals may need to undertake exercise where their body mass is supported during the activity, such as in swimming, the use of seated or recumbent cycle ergometers or resistance training. Such forms of exercise are unlikely to be sustainable over long periods of time for many sedentary overweight people, especially children, as they may well find them boring and unsatisfying, even though some members of the population do exercise regularly in this way. When engaging individuals in physical activity it is important to establish their likes and dislikes and work with them in terms of behaviour management to set achievable short term goals. In our experience this approach may, for example, move some adults from non-weight bearing exercise to a mixture of active transport and active leisure and some children into recreational or competitive sport.

The importance of physical activity to health

There are a number of health benefits associated with regular physical activity, these include:

- reduced risk of coronary heart disease and stroke;
- better control of blood pressure;
- increased aerobic or endurance fitness and capacity to cope with extra physical demands;
- prevention of osteoporosis;
- maintenance of muscle strength and joint flexibility;
- alleviation of some disabilities;
- reduced stress, enhanced mood and self esteem;
- maintenance of a full and active quality of life well into older age;
- social benefits associated with an active lifestyle;
- reduced risk of the metabolic syndrome;

- management of type 2 diabetes;

- management of body weight and hence reduced risk of obesity and related diseases.
  (Activity and Health Research, 1992; Blair and Brodney, 1999; Bouchard and Blair, 1999; Rissanen and Fogelholm, 1999; Ross and Janssen, 1999; WHO, 1997)

Although obesity and type 2 diabetes are the major focus of this chapter, they are both closely related to the metabolic syndrome, where responses to physical activity or exercise are beneficial to improved metabolic and haematological control, fat loss, and an increase in muscle mass.

Physical activity and type 2 diabetes

The ACSM position stand on exercise and type 2 diabetes states that 'physical activity is an under-utilized mode of therapy for type 2 diabetes, often due to a lack of understanding' (Albright et al., 2000). A range of studies have shown that physical activity and exercise can have a significant impact on both treating and preventing or delaying the onset of type 2 diabetes. Given the relatively low cost of physical activity participation it is difficult to see why it is such an underused resource. A range of factors effect the utilization of physical activity, these include: a lack of understanding about exercise, a reluctance of patients to engage in physical activity as it adds a further variable when trying to control blood glucose levels, but arguably most importantly, long-term intervention studies have shown that lifestyle change in the form of promoting sustained changes in physical activity is difficult to achieve (Albright et al., 2000).

The specific benefits of physical activity to improved glucose tolerance and control are associated with regular bouts of exercise that repeatedly provoke the acute effects of a single bout. These and other improvements in metabolic control associated with physical activity are not only important to those with type 2 diabetes but also to the sedentary and overweight, and those who have the metabolic syndrome. Significant improvements in metabolic fitness have been associated with increased physical activity that may not be sufficient in intensity to increase the more traditional measures of fitness such as maximal oxygen uptake ($\dot{V}_{O_2}$ max, the maximum rate at which an individual can take up and utilize oxygen while breathing air at sea level (Astrand and Rodahl, 1986)). However, sustained changes in activity levels are required for the benefits of exercise or physical activity to positively affect insulin action (Ivy et al., 1999; Albright et al., 2000; ADA, 2002). According to the ACSM (2000) favourable changes in glucose tolerance and insulin sensitivity usually deteriorate within 72 h or the last exercise session. Therefore sustained changes in daily physical activity are required to ensure the repeated stimulus associated with the acute effects of exercise.

Several long-term studies have shown improvements in glycaemic control (Heath *et al.*, 1991; Vanninen *et al.*, 1992). These improvements in carbohydrate metabolism and insulin sensitivity were also shown to be maintained for at least five years in those patients that continued to participate in physical activity and exercise. Improvements in HbA1c were around 10–20 per cent, compared to baseline. The improvements in glycaemic control were greatest in those patients with mild type 2 diabetes, and those who were likely to be most insulin resistant (Saltin *et al.*, 1979; Ruderman *et al.*, 1979; Schneider *et al.*, 1992). The mechanisms of this improved control are poorly understood, what is known is that exercise increases the number of glucose transporter proteins (GLUT 4) in the plasma membrane. Although Chipkin *et al.* (2001) also highlighted that in poorly controlled diabetic patients, the ability of exercise to stimulate GLUT4 transporters is decreased.

In addition to the independent benefit of physical activity to cardiovascular health, the combined benefits to blood lipid profile, haematological profile and blood pressure further support the use of physical activity and exercise for the type 2 diabetic patient (Krotkiewski *et al.*, 1979; Schneider *et al.*, 1986; Hagberg *et al.*, 1989).

A number of reviews have shown that programmes that include a prescription of exercise involving 60–85 per cent $\dot{V}_{O_2}$ max lasting 30–60 min three to four times per week for 6–12 weeks achieve significant improvements in $\dot{V}_{O_2}$ max (ADA/ACSM, 1997; Chipkin *et al.*, 2001). Other studies have also shown that diabetic patients have lower aerobic fitness than sedentary non-diabetic individuals, which would increase the magnitude of improvement in fitness with regular physical activity or exercise, but will require a gentle progression in exercise intensity, duration and frequency from the sedentary state.

Physical activity and obesity

Exercise is the most variable component of energy expenditure; it is therefore clear to see why exercise has been adopted as a component to treat overweight and obesity. Indeed, exercise or physical activity is promoted within a range of guidelines for the prevention and treatment of overweight and obesity (WHO, 1997; NIH, 1998). Understanding the impact of physical activity and exercise on obesity and associated variables is important, as an increase in physical activity not only has significant positive effects on body mass and body fat mass, but also on a range of other variables associated with health (Blair and Brodney, 1999). Physical activity has been suggested to have favourable effects on: weight loss, decreased fat percentage, decreased skinfold thickness, android disease, decreased risk of coronary heart disease (CHD), improved glucose metabolism, increased basal metabolic rate (BMR), prevention of loss of fat free mass (FFM), increased dietary thermogenesis, reduced blood pressure, improved cardiovascular fitness, and benefits to psychosocial health (WHO 1997; Blair & Brodney,

Table 8.1   Relative risk by categories of percentage body fat for fit and unfit groups of men

Lean (<17% body fat)	Fit = 1.0	Unfit = 3.16 (1.12–8.92)
Normal (17–25% body fat)	Fit = 1.43 (0.77–2.67)	Unfit = 2.94 (1.48–5.83)
Obese (>25% body fat)	Fit = 1.35 (0.66–2.76)	Unfit = 4.11 (2.20–7.68)

Adapted from Lee *et al.*, 1999. Reproduced with permission by the *American Journal of Clinical Nutrition*. © Am J Clin Nutr. American Society for Clinical Nutrition.

1999; Bouchard and Blair, 1999; Rissanen and Fogelholm, 1999; Ross and Janssen, 1999).

A review by Blair and Brodney (1999) suggested that the negative health consequences of obesity are more associated with low physical fitness (maximal exercise treadmill test, a proxy measure of physical activity) than obesity *per se* (based on BMI and per cent body fat). Physical fitness was used as a marker of physical activity as it is notoriously difficult to assess physical activity in free-living individuals. However, physical fitness has been shown to be a valid surrogate for physical activity, given the strong relationships demonstrated between fitness, physical activity and reduced mortality (Stofan *et al.*, 1998). Blair and Brodney (1999) showed that the risk of CHD in active overweight or obese males (fat but fit individuals) was the same as normal-weight active control subjects, while the risk associated with the sedentary normal weight controls was greater. Further evidence from the same group of researchers (Lee *et al.*, 1999) supported these findings with a study of 21 925 men aged 30–83 years conducted between 1971 and 1989, which showed that the relative risk (RR) of cardiovascular disease mortality was not significantly different for fit and lean, normal and fit or obese and fit, whereas for the same percentage body fat categories the unfit had significantly higher relative risk (Table 8.1).

Energy balance

The energy balance equation is often used to explain the basis on which weight will either be maintained (energy input = energy output), gained (energy input > energy output) or lost (energy input < energy output). To achieve a desirable outcome in terms of weight loss for the overweight or obese the energy balance equation needs to be unbalanced by increasing energy expenditure, decreasing energy intake or some combination of the two, known as a state of negative energy balance. We will not deal with the issues of decreasing energy intake and changing the composition of the diet in this chapter, but it is well understood that the most successful intervention programmes for weight loss are those that incorporate dietary modification and an increase in habitual physical activity or exercise managed through behaviour change.

It is therefore, on the face of it, a simple task to estimate energy intake and energy expenditure, make appropriate alterations to both and observe the ensuing weight loss. It is of course not that simple for those who are chronically overweight or obese, many of which have type 2 diabetes. The precise contributions of sedentary living and excessive food intake to the development of obesity are poorly understood from a population perspective and will differ in degree on an individual basis. However, epidemiological evidence supports the view that changes in calories consumed has on average fallen slightly (Prentice and Jebb, 1995), certainly not increasing to account for the continued increase in prevalence of overweight and obesity that we are observing. These observations support the contention that we are much more sedentary than we used to be. Whilst genetic predisposition will interact with environmental factors, genetics cannot explain the increased prevalence of overweight and obesity over such a short period of time.

Energy expenditure

Energy expenditure includes: BMR, the thermogenic effect of food (TEF) and physical activity. BMR is the main component of energy expenditure in the average person and is the energy expenditure for maintenance processes. BMR is measured under very strict laboratory conditions that include a 12-h fast and rest, making early morning a good time to make such measurements. Any measure to estimate BMR not made under such strict conditions is referred to as resting metabolic rate (RMR). Energy expenditure associated with physical activity is quantified and discussed in the literature in various forms using energy units such as the kilocalorie or the Joule (SI unit) and other dimensionless quantities which are multiples of BMR (the PAL or the MET). Although the Joule is the SI unit of energy, the kilocalorie is still in common use partly because of the physics related to its definition and mostly because of its use in everyday life in terms of dieting (i.e. calorie counting). There are 4186 J in 1 kcal and both units normally appear on food labels. A MET is defined as the energy requirement for BMR, PAL stands for physical activity level and is also a multiple of BMR, where in both cases 1 MET and a PAL of 1 are both equivalent to the energy requirement of BMR.

Ainsworth *et al.* (2000) have presented a comprehensive compendium of physical activities classified in terms of intensity according to the number of METS of energy required. Total energy expenditure expressed as $kcal \cdot day^{-1}$ is divided by BMR to determine the value for PAL. PALs therefore express the proportion of total energy expenditure that is expended in physical activity, including energy expended in the thermic response to food. BMR increases with size, but the PALs of heavier individuals may not differ significantly in weight bearing exercise to those of normal weight individuals because the energy cost of movement also increases with size. A sedentary person would have a PAL of about 1.4, while an individual engaged in a lot of physical activity would have a PAL of about 2, whereas endurance trained athletes may have a PAL in excess of 4 (Ferro-Luzzi and Martino, 1996). Values for energy expenditure are also expressed in absolute terms (kcal, J) or relative to time (kcal·min^{-1}, W) or time and body mass (kcal·kg^{-1}·min^{-1}, W·kg^{-1}·min^{-1}). McArdle *et al.* (1996) provide estimates of energy expenditure values for a range of activities in kcal·kg^{-1}·min^{-1}.

Physical activity is the most variable component of daily energy expenditure. Ravussin and Swinburn (1992) suggested that physical activity typically represents between 20 and 40 per cent of daily energy expenditure. Other studies assessing the energy expenditure of individuals in a respiratory chamber have shown there are large differences in individuals with respect to spontaneous physical activity (SPA), which range from 100 to 800 kcal·day^{-1} (Ravussin, 1995).

A major feature of the most recent recommendations for adults and children in the UK and in the USA is the emphasis that is placed on moderate intensity exercise. In the recommendations outlined above examples of moderate exercise are given that can be easily understood by members of the public and health professionals. However, the use of such qualitative descriptors in describing energy expenditure associated with physical activity can be confusing given the range of intensities of physical activity that have been used in the physical activity research literature for moderate exercise (ACSM, 1998). In the current American recommendations moderate intensity exercise is defined as 3 to 6 METS, which equates to the energy requirements of walking at 3 and 4 mph respectively. Light activities are described as requiring <3 METS and heavy or vigorous activities are those requiring >6 METS. This is not the case for all studies so it is important to look for definitions of such qualitative descriptors when assessing research literature concerned with physical activity interventions.

Prescribing exercise using relative exercise intensity

To add to the confusion the same qualitative descriptors of light, moderate and vigorous are often used to describe relative exercise intensity, that is the exercise intensity relative to maximal heart rate predicted for age or predicted maximal oxygen consumption (or directly measured, but not normally for obese or type 2 diabetics). For example, two individuals can be exercising at the same absolute energy expenditure, say walking together at a speed of 3 mph (4.8 km·h^{-1}, 3 METS). The least fit obese person may be working at a vigorous exercise intensity relative to their aerobic fitness (defined as >60% of $\dot{V}_{O_2}$ max, ACSM, 1998), whilst the fitter individual may be working at a light exercise intensity relative to their aerobic fitness (<40% of $\dot{V}_{O_2}$ max). Table 8.2 shows a comparison of absolute and different relative exercise intensities that are used together with qualitative descriptors, but these are not consistently applied in the physical activity literature. Table 8.3 shows examples of activities that expend 150 kcal.

$\dot{V}_{O_2}$ max is the maximum rate at which an individual can take up and utilize oxygen while breathing air at sea level (Astrand and Rodahl, 1986). It has traditionally been used as the criterion standard of cardiorespiratory fitness,

Table 8.2 Examples of absolute and relative exercise intensity (based on Heyward, 1998)

Qualitative descriptor	Relative exercise intensity			Absolute exercise intensity	
	$\%\dot{V}_{O_2}$ max or %HRR	%HR max	RPE (6–20 scale)	METs	
				20–39 years	40–64 years
Light	40	63	10	4.2	4.0
Moderate	50	69	11	5.5	5.0
Moderate	60	76	12	7.2	6.0
Hard	70	82	14	8.4	7.0
Hard	80	89	15	9.5	8.0
Very hard	85	92	16	10.2	8.5
Very hard	90	95	18	10.8	9.0
Maximal	100	100	20	12.0	10.0

Table 8.3 Examples of activities that expend 150 kcal for an average 70 kg adult

Descriptor of intensity	Activity	Approximate duration (min)
Light	Typing	85–90
Light	Sitting playing with child	50–60
Light	Washing and polishing a car	45–60
Light	Washing windows or floors	45–60
Light	Playing volleyball	45
Light	General gardening	30–45
Light	Volleyball (non-competitive)	43
Light	Wheeling a wheelchair	30–40
Light	Walking 1.75 miles at 3 mph	35
Moderate	Basketball (shooting baskets)	30
Moderate	Cycling 5 miles at 10 mph	30
Moderate	Dancing fast (social)	30
Moderate	Pushing a pushchair 1.5 miles	30
Moderate	Raking leaves	30
Moderate	Water aerobics	30
Moderate	Swimming lengths	20
Moderate	Wheelchair basketball	20
Moderate	Game of basketball	15–20
Moderate	Cycling 4 miles at 16 mph	15
Moderate	Skipping	15
Moderate	Running 1.5 miles at 6 mph	15
Moderate	Shovelling snow	15
Moderate	Climbing stairs	15
Hard	Jogging at 5 mph	18
Hard	Field hockey (game)	16

Adapted from *Clinical Guidelines*, NIH (1998) and Surgeon General's Report (1996).

as it is considered to be the single physiological variable that best defines the functional capacity of the cardiovascular and respiratory systems. Measurements of $\dot{V}_{O_2}$ max indicate aerobic potential and to a lesser extent training status. The sensitivity of $\dot{V}_{O_2}$ max to the establishment of regular physical activity is strongly related to the degree of development that may ultimately be realized, which reflects a combination of endowment and habitual physical activity. Individual $\dot{V}_{O_2}$ max values are used to provide one form of relative exercise intensity (Table 8.2) where absolute exercise intensity in the form of oxygen uptake is expressed as a percentage of the individual's $\dot{V}_{O_2}$ max, as in the example of the two individuals walking together at the same walking speed.

Heart rate is a common method used for setting relative exercise intensity. There are three ways in which this can be done, but all are based on the assumption that heart rate is a linear function of exercise intensity, which it is throughout most of the submaximal range, but not necessarily at very low or high exercise intensities (Astrand and Rodahl, 1986). Using data from a progressive, incremental steady state exercise test, heart rate at the end of each stage can be plotted against oxygen uptake or MET values (Figure 8.1). Maximum heart rate can be predicted by using 220-age (years), but this can be in error by $\pm$ 10 beats·min^{-1}. $\dot{V}_{O_2}$ max can then be predicted by either extrapolation of the heart rate oxygen uptake line to predicted maximum heart rate (Harrison *et al.*, 1980) or a nomogram can be used to estimate it (Astrand and Ryhming, 1954). It should be noted that the standard error of predicting maximal oxygen uptake using the nomogram is up to 15 per cent in moderately trained individuals of different ages (Astrand and Rodahl, 1986). Indeed, the authors concluded that this drawback holds true for any submaximal cardiorespiratory test. $\dot{V}_{O_2}$ max can be measured directly but this procedure requires maximal exercise to volitional exhaustion. It is not recommended as a positive experience for obese or type 2 diabetics and will often be so symptom limited in terms of effort and discomfort that the measurement will not represent a valid assessment of $\dot{V}_{O_2}$ max.

The $\dot{V}_{O_2}$ max and maximum heart rate values are then used to calculate the training zone for aerobic exercise known to promote a training response in terms of increasing cardiorespiratory fitness (60–85 per cent of $\dot{V}_{O_2}$ max, Heyward, 1998). For example, given a predicted $\dot{V}_{O_2}$ max of 21 ml·kg^{-1}·min^{-1} (which is equivalent to 6 METS, 1 MET is approximately equivalent to 3.5 ml·kg^{-1}·min^{-1} of oxygen uptake) and a maximum heart rate of 195 beats·min^{-1} (age 25 years) the target heart rate zone or MET zone would be 112 to 162 beats·min^{-1} or 3.6 to 5.1 METS, respectively (Figure 8.1). It is important to note that heart rate response to exercise is dependent on the mode of exercise. Therefore, if exercise testing is undertaken partly for the purpose of setting relative exercise intensity for training, the same mode of exercise should be used in both where possible. If this is not possible a mode that elicits similar heart rate responses should be used. Readers interested in more detail on exercise testing and prescription are directed to Heyward (1998) and Cooke (2001).

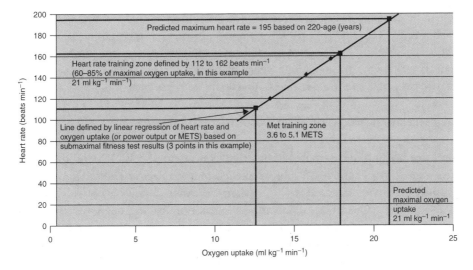

Figure 8.1 Heart rate training zone defined by results from a submaximal exercise test.

The second of the common procedures for determining target heart rates for training is to use the Karvonen percentage of heart rate range. This method uses the resting heart rate (HR rest) and the heart rate range (HRR), which is the difference between maximum (HR max) and resting heart rate. Maximum heart rate must therefore be predicted by use of a formula such as 220-age.

$$\text{Target heart rate} = (\%HRR/100) \times (\text{HR max} - \text{HR rest}) + \text{HR rest}$$

The ACSM (1995) recommends using 50 to 85 per cent HRR. Using the 25-year-old individual as an example again and given a resting heart rate of 72 beats·min^{-1}, the target heart rate for training at 50 per cent HRR would be given by:

$$\text{Target heart rate} = (50/100) \times (195 - 72) + 72,$$

$$\text{which gives a target heart rate of 134 beats·min}^{-1}$$

Comparing this value with the target heart rate zone in Figure 8.1 shows this value to be in the middle of the heart rate zone. Given the comments already made regarding the typical sedentary nature of the lifestyle of the obese or type 2 diabetic, it is always better to start off at very low exercise intensities and then progress according to the principle of progressive overload. As the individual adapts their functional capacity to cope easily with the exercise challenge, so the exercise challenge is extended slightly.

The third common procedure for estimating target heart rates for setting relative exercise intensity is to use percentage of predicted maximal heart rate (again using the formula 220-age). This method makes use of the strong linear relationship between percentage heart rate max and percentage $\dot{V}_{O_2}$ max (Table 8.2). The ACSM (1995) recommends prescribing target heart rates between 60 and 90 per cent of HR max, depending on the fitness of the individual. Returning to our 25-year-old individual and selecting 60 per cent of HR max, the target heart rate is given by:

Target heart rate = (%HR max/100) × HR max,   which gives 117 beats·min^{-1}

This method produces a target heart rate close to the bottom of the target heart rate zone. Compared to the Karvonen method the per cent HR_{max} method produces a lower target heart rate when the same relative exercise intensity is used. The ACSM (1995) recommends multiplying the heart rate from the per cent HR_{max} method by 1.15 to obtain a more accurate target heart rate. However, this method therefore has advantages for use with obese and type 2 diabetics as it provides a conservative estimate of the target heart rate using a simple procedure without the need for exercise testing. It should be noted that the use of any heart rate method for setting relative exercise intensity has limitations based on the use of predictions of maximal heart rate, assumptions regarding the relationship between percentage heart rate and percentage $\dot{V}_{O_2}$ max, the influence of exercise mode, environmental factors and emotional state, together with the effects of some forms of medication on heart rate response.

An alternative to using heart rate for setting and monitoring exercise intensity is rating of perceived exertion (RPE). RPE scales (see Table 8.2) are reported as valid and reliable for assessing the level of exertion during aerobic exercise (Borg and Linderholm, 1967; Birk and Birk, 1987; Dunbar et al., 1992). The original basis of the RPE scale shown in Table 8.2 was that if you multiply the RPE value by 10 it would produce an approximation to the exercise heart rate. Dunbar et al. (1992) suggest that RPEs of 11 and 16 closely approximate 50 and 85 per cent HRR. Heyward (1998) suggests the use of MET values corresponding to RPEs of 12 (somewhat hard) and 16 (hard) to set the minimum and maximum training intensities for aerobic exercise.

Even if some forms of heart rate training zone or values are estimated they must not form the sole focus of monitoring relative exercise intensity. How the individual is feeling and how hard they perceive the effort to be is more important. It is better to start off with short periods of enjoyable and achievable exercise when working with previously sedentary individuals, but especially with the obese or type 2 diabetic. Use of heart rate or RPE values for the obese or type 2 diabetic should be at the lowest recommended values to start with. This is recognized as important by the ACSM (1995) as they state that poorly conditioned individuals may be able to exercise at a low intensity (40 per cent $\dot{V}_{O_2}$ max) for only about 10 min (see the next section for exercise tolerance values for obese adults and children). The obese or type 2 diabetic person may therefore need to perform short bouts of exercise throughout the day to accumulate half an hour of regular habitual physical activity. The exercise intensity, duration and frequency can then be progressively increased as the functional capacity of the individual increases, building up to achieving the general recommendations for physical activity and beyond, if the individual is provided with the appropriate guidance and support and is able to take part regularly in some form of physical activity that they find enjoyable and fulfilling.

The combination of a lack of valid methods of assessment and the complex interactions between physical activity, energy intake and energy balance, complicate the accurate determination of energy balance in obesity (Ravussin and Swinburn, 1992; Goran, 1998; DeLany, 1998; Roberts and Leibel, 1998). The number of components that influence energy expenditure further complicates this issue. Blaak *et al.* (1992) suggested that the differences observed between some training studies with regard to weight loss induced by exercise are limited due to the concomitant changes in other elements of lifestyle outside of the training prescribed. Blaak *et al.* (1992) found that there was an increase in overall energy expenditure and little change in spontaneous physical activity.

Exercise tolerance and cardiorespiratory fitness in overweight and obese adults and children

There is very little data published on the exercise tolerance of obese adults. We tested 19 obese adults (4 males and 15 females aged 40.3 ± 13.5 years) for exercise tolerance (Gately *et al.*, 1997). Mean body mass and BMI of the group was 112.6 ± 18.9 and $37.9 \pm 10.6 \, \text{kg/m}$, respectively. Exercise tolerance was assessed using the treadmill walking test protocol developed for the Allied Dunbar National Fitness Survey (ADNFS; Activity and Health Research, 1992). Exercise tolerance was low as identified by a symptom limited mean peak $\dot{V}_{O_2}$ of $2.05 \pm 0.51 \, \text{l·min}^{-1}$ or $19.62 \pm 5.45 \, \text{ml·kg}^{-1} \cdot \text{min}^{-1}$ for the females and $2.15 \pm 1.06 \, \text{l/min}$ or $16.28 \pm 8.56 \, \text{ml·kg}^{-1} \cdot \text{min}^{-1}$ for males, respectively. Average values for the ADNFS for females and males aged 35 to 44 years were 34.8 and $45.5 \, \text{ml·kg}^{-1} \cdot \text{min}^{-1}$ respectively. Even comparing the values with the 5th percentile from the ADNFS ($24.5 \, \text{ml·kg}^{-1} \cdot \text{min}^{-1}$ for the females and $34.2 \, \text{ml·kg}^{-1} \cdot \text{min}^{-1}$ for the males respectively) the values for the obese are significantly lower (20 and 54 per cent for the females and males, respectively). This comparison demonstrates that relative to the average or unfit adult, who is not taking sufficient physical activity to gain the associated health benefits, the obese or type 2 diabetic adult is likely to be starting from a position of extremely limited exercise tolerance, especially when considering the challenge of weight bearing exercise such as walking.

The criterion for defining the endpoint of the walking test is normally the achievement of 85 per cent of age related maximum heart rate. However, all participants stopped walking before the target heart rate was achieved. Most gave the reason of pain in the lower legs, normally in the calves, as the reason for stopping the test. Their mean test time of 9.83 ± 2.30 min equates to walking at 5 km·h^{-1} at a gradient of 10 per cent, and they produced a mean peak respiratory exchange ratio of 1.10 ± 0.10 (RER $= \dot{V}_{CO_2}/\dot{V}_{O_2}$; a value of 1.0 indicates that anaerobic metabolism predominates). Overall, these data illustrate that exercise tolerance is severely restricted in these obese subjects. They required greater than 50 per cent of their peak $\dot{V}_{O_2}$ (60 per cent max. HR) to be able to walk at 4.8 km·h^{-1} on the flat. Walking therefore constitutes a major exercise challenge for these participants, illustrating the need for specialist prescription of exercise for the chronically obese, sedentary type 2 diabetic population involving non-weight-bearing activity in the early stages. Walking as a form of physical activity to meet the recommendations for weekly moderate physical activity is therefore not likely to be an immediate or short-term goal for such adults, but one they might aspire to as a medium term objective. Different forms of non-weight-bearing exercise such as swimming (although this has obvious problems regarding use of public swimming pools in terms of psychological and emotional stress for many obese individuals), recumbent or seated cycle ergometry or resistance training may be required in combination with simple physical activity challenges around the home, before many individuals can begin to work towards regular sustained walking as a daily physical activity. It is important to ensure that the physical activity suggested is acceptable and achievable for the individual, hopefully in a setting where they have appropriate social support and encouragement and can get a sense of achievement, satisfaction and enjoyment from their hard work.

Our data on overweight and obese children (OWC) tested with the same treadmill walking test shows that they also have impaired exercise tolerance. We tested 65 overweight and obese children (28 males and 37 females aged 14.04 ± 2.06 years, body mass 87.9 ± 27.6 kg) and found significantly ($P < 0.001$) lower (39 per cent) levels of relative submaximal aerobic fitness compared to 63 normal weight children (NWC; 30 males and 33 females aged 14.22 ± 1.07 years, body mass 55.03 ± 11.43 kg,). Peak $\dot{V}_{O_2}$ at 85 per cent max. HR was 23.28 ± 5.84 ml·kg^{-1}·min^{-1} for the OWC group compared with 38.26 ± 9.32 ml·kg^{-1}·min^{-1} for the NWC. Significant ($P < 0.05$) differences were also noted in peak RER (0.94 ± 0.13 OWC compared to 1.07 ± 0.26 NWC; $P < 0.05$), mean test time (12.66 ± 1.59 min OWC compared to 16.03 ± 1.14 min NWC, $P < 0.001$) and rate of perceived exertion (RPE; 16.65 ± 2.47 OWC compared to 14.78 ± 1.64 NWC, $P < 0.05$). These data show that overweight and obese children have 38 per cent lower levels of exercise tolerance, as measured by a submaximal cardiorespiratory fitness test, compared to normal weight children. As with the adults data, consideration of these findings are important when prescribing exercise for overweight and obese children. However, comparing the weight-adjusted oxygen uptake values shows that the obese adult sample had, on average, 20 per cent lower cardiorespiratory fitness scores per kilogram body mass than the children.

Guidelines for exercise and activity prescription (including practical issues of clinical management for diabetics and the obese)

There is a concern that sedentary people engaging in physical activity may increase their risk of sudden cardiac death (Surgeon General's Report, 1996). However, Albert *et al.* (2000) concluded that there is a transient increase in risk but that habitual vigorous exercise had a low risk (1 sudden death per 1.51 million episodes of exertion).

Evaluation of the type 2 diabetic patient prior to physical activity prescription

A key factor in the prescription of exercise to the diabetic patient is the associated considerations for the outcomes of the diabetic disease state. Therefore prior to exercise prescription a detailed medical history and assessment of a range of physical factors, which includes the heart, blood vessels, eyes, kidneys, nervous system and feet, should be undertaken. The age of the patient, duration of diabetes and extent of co-morbidity will effect the appropriate choice of prescription options. A joint position statement by the ADA/ACSM (1997) suggested that a graded exercise test may be helpful prior to beginning an exercise programme if a patients is at high risk of cardiovascular disease, based on the following criteria:

- age >35 years;
- type 2 diabetes >10 years duration;
- presence of any additional risk factor for coronary artery disease;
- presence of microvascular disease (retinopathy or nephropathy, including microalbuminuria);
- peripheral vascular disease;
- autonomic neuropathy.

Further tests with imaging techniques may also be appropriate for some patients. The position statement also suggests that for patients embarking on low intensity forms of exercise (<60 per cent of maximal heart rate) the general practitioner/physician should use clinical judgement in deciding whether to recommend an exercise stress test (ADA/ACSM, 1997) The following factors should be considered during the prescription of exercise to the type 2 diabetic.

Acute control of blood glucose

Hypoglycaemia is a potential complication for the exercising diabetic. The risk of hypoglycaemia is highest when insulin levels reach a peak at the same time as activity is undertaken, as well as glucose availability from food intake during exercise. A number of considerations are important in order to prevent hypoglycaemia during exercise, these include the form and the location of the insulin administration. Regular physical activity participation would promote better glycaemic control to prevent hypoglycaemia, as the patient will be more able through improved experience to achieve glycaemic control. Chipkin *et al.* (2001) suggested that the following should be undertaken by the exercising diabetic: blood glucose levels should be measured before, during and after exercise, easily absorbable carbohydrates should be available during exercise, extra carbohydrate should be taken for unplanned exercise and insulin dosages should be decreased by 50 per cent for planned exercise.

Minimizing foot trauma

It is essential to consider the health of the feet of the patient prior to engaging in exercise or physical activity, this is especially important for patients with peripheral neuropathy. Appropriate footwear, socks and care of feet before and after the exercise bout is important. Daily visual checks by the patient and regular checks by a health professional are also important (Chipkin *et al.*, 2001; ADA, 2002). Furthermore, weight bearing exercise may not be appropriate for some patients with severe peripheral neuropathy.

Nephropathy

According to Chipkin *et al.* (2001) little is known about the effects of exercise on long term renal function. In addition, dialysis limits exercise capacity, although some researchers have successfully provided suitable exercise programmes (Burke *et al.*, 1987).

Autonomic neuropathy

Sudden death and painless myocardial ischemia have been observed in both type 1 and type 2 diabetic patients (ADA/ACSM, 1997). In addition, during exercise patients with autonomic neuropathy have lower stroke volumes and decreased ejection fractions. Hypo- or hypertension are also possible in patients with autonomic neuropathy following vigorous exercise, particularly when they are at the start of an exercise programme.

Research evidence on the role of physical activity in the prevention and treatment of obesity and type 2 diabetes

Physical activity and the prevention of weight gain

With the use of doubly labelled water researchers have been able to determine the relationship between physical activity and typical patterns of unhealthy weight gain in adults. Schulz and Schoeller (1994) examined the relationship between percentage body fat and non-basal energy expenditure and proposed that a PAL of 1.75 to 1.80 should be a threshold target for the population as a whole. Black *et al.* (1996) using data on 574 free-living individuals stated that their modal physical activity level (PAL) was between 1.55 to 1.65 for both men and women. Thus, to raise the PALs of these individuals to a value that would prevent unhealthy weight gain would require an increase of 0.3 PAL, which relates to moderate exercise lasting between 30–60 min four to five times per week.

Although such guidelines are useful for quantifying levels of physical activity for the population, studies using such levels of physical activity prescription have been limited in their ability to achieve weight management. Seidell (1998) has shown, based on crude estimates, that the increased prevalence of obesity in the Netherlands related to approximately 1 kg gain over a 10 year period (i.e. $2 \, kcal \cdot day^{-1}$). The requirement for such a small amount of daily energy imbalance to make a difference in preventing weight gain or providing weight maintenance, demonstrates the challenge of making small but sustainable changes in behaviour. One problem associated with prescribing and monitoring small changes in energy balance is the difficulty of measuring energy intake and energy expenditure with sufficient accuracy during monitoring and evaluation of intervention programmes. Common use of techniques that rely on self-report is also problematic given the well established inaccuracies associated with such techniques.

Three prospective cohort studies have highlighted the positive impact of physical activity on preventing weight gain in adults (Haapanen *et al.*, 1997; Coakley *et al.*, 1998; Schmitz *et al.*, 2000). Haapanen *et al.* (1997) used a clinically significant body mass gain defined as 5 kg or more over the 10-year follow-up period as a main outcome measure and leisure time physical activity was determined from self-administered questionnaires. Using logistic regression analysis they showed that the men and women with no regular weekly physical activity at the end of the follow up period had an odds ratio of 2.59 (95 per cent confidence interval (CI) 1.69–3.97) and 2.67 (1.65–4.31), respectively for clinically significant weight gain compared to the most active groups. They concluded that regular physical activity prevents body mass gain and physical inactivity is a risk factor for body mass gain and obesity among adults.

Table 8.4   Mean change (post − pre) in vigorous physical activity levels and corresponding change in body mass for the four groups in the CARDIA study

Group	% Change in vigorous physical activity levels (>6 METS)*		% Change in body mass	
	Absolute change (exercise units)	% Change	Absolute change (kg)	% Change
Black women	−43	−26	11.5	17
White women	−78.9	−30	6.8	11
Black men	−67.8	−18	10.5	14
White men	−79	−23	7.7	10

*Data were self reported levels by questionnaire.

Coakley *et al.* (1998) examined the effect of changing exercise, TV viewing, smoking and eating habits on 4-year change in body mass in a cohort of 19 478 US male health professionals. They showed that for middle-aged men vigorous physical activity was associated with weight reduction and TV viewing and eating between meals was associated with weight gain. Over the 4-year follow up period middle aged men who increased their physical activity, decreased TV viewing and stopped eating between meals lost an average of 1.4 kg (95 per cent CI −1.6 to −1.1 kg), compared to a weight gain of 1.4 kg in the overall population. The prevalence of obesity in middle-aged men was lowest among those who maintained a relatively high level of vigorous physical activity, compared to those who were relatively sedentary. Coakley *et al.* (1998) concluded that an improvement in a number of healthy habits, particularly increasing vigorous physical activity, as well as decreasing TV viewing and changing eating habits results in weight maintenance or a modest weight loss over 4 years.

Schmitz *et al.* (2000), reporting data from the Coronary Artery Risk Development In Young Adults (CARDIA) study, showed an inverse relationship between change in physical activity and change in body mass over a 10-year follow-up period (Table 8.4). All three of these large prospective studies support the hypothesis that regular physical activity prevents body mass gain and physical inactivity is a risk factor for body mass gain and obesity amongst adults.

Physical activity and the treatment of overweight and obesity

There have been a number of review articles that have demonstrated greater success with the inclusion of physical activity in the treatment of overweight and obesity (Miller *et al.* 1997, 1995; Ballor and Poehlman, 1995; Epstein and Myers, 1998). It is clear from a variety of intervention studies that acute treatments lead to significant weight loss (Ballor and Poehlman, 1995; Miller *et al.*, 1997; Epstein and Myers, 1998) but weight loss maintenance tends to be limited (Garner and Wooley, 1991; Miller, 1999).

Studies comparing the outcomes of diet only versus exercise only interventions, show that the ability of exercise only interventions to achieve weight loss is very limited (Garrow and Summerbell, 1995; Miller *et al.*, 1997). Miller *et al.* (1997) compared diet only, exercise only and diet plus exercise interventions, the outcomes of which were average weight losses of $10.7 \pm 0.5\,$kg, $2.9 \pm 0.4\,$kg and $11.0 \pm 0.6\,$kg respectively for short duration interventions lasting 15.6 ± 06 weeks. Miller *et al.* (1997) also reported 1-year follow-up data for the diet only and diet plus exercise programmes, they achieved a weight loss maintenance of 6.6 $\pm 0.5\,$kg and $8.6 \pm 0.8\,$kg respectively. Ballor and Poehlman (1995) showed that minimal changes in body mass were achieved by studies using physical activity or exercise to induce change in body mass over 12 ± 1 years. Physical activity was separated into run/walk, cycling or resistance training, the outcomes in terms of changes in body mass were -1.3 ± 0.2, -1.1 ± 0.4 and $1.2 \pm 0.2\,$kg respectively. Ballor and Poehlman (1995) showed that weight training tends to preserve lean tissue, which is important during dietary intervention programmes.

However, encouraging data from the National Weight Control Registry (USA) (Klem *et al.*, 1997) shows that inclusion of physical activity is particularly important in promoting weight loss maintenance compared to dietary restriction alone. Despite long histories of overweight and obesity, the 629 women and 155 men in the registry lost an average of 30 kg and maintained a required minimum weight loss of 13.6 kg for 5 years. Just over half lost weight through formal programmes, the remainder lost weight on their own. Both groups reported using diet and physical activity to lose weight. It is important to note that almost 77 per cent of the sample reported that a triggering event in their lives had preceded their weight loss. Current physical activity was reported to be very high relative to current population guidelines in both the USA and the UK, at 404 kcal·day^{-1}. Klem *et al.* (1997) were surprised that 42 per cent of the sample reported that maintaining their weight loss was less difficult than losing the weight. Nearly all the sample reported that weight loss had led to improvements in their level of energy, physical mobility, general mood, self-confidence and physical health.

A meta-analysis by Anderson *et al.* (2001) based on 29 studies with a 5-year follow up of structured weight loss programmes showed that an average weight loss of 3.0 kg or 23 per cent of initial weight loss was maintained. The authors concluded that although this is positive much more research is required to optimize the outcomes of lifestyle intervention programmes. Anderson *et al.* (2001) also reported that weight loss maintenance was significantly greater when participants exercised more. The increasing prevalence and associated magnitude of obesity suggests that these small gains reported for structured weight loss programmes are of limited value given the scale of this public health problem. The treatment options in these programmes were varied, whereas the studies reviewed by Miller *et al.* (1997) only included those that used aerobic exercise.

Dunn *et al.* (1998) compared a lifestyle physical activity programme with a structured exercise programme in adults ($n = 235$), at 6 months both groups had increased their energy expenditure (mean ± SE) $1.53 \pm 0.19 \, kcal \cdot kg^{-1} \cdot day^{-1}$ for the lifestyle group and $1.53 \pm 0.19 \, kcal \cdot kg^{-1} \cdot day^{-1}$ structured exercise group. Both groups had a significant increase in cardiorespiratory fitness (maximal treadmill test) and the increase in the structured group was significantly ($P < 0.01$) greater, $3.64 \pm 0.33 \, ml \cdot kg^{-1} \cdot min^{-1}$ and $1.58 \pm 0.33 \, ml \cdot kg^{-1} \cdot min^{-1}$ for the structured and lifestyle groups respectively. Dunn et al. (1998) suggested that the key outcome was the emphasis on behavioural skill building rather than exercise prescription, as for the lifestyle group this was equally as effective at achieving increases in physical activity.

Physical activity and obesity treatment in children

A review by Epstein and Goldfield (1999) has outlined the important elements of intervention programmes for overweight and obese children. The only area where there was a sufficient number of studies to make a quantitative analysis led to the conclusion that diet plus exercise programmes achieved greater weight loss. Two studies have shown that subjects involved in a diet only intervention were less successful than subjects involved in diet plus exercise (Epstein et al., 1985) ($-3.8 \, kg$ diet only versus $-6.8 \, kg$ diet and exercise) and Hills and Parker (1988) ($-2.6 \, kg$ diet only versus $-5.5 \, kg$ diet and exercise)). Gutin et al. (1999) has shown that exercise only interventions can produce improvements in: body composition ($-2.2 \, kg$), fitness (-3.8 bpm at 48 w during a cycle ergometer test) and biochemical profiles (TAG ($1.15 \pm 0.01 \, mmol/l$ pre; $0.95 \pm 0.01 \, mmol \cdot l^{-1}$ post; intervention group compared to $0.98 \pm 0.01 \, mmol \cdot l^{-1}$ pre; $1.10 \pm 0.01 \, mmol \cdot l^{-1}$ post; control group) and fasting insulin ($155.5 \pm 7.9 \, pmol \cdot l^{-1}$ pre and $140.6 \pm 7.9 \, pmol \cdot l^{-1}$ post for the intervention group compared to $170.9 \pm 7.9 \, pmol \cdot l^{-1}$ pre and $176.5 \, pmol \cdot l^{-1}$ post for the control group) although body mass increased ($1.1 \, kg$).

Further analysis of the studies in Epstein's review showed that a range of exercise programmes were used. Most studies used aerobic exercise in the form of walking, jogging or cycling (Sasaki et al., 1987; Rocchini et al., 1988; Epstein et al., 1994; Gutin et al., 1995; Owens et al., 1999). Sasaki et al. (1987) used running at lactate threshold adjusted monthly to ensure a consistent relative level of exercise intensity. Some studies used sports and games based activities, but the aim was still to maintain a high-energy expenditure during these sessions (Rocchini et al., 1988; Owens et al., 1999). Epstein et al. (1982) reported the effects of lifestyle change compared to programmed aerobic exercise, with or without diet, on weight, fitness and adherence in overweight and obese children. The 8-week interventions induced equivalent changes in weight, while fitness changes were greater in the programmed aerobic exercise group. During the follow-up period the lifestyle change group maintained their weight loss and fitness levels better than the programmed aerobic exercise group.

Several researchers have promoted the use of strategies to decrease sedentary behaviours or lifestyle activities (such as limiting access to TV and computer games) (Epstein *et al.*, 1994, 1995; Gutin *et al.*, 1995). Epstein *et al.* (1995) randomly assigned children to one of three groups: reinforcing decreased sedentary activity (sedentary); reinforcing increased physical activity (exercise); or reinforcing decreased sedentary activity and increased physical activity (combined). After the 4-month intervention the group who were reinforced only for decreasing sedentary activity were more successful (-13.2 kg (exercise), -19.9 kg (sedentary) and -17.0 kg (combined)) than the other two groups. Epstein *et al.* (1995) have suggested that one possible explanation for the greater success of reducing sedentary behaviour is that the children are provided with choice and control. Choice and control are powerful psychological variables that have been shown to influence exercise adherence (Thompson and Wankel, 1980). Epstein and Myers (1998) concluded that increased physical activity is critical to long-term success in weight control for children.

Physical activity and the prevention of type 2 diabetes

Several prospective studies have shown that physical activity does play an important role in the prevention of type 2 diabetes. A study by Helmrich *et al.* (1991) at the University of Pennsylvania found that at 14-year follow-up every 500 kcal of additional leisure time physical activity each week was associated with a 6 per cent reduction in diabetes risk. In addition, levels of exercise were also assessed, such that those that participated in moderate to vigorous exercise had a 35 per cent lower risk of type 2 diabetes compared to sedentary patients. Those with the highest risk for the development of type 2 diabetes achieved the most by their participation in physical activity and exercise, as they decreased their risk the most.

Manson *et al.* (1991) in the Nurses study showed, that those women reporting participation in vigorous physical activity (long enough to produce a sweat) at least once per week had a 16 per cent lower risk of diabetes at 8-year follow-up, compared to those who did not engage more than once a week. A further study by Manson *et al.* (1992) in men also showed a protective effect of physical activity. In a study of 21 271 male physicians, those engaging in vigorous exercise at least once per week had a 29 per cent lower risk of diabetes compared to those engaging in vigorous activity less than once per week.

In the Nurses Health Survey, Hu *et al.* (1999) compared the effect of walking with that of vigorous activity on risk of diabetes in 70 102 participants. At the 8-year follow-up those in the highest quintile of physical activity had a 26 per cent decrease in risk of diabetes compared to the women in the lowest quintile. Given such strong prospective evidence the ability of physical activity to prevent diabetes should be considered with the utmost importance.

A study by Eriksson and Lindgarde (1998) achieved success in reducing mortality over 12 years in subjects with impaired glucose tolerance, treated with diet and exercise.

Physical activity in the treatment of type 2 diabetes

The Diabetes Prevention Programme Research Group (2002) achieved significant reductions in the incidence of type 2 diabetes in a lifestyle intervention group (58 per cent reduction) (goals to reduce body mass by 7 per cent and achieve at least 150 min of physical activity per week). This was in comparison to both a metformin (850 mg twice daily) intervention group that also produced a significant reduction of 31 per cent, and a placebo group during the 2.8-year period of treatment. The research group identified these two forms of treatment as 'highly effective means of delaying or preventing type 2 diabetes.' Tuomilehto *et al.* (2001) showed similar results in the incidence of diabetes in a sample of 522 middle-aged overweight subjects treated with a lifestyle intervention programme (5 per cent weight loss, total intake of fat <30 per cent of energy consumed, intake of saturated fat to <10 per cent of energy consumed, and increase in fibre intake to at least 15 g per 1000 kcal and at least 30 min of moderate exercise each day). The risk of diabetes was reduced by 58 per cent in the intervention group.

A meta-analysis by Brown *et al.* (1996) involving 89 studies and 1800 subjects, examined the outcomes of strategies to achieve weight loss and improved metabolic control (change in glycosylated haemoglobin) in obese diabetic patients. In this analysis diet alone achieved the greatest weight loss and improvement in metabolic control (-20 lb and -2.7 per cent glycosylated haemoglobin)), behavioural programmes alone also achieved significant improvements (-6.4 lb and -1.5 per cent). Exercise studies also achieved improvements but they were not statistically significant (-3.4 lb and -0.8 per cent). Behaviour and diet therapies achieved statistically significant improvements (-8.5 lb and -1.6 per cent) but these changes were not as high as diet-only programmes. However, as with most of the reviews on weight loss maintenance in the obese, the author concluded that most of the studies were limited with a general a lack of reported data on long-term follow-up.

Although relatively little research has been conducted on the impact of intensity of intervention on treatment outcomes, McAuley *et al.* (2002) compared a modest treatment (similar to current standard treatment programmes) and a more intensive treatment programme. The more intensive treatment programme produced a more significant improvement in insulin sensitivity (23 per cent, $P = 0.006$ (intensive intervention group) versus 9 per cent $P = 0.23$ (modest/standard intervention group and for aerobic fitness (11 per cent increase in intensive group, $P = 0.02$ versus 1 per cent in the modest group, $P = 0.94$). The more intensive treatment included goals to achieve both greater dietary change than the modest treatment group and the 1990 ACSM guidelines for developing and maintaining cardiorespiratory and muscular fitness. The differences in response of these groups and the lack of improvement in insulin sensitivity for standard treatment shown in this study highlight the significant challenge ahead with the increasing prevalence of type 2 diabetes. Agurs-Collins *et al.* (1997)

also showed that a more intensive intervention programme (12 weekly group sessions, 1 individual session and 6 biweekly group sessions) was effective in improving glycaemic and blood pressure control compared to usual care (1 class and 2 informational mailings). However, the author stated that the decrease in HbA1c was generally independent of the relatively modest changes in dietary intake, weight, and activity and may reflect indirect programme effects on other aspects of self care.

According to the ADA/ACSM (1997) position statement, all patients with diabetes can use resistance training, although as with general training recommendations the resistance training programme should relate to the ability, experience and fitness of the diabetic patient.

Physical activity and the behavioural treatment of obesity

The behavioural treatment of obesity refers to a set of principles and techniques designed to help overweight and obese individuals reverse their maladaptive eating, activity and thinking habits (Wadden and Foster, 2000).

A number of important factors that effect physical activity behaviour change have been highlighted by researchers; these include:

- Personal and environmental factors: factors such as transport policy, urban planning, TV and advertising are important considerations, as are barriers to people contemplating physical activity, exercise and sports participation (Dishman, 1994; Sallis and Owen, 1997).

- Choice is a powerful psychological variable that can influence a variety of outcomes, including adherence to exercise and physical activity (Rodin *et al.*, 1985).

- Social support is an important determinant in physical activity participation (Sallis and Owen, 1997).

- Safety and the environment: Sallis and Owen (1997) have suggested that time spent outdoors was the single best correlate of physical activity for children. However, many parents keep their children indoors because of concern about safety and lack of space and facilities near homes. A consideration for children is not only their physical safety, but their psychological safety is also of paramount importance. The evidence on the psychological co-morbidities associated with obesity is high (Gortmaker *et al.*, 1993; Sullivan *et al.*, 1993).

- Personal factors: Fox (1988) has suggested a need to include children's perceptions in the development of intervention programmes, which is equally important for adults. Studies have been conducted to identify reasons for participation in physical activity (Gould, 1984; Wankel and Kreisel, 1985; Parker, 1991; Stucky-Ropp and Dilorenzo, 1993; Bar-Or and Baranowski, 1994). For example, Gould (1984) assessed a sample of 347 young people aged 8–16 years using a questionnaire. He concluded that children's primary reason for participation in exercise is 'to have fun' followed by 'improve skills' and 'learn new skills'. This conclusion is supported by Sallis and Owen (1997).

For a thorough consideration of the role of behavioural approaches in the treatment of obesity the reader is referred to the preceding chapter and a number of reviews of this subject (Wadden *et al.*, 1999; Faith *et al.*, 2000; Wadden and Foster, 2000).

Linking research and practice

Our team has developed the Carnegie International Camp, a summer residential fun-type skill-based intervention programme that combines physical activity, diet and behaviour modification. The programme has been developed during our 8 years' evaluative research of residential treatment programmes for children. The programme is based on the basic principle that in order to engage children in persistent behaviour change, children should be given positive experiences of physical activity and healthy eating. It is our view that most treatment programmes do not adopt such an approach, but rather they prioritize the determination of the dietary restriction and physical activity levels to achieve a specific energy imbalance. Few studies consider the elements of the process of behaviour change for overweight and obese people engaged in weight loss strategies. We believe that understanding the process of intervention is critical to the successful treatment of this disease. There are some common principles in successful weight loss intervention but they need to be flexible and enable the intervention to be tailored to the individual. General advice and guidelines will therefore not work for many people. Our experience supports the work of McAuley *et al.* (2002) that showed that more intensive treatments produced better outcomes than so called standard treatments for type 2 diabetes. Clearly, more research is required in order to determine how different interventions can be applied efficaciously in different settings for different target groups, but research seems to suggest that more resources are needed to offer more intensive treatment and support to deal with both obesity and type 2 diabetes.

To illustrate the link between our research and practice we have included: (1) a case study of a child who has attended the UK camp programme; (2) data from one summer programme in the UK.

Case study

Table 8.5 shows that this child lost significant amounts of body mass, body fat, waist circumference and significantly improved his cardiorespiratory fitness following the six week camp programme. These changes were improved further

Table 8.5 Baseline, post camp and 2-year follow-up data for a child who attended the 6 week camp programme

Variable	Baseline Week 0	Post Week 6	Pre Week 52	Post Week 58	Pre Week 104
Age (years)	15.5		16.5		17.5
Stature (m)	1.77	1.77	1.78	1.78	1.80
Body mass (kg)	107.2	99.9	102.8	100.0	89.4
BMI (kg·m^{-2})	34.22	31.93	32.52	31.56	27.59
% Body fat	36.8	30.7	31.5	32.4	17.7
Waist circumference (cm)	113	105	98.45	93.6	88
$\dot{V}_{O_2}$ at 85% MHR ml·kg^{-1}·min^{-1}	30.25	31.10	36.7	38.73	40.25

Baseline and 2-year follow-up photo's of the case study

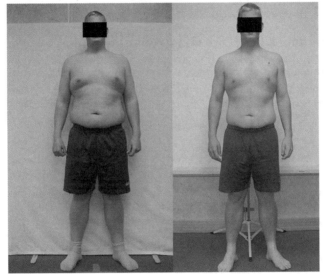

during the two year follow up period. Clearly a reduction in body mass of 18 kg and a reduction of 19% in body fat demonstrate a highly effective programme for this individual.

Qualitative information from the case study

This young man identified that following the camp programme, he had developed a range of skills that enabled participation in more lifestyle physical activity (increasing every day activities such as walking to school, taking the stairs) and strongly pursued the sports that he felt he was good at. He also reported that the programme had encouraged and helped him understand training principles, which led to participation in weight training and cardiovascular training to improve performance in his chosen sport of rugby. In terms of diet, he reported few changes but acknowledged that participation in sport helped regulate his eating patterns. He also reported little change in his sedentary behaviours, but following discussions with him, it was clear that his sedentary behaviours had indeed reduced as he spent less time watching TV and also highlighted spending more time out with his friends.

Such qualitative information regarding the influence of treatment programmes is critical to the further development of effective intervention programmes for overweight and obese people. As clinicians and practitioners, many of us modify our practices based on feedback from the patient. Our research has actively pursued the collection of this information as it is critical to the further development of our treatment model, but also the development of effective, treatment programmes for the obese in general. In fact, many of the issues raised by the children are similar, but there are also issues that separate children and therefore the individual nature of their treatment.

Some group data from residential weight-loss-camps

The case study illustrates only one individual set of results. We have therefore included some group data we have collected from two residential camps, one in the US (Table 8.6) and one in the UK (Table 8.7).

We have also published 1-year follow-up data on children who have attended the US camp programme (Table 8.8, Gately *et al.* 2000). These data show longer-term outcomes of the intervention programme, with 89 per cent of the children having a lower standardized BMI at 1-year follow-up compared to baseline. Whilst the residential camp setting is different to the everyday environment that the children are used to it does provide a good opportunity for us to learn about the elements of intervention treatment and behaviour change

Table 8.6 Mean ± standard deviation pre, post, and change for all variables for campers during one US summer programme

Campers ($n = 283$)	Pre	Post	Change
Age (years)	13.6 ± 1.8		
Stature (m)	1.59 ± 0.1		
Body mass (kg)	82.1 ± 21.4	75.5 ± 20.0	−6.6 ± 3.39***
Body mass index (kg·m^{-2})	32.7 ± 7.26	30.0 ± 6.8	−2.7 ± 1.3***
% Body fat ($n = 190$)	35 ± 9	32 ± 8	−2 ± 3***
FM (kg) ($n = 190$)	29.8 ± 13.4	25.4 ± 11.4	−4.5 ± 2.8***
FFM (kg) ($n = 190$)	52.3 ± 11.6	50.1 ± 9.4	−2.2 ± 2.5***
Waist circumference (cm) ($n = 283$)	93.2 ± 15.0	87.3 ± 13.5	−7.05 ± 4.84***
Hip circumference (cm) ($n = 283$)	109.5 ± 14.8	104.5 ± 14.0	−5.97 ± 4.92***
Aerobic fitness (l·min^{-1}) ($n = 50$)	3.83 ± 0.78	4.19 ± 0.95	0.37 ± 0.45***

Data collected on US camp programme, unpublished.
*** = $P < 0.001$, ** = $P < 0.01$, * = $P < 0.05$, paired *t*-test (pre, post).

Table 8.7 Mean ± standard deviations pre, post and change for all variables for campers during one UK summer programme

Campers ($n = 65$)	Pre	Post	Change
Age (years)	14.0 ± 2.1		
Stature (m)	1.62 ± 0.1		
Body mass (kg)	87.9 ± 27.6	82.5 ± 25.8	−5.3 ± 3.1***
BMI (kg·m^{-1})	32.7 ± 6.9	30.6 ± 6.5	−2.0 ± 1.1***
% body fat	47 ± 6	43 ± 7	−4 ± 4***
FM (kg)	42.6 ± 16.3	35.9 ± 13.5	−5.7 ± 5.1***
FFM (kg)	45.4 ± 12.2	45.9 ± 13.1	0.4 ± 3.5
WC (cm)	94.0 ± 14.7	89.4 ± 13.5	−4.6 ± 3.2***
HC (cm)	112.1 ± 15.7	108.2 ± 15.8	−4.0 ± 3.1***
V_{O_2} @85% MHR (l·min^{-1})	2.00 ± 0.57	2.26 ± 0.63	0.26 ± 0.33***
V_{O_2} @85% MHR (ml·kg^{-1}·min^{-1})	23.3 ± 5.8	28.0 ± 5.9	4.7 ± 4.0***
Global self worth	2.51 ± 0.64	2.86 ± 0.55	0.34 ± 0.6.0 ***

Data collected on UK camp programme, unpublished;
$*** = P < 0.001$, $** = P < 0.01$, $* = P < 0.05$, paired t-test (pre, post).

Table 8.8 Acute (8-week) and 1-year follow-up outcomes of a residential weight loss programme

Variables	Baseline (Week 0)	Post camp (Week 8)	One year follow up (Week 52)
Stature (m)	1.58 ± 0.12		1.64 ± 0.11‡
Body mass (kg)	83.5 ± 26.66	72.3 ± 23.6***	82.2 ± 25.9†
BMI (kg·m^{-2})	32.7 ± 7.2	28.3 ± 6.4***	30.1 ± 7.0†‡
Standardized BMI	3.61 ± 1.9	2.43 ± 1.64***	2.73 ± 1.93†‡

$*** = P < 0.01$ difference between week 0 and week 8.
$† = P < 0.01$ difference between week 8 and week 52.
$‡ = P < 0.05$ difference from week 0 to week 52.

that are effective in terms of changes in both body mass and body composition, but also in terms of the children who continue to work with us to improve our programme. The acute and 1-year follow-up data on changes in standardized BMI are certainly encouraging. We are now transferring many of the successful principles and practices of the camp programme to more regular intervention treatments that are more accessible to a wider range of children.

Summary

This chapter has considered the role that physical activity can play in both the prevention and treatment of obesity and type 2 diabetes. It combines a summary of research evidence pertinent to understanding the relationships between physical activity, obesity and type 2 diabetes and practical guidance related to increasing physical activity in sedentary individuals. The following is a summary of the key points from the chapter:

- Regular habitual physical activity makes a significant contribution to a healthy lifestyle.

- Physical activity is an important component in both the prevention and treatment of obesity and type 2 diabetes.

- Achievement of current population recommendations for physical activity will make a significant contribution to energy balance and metabolic control in the obese and type 2 diabetic populations.

- Physical activity and fitness are important for decreasing the risk profile and improving health status independently of weight loss, although also decreasing excess body fat is still preferable.

- Any increase in physical activity is to be encouraged and positively reinforced in the sedentary population as sustained increases in physical activity through walking and other achievable activities has been shown to improve metabolic control, lipid profiles and blood pressure independently of improvements in traditional measures of cardiorespiratory fitness such as V_{O_2} max.

- Physical activity is most effective as a treatment intervention when applied together with improvements in eating behaviour set in the framework of sustainable behaviour modification of lifestyle.

- Physical activity helps maintain fat-free mass during calorific restriction.

- Physical activity can increase basal metabolic rate through increasing muscle mass.

- Increasing physical activity will produce functional adaptations in the body that improve the risk profile and health status of the participant in terms of overweight, obesity and type 2 diabetes.

- Achievement of current population guidelines for physical activity may represent a relatively long-term goal for the chronically obese and long-term sedentary type 2 diabetic due to their severely limited exercise tolerance.

- Non-weight-bearing physical activity in short bouts of a few minutes regularly throughout the day will be needed in the most sedentary and obese individuals due to poor exercise tolerance in comparison with normal weight sedentary peers.

- The chronically obese and type 2 diabetics should be evaluated and monitored by their clinicians both before embarking on and during regular habitual physical activity.

- Most obese and type 2 diabetics will have led a sedentary existence for some considerable time, often many years, therefore treatments incorporating physical activity must be realistic in setting and managing expectations in participants.

- Substantial and sustained weight loss is often triggered by a key event so it will not work in all cases.

- Substantial weight loss and sustained weight maintenance are commonly associated with a sustainable increase in daily habitual physical activity.

- Many overweight and obese people like physical activity and sport, but not all do. Individual needs, lifestyle and enjoyment must be considered when attempting to increase physical activity in a sustainable way.

- Achievement of current physical activity recommendations will not be sufficient in energy expenditure terms to offset the energy intake of many individuals, the result of which is seen in the continued increase in prevalence of overweight and obesity.

- Increasing physical activity must be achievable within the lives of the participants in such a way that they can enjoy it and see it as sustainable.

- Increasing physically activity must be targeted to the needs of the individual with appropriate support and guidance, simply telling people to eat less and take more exercise does not work.

- Barriers and determinants of a physically active lifestyle will vary from person to person. Addressing the issues of enjoyment, physical competence in terms of improved skills, choice, opportunity, empowerment, social and emotional support are more likely to lead to sustainable lifestyle change, including increased activity than energy balance *per se.*

References

Activity and Health Research (1992) *Allied Dunbar National Fitness Survey: Main Findings.* Health Education Authority and Sports Council.

Agurs-Collins TD, Kumanyika SK, Ten Have TR and Adams-Cambell LL (1997) A randomised controlled trial of weight reduction and exercise for diabetes management in older African-American Subjects. *Diabetes Care* **20**: 1503–11.

Albert CM, Mittleman MA, Chae CU *et al.* (2000) Triggering of sudden death from cardiac causes by vigorous exertion. *N Engl J Med* **343**: 1355–61.

Albright A, Franz M, Hornsby G *et al.* (2000) American College of Sports Medicine position stand on exercise and Type 2 diabetes. *Med Sci Sports Exerc* **32**: 1345–60.

Ainsworth BE, Haskell WL, Whitt MC *et al.* (2000) Compendium of physical activities: an update of activity codes and MET intensities. *Med Sci Sports Exerc* **32**(9 Suppl): S498–S504.

American College of Sports Medicine (1995) *ACSM's guidelines for exercise testing and prescription.* Williams & Wilkins, Baltimore.

American College of Sports Medicine (1998) *Resource manual for guidelines for exercise testing and prescription*, 3rd edn. Williams & Wilkins, Baltimore.

American College of Sports Medicine and American Diabetes Association joint position statement (1997) Diabetes mellitus and exercise. *Med Sci Sports Exerc* **29**(12): i–vi.

American Diabetes Association (2002) The prevention or delay of type 2 diabetes. *Diabetes Care* **25**: 742–9.

Anderson JW, Konz EC, Frederich RC and Wood CL (2001) Long-term weight loss maintenance: a meta-analysis of US studies. *Am J Clin Nutr* **74**: 579–84.

Astrand PO and Ryhming I (1954) A nomogram for the calculation of aerobic capacity (physical fitness) from pulse rate during submaximal work. *J Appl Physiol* **7**: 218.

Astrand PO and Rodahl K (1986)   *Textbook of Work Physiology, Physiological Bases of Exercise*, 3rd edn. McGraw-Hill, New York.

Ballor DL and Poehlman ET (1995) A meta-analysis of the effects of exercise and/or dietary restriction on resting metabolic rate. *Eur. J. Appl Phys* **71**: 535–42.

Bar-Or O and Baranowski T (1994) Physical activity, adiposity and obesity among adolescents. *Pediats Exerc Sci* **6**: 348–360.

Biddle S, Sallis J and Cavill N (eds) (1998) *Young and Active? Young People and Health-enhancing Physical Activity – Evidence and Implications*. Health Education Authority, London.

Birk TJ and Birk CA (1987) Use of ratings of perceived exertion for exercise prescription. *Sports Med* **4**: 1–8.

Blaak EE, Westerterp KR, Bar-Or O *et al.* (1992) Total energy expenditure and spontaneous activity in relation to training in obese boys. *Am J Clin Nutr* **55**: 777–82.

Black AE, Coward WA, Cole TJ and Prentice AM (1996) Human energy expenditure in affluent societies: an analysis of 574 doubly-labelled water measurements. *Eur J Clin Nutr* **50**: 72–92.

Blair SN and Brodney S (1999) Effects of physical inactivity and obesity on morbidity and mortality: current evidence and research issues. *Med. Sci. Sports Exerc* **31**: S646–S662.

Borg GV and Linderholm H (1967) Perceived exertion and pulse rate during graded exercise in various age groups. *Acta Med Scand* **472**(Suppl): 194–206.

Bouchard C and Blair SN (1999) Roundtable introduction, introductory comments for the consensus on physical activity and obesity. *Med Sci Sports Exerc* **31**: S498–501.

Brown SA, Upchurch S, Anding R *et al.* (1996) Promoting weight loss in type 2 diabetes. *Diabetes Care* **19**: 613–24.

Burke EJ, Germain MJ, Fitzgibbons JP *et al.* (1987) A comparison of the physiologic effects of submaximal exercise during and off hemodialysis treatment. *J Cardiopulm Rehab* **7**: 68–72.

Casperson CJ, Powell KE and Christenson GM (1985) Physical activity, exercise and fitness. *Publ Health Rep* **100**: 125–31.

Chipkin SR, Klugh SA and Chasan-Taber L (2001) Exercise and diabetes. *Cardiol Clin* **19**: 489–505.

Coakley EH, Rimm EB, Colditz G *et al.* (1998) Predictors of change in men: Results from the health professionals follow up study. *Int J Obes* **22**: 89–96.

Cooke CB (2001) Metabolic rate and energy balance. In Eston R and Reilly T (eds) *Kinanthropometry and Exercise Physiology Laboratory Manual: Test Procedures and Data*. Volume 2: *Exercise Physiology*, 2nd edn. Routledge, London.

DeLany JP (1998) Role of energy expenditure in the development of paediatric obesity. *Am J Clin Nutr* **68**: 950–5.

Diabetes prevention program research group. (2002) Reduction in the incidence of type 2 diabetes with lifestyle intervention or metformin. *N Engl J Med* **346**: 393–403.

Dishman RK (1994) *Advances in Exercise Adherence*. Human Kinetics, Champaign.

Drake AJ, Smith A, Betts PR *et al*. (2002) Type 2 diabetes in obese white children. *Arch Dis Child* **86**: 207–8.

Dunbar CC, Robertson RJ, Baun R *et al*. (1992) The validity of regulating exercise intensity by ratings of perceived exertion. *Med Sci Sports Exerc* **24**: 94–9.

Dunn AL, Garcia ME, Marcus BH *et al*. (1998) Six-month physical activity and fitness changes in project active, a randomised trial. *Med Sci Sports Exerc* **30**: 1076–83.

Epstein LH and Myers MD (1998) Treatment of pediatric obesity. *Paediatrics* **101**: 554–71.

Epstein LH and Goldfield GS (1999) Physical activity in the treatment of childhood over-weight and obesity: Current evidence and research issues. *Med Sci Sports Exerc* **31**: S553–S559.

Epstein LH, Wing RR, Koeske R *et al*. (1982) A comparison of lifestyle change and pro-grammed aerobic exercise on weight and fitness changes in obese children. *Behav Ther* **13**: 651–65.

Epstein LH, Wing RR, Koeske R and Valoski A (1985) A comparison of lifestyle exercise, aerobic exercise and calisthenics on weight loss in obese children. *Behav Ther* **16**: 345–56.

Epstein LH, Valoski A, Wing RR and McCurley J (1994) Ten-year outcomes of behavioural family-based treatment for childhood obesity. *Health Psychol* **13**: 373–83.

Epstein LH, Valoski LS, McCurley J *et al*. (1995) Effects of decreasing sedentary behaviour and increasing activity on weight change in obese children. *Health Psychol* **14**: 109–15.

Eriksson KF and Lindgarde F (1998) No excess 12 year mortality in men with impaired glucose tolerance who participated in the Malmo preventive trial with diet and exercise. *Diabetologia* **41**: 1010–16.

Faith MS, Fontaine KR, Cheskin LJ and Allison DB (2000) Behavior approaches to the problems of obesity. *Behav Modific* **24**(4): 459–93.

Ferro-Luzzi A and Martino L (1996) Obesity and physical activity. In *The Origins and Consequences of Obesity: Ciba Foundation Symposium 201*. Chichester, UK, John Wiley & Sons.

Fox K (1988) Children's participation motives. *Br J Phys Educ* **19**: 79–82.

Freedman DS, Dietz WH, Srinivasan SV and Berenson GS (1999) The relation of overweight to cardiovascular risk factors among children and adolescents: the Bogalusa Heart Study. *Pediatrics* **103**: 1175–82.

Freedman DS, Khan LK, Dietz WH *et al*. (2001) Relationship of childhood obesity to coronary heart disease risk factors in adulthood: the Bogalusa Heart Study. *Pediatrics* **108**(3): 712–18.

Garner DM and Wooley SC (1991) Confronting the failure of behavioural and dietary treatment for obesity. *Clin Psychol Rev* **11**: 729–80.

Garrow JS and Summerbell CD (1995) Meta-analysis: effects of exercise, with or without dieting, on the body composition of overweight subjects. *Eur J Clin Nutr* **49**: 1–10.

Gately PJ, Cooke CB, Barth JH and Butterly RJ (1997) Exercise tolerance in a sample of morbidly obese subjects. *Proceedings of the European Congress on Obesity*, Trinity College, Dublin, Ireland.

Gately PJ, Cooke CB, Butterly RJ *et al*. (2000) The effects of a children's summer camp programme on weight loss, with a 10 month follow up. *Int J Obes* **24**: 1445–52.

Goran MI (1998) Measurement issues related to studies of childhood obesity: Assessment of body composition, body fat distribution, physical activity and food intake. *Paediatrics* **101**: 505–19.

Gortmaker SL, Must A, Perrin JM *et al*. (1993) Social and economic consequences of overweight in adolescent and young adulthood. *N Engl J Med* **329**: 1008–12.

Gould D (1984) Psychosocial development and children's sport. In Thomas JR (ed.) *Motor Development During Childhood and Adolescence*. Burgess, Minneapolis, MN.

Gutin B, Cucuzzo N, Isalm S *et al.* (1995) Physical training improves body composition of black obese 7- to 11-year-old girls. *Obes Res* **3**(4): 305–12.

Gutin B, Owens S, Okuyama T *et al.* (1999) Effect of physical training and it's cessation on percent body fat and bone density of children with obesity. *Obes Res* **7**(2): 208–14.

Haapanen N, Miilumnpalo S, Pasanen M, Oja P and Vuori I (1997) Association between leisure time physical activity and 10 year body mass change among working aged men and women. *Int J Obes* **21**: 288–96.

Hagberg JM, Montain ST, Martin MH and Ehsani AA (1989) Effect of exercise training in 60 to 69 year old persons with essential hypertension. *Am J Cardiol* **64**: 348–53.

Harrison MH, Bruce DL, Brown GA and Cochrane LA (1980) A comparison of some indirect methods of predicting maximal oxygen uptake. *Aviat Space Environ Med* **51**: 1128.

Heath GW, Wilson RH, Smith J and Leonard BE (1991) Community based exercise and weight control: Diabetes risk reduction and glycemic control in Zuni Indians. *Am J Clin Nutr* **53**: S1642–S1646.

Helmrich SP, Ragland DR, Leung PW and Paffenbarger RS Jr (1991) Physical activity and reduced occurrence of non-insulin dependant diabetes mellitus. *N Eng J Med* **325**: 147–52.

Heyward V (1998) *Advanced Fitness Assessment and Exercise Prescription*, 3rd edn. Human Kinetics, Champaign.

Hills AP and Parker AW (1988) Obesity management via diet and exercise intervention. *Child Care Health Develop* **14**: 409–16.

Hu FB, Sigal RJ, Rich-Ewards JW *et al.* (1999) Walking compared with vigorous physical activity and risk of type 2 diabetes in women. *JAMA* **282**(5): 1433–7.

Ivy JL, Zderic TW and Fogt DL (1999) Prevention and treatment of non-insulin-dependant diabetes mellitus. *Exerc Sports Sci Rev* **47**: 37–44.

Joint Health Surveys Unit (1999) *Health Survey of England*, 1998. The Stationery Office, London.

Klem ML, Wing RR, McGuire MT *et al.* (1997) A descriptive study of individuals successful at long-term maintenance of substantial weight loss. *Am J Clin Nutr* **66**: 239–46.

Krotkiewski M, Mandroukas K and Sjostrom L (1979) Effects of long term physical training on body fat, metabolism and blood pressure in obesity. *Metabolism* **28**: 650–8.

Lee C, Blair SN and Jackson AS (1999) Cardiorespiratory fitness, body composition, and all cause and cardiovascular disease mortality in men. *Am J Clin Nutr* **69**: 373–80.

Manson JE, Rimm EB, Stampfer MJ *et al.* (1991) Physical activity and incidence of non-insulin dependant diabetes mellitus in women. *Lancet* **338**: 774–8.

Manson JE, Nathan DM, Krolewski AS *et al.* (1992) A prospective study of exercise and incidence of diabetes among US male physicians. *JAMA* **268**: 63–7.

McArdle WD, Katch FI and Katch VL (1996) *Exercise Physiology, Energy, Nutrition and Human Performance*, 4th edn. Williams & Wilkins, Baltimore.

McAuley KA, Williams SM, Mann JI *et al.* (2002) Intensive lifestyle changes are necessary to improve insulin sensitivity. *Diabetes Care* **25**: 445–52.

Miller WC, Koceja DM and Hamilton EJ (1997) A meta-analysis of the past 25 years weight loss research using diet, exercise or diet plus exercise intervention. *Int J Obes* **21**: 941–7.

Miller WC (1999) How effective are traditional dietary and exercise interventions for weight loss? *Med Sci Sports Exerc* **31**(8): 1129–34.

National Institutes of Health (1998) National Heart, Lung and Blood Institute: *The practical guide. Identification, evaluation, and treatment of overweight and obesity in adults.* NIH publication, Bethesda MD.

Owens S, Gutin B, Allison J *et al.* (1999) Effect of physical training on total and visceral fat in obese children. *Med Sci Sports Exerc* **31**: 143–8.

Parker DL (1991) Juvenile obesity. The importance of exercise and getting children to do it. *Phys Sports Med* **19**: 113–25.

Physical Activity Task Force (1995) *More People More Active More Often–Physical Activity in England A Consultation Paper*. Department of Health, London.

Prentice AM and Jebb SA (1995) Obesity in Britain: gluttony or sloth? *Br Med J* **311**: 437–9.

Ravussin E (1995) Energy expenditure and body weight. In Brownell KD and Fairburn CG (eds) *Eating Disorders and Obesity*. The Guilford Press, New York.

Ravussin E and Swinburn BA (1992) Pathophysiology of obesity. *Lancet* **340**: pp. 404–408.

Rissanen A and Fogelholm M (1999) Physical activity in the prevention and treatment of other morbid conditions and impairments associated with obesity: current evidence and research issues. *Med. Sci. Sports Exerc* **31**: S635–S645.

Roberts SB and Leibel RL (1998) Excess energy intake and low energy expenditure as predictors of obesity. *Int J Obes* **22**: 385–6.

Rocchini AP, Katch V, Anderson J *et al*. (1988) Blood pressure in obese adolescents: effect of weight loss. *Paediatrics* **82**: 16–23.

Rodin J, Silberstein LR and Striegel-Moore RH (1985) Women and weight: a normative discontent. *Nebr Symp Motiv* **32**: 20–35.

Rosenbaum M and Leibel RL (1998) The physiology of body weight regulation: Relevance to the etiology of obesity in children. *Paediatrics* **101**: 525–40.

Ross R and Janssen I (1999) Is abdominal fat preferentially reduced in response to exercise-induced weight loss? *Med Sci Sports Exerc* **31**: S568–S572.

Ruderman NB, Ganada OP and Johansen K (1979) The effect of physical training on glucose tolerance and plasma lipids in maturity-onset diabetes. *Diabetes* **28**: 89–94.

Sallis JF and Owen N (1997) *Physical Activity and Behavioural Medicine*. Sage, California.

Saltin B, Lindgarde F, Houston M *et al*. (1979) Physical training and glucose tolerance in middle-aged men with chemical diabetes. *Diabetes* **28**: 30–79.

Sargeant LA, Wareham NJ and Khaw KT (2000) Family history of diabetes identifies a group at increased risk for the metabolic consequences of obesity and physical inactivity in EPIC-Norfolk: a population based study. *Int J Obes* **24**: 1333–9.

Sasaki J, Shindo M, Tanaka H *et al*. (1987) A long term aerobic exercise program decreases the obesity index and increases the high density lipoprotein cholesterol concentration in obese children. *Int J Obes* **11**: 339–45.

Seidell JC (1998) Epidemiology: definition and classification of obesity. In Kopelman PG and Stock MJ *Clinical Obesity*. Blackwell Science, London.

Schmitz KH, Jacobs DR, Leon AS *et al*. (2000) Physical activity and body weight associations over ten years in the CARDIA study. *Int J Obes* **24**: 1475–87.

Schneider SH, Vitug A and Ruderman AB (1986) Atherosclerosis and physical activity. *Diabetes Metab Rev* **1**: 445–81.

Schneider SH, Khachadurian AK and Amorosa LF *et al*. (1992) Ten-year experience with an exercise-based outpatient lifestyle modification program in the treatment of diabetes mellitus. *Diabetes Care* **15**: 1800–10.

Schulz LO and Schoeller DA (1994) A compilation of total daily energy expenditures and body weights in healthy adults. *Am J Clin Nut* **60**: 676–81.

Stofan JR, Dipietro L, Davis D *et al*. (1998) Physical activity patterns associated with cardiorespiratory fitness and reduced mortality: The aerobics center longitudinal study. *Am J Publ Health* **88**: 1807–13.

Stucky-Ropp RC and Dilorenzo TM (1993) Determinants of exercise in children. *Prev Med* **22**: 880–9.

Surgeon General's Report (1996) *Physical activity and health: a report of the surgeon general*. US Department of Health and Human Services, Washington, DC.

Sullivan M, Sullivan M, Karlsson J *et al*. (1993) Swedish obese subjects (SOS) – an intervention study of obesity. Baseline evaluation of health and psychosocial functioning in the first 1743 subjects examined. *Int J Obes* **17**: 503–12.

Thompson CE and Wankel LM (1980) The effects of perceived activity choice upon frequency of exercise behaviour. *J App Soc Psyc* **10**: 436–43.

Tuomilehto J, Lindstrom J, Eriksson JG *et al.* (2001) Prevention of type 2 diabetes mellitus by change in lifestyle among subjects with impaired glucose tolerance. *N Engl J Med* **344**: 1343–50.

Vanninen E, Uusitupa M and Siitonen O (1992) Habitual physical activity, aerobic capacity, and metabolic control in patients with newly diagnosed type 2 diabetes mellitus: Effect of a 1 year diet and exercise intervention. *Diabetologia* **35**: 340–6.

Wadden TA and Foster GD (2000) Behavioral treatment of obesity. *Med Clin N Am* **84**(2): 441–61.

Wadden TA, Sarwer DB and Berkowitz RI (1999) Behavioural treatment of the overweight patient. *Baillière's Clin Endocrinol Metab* **13**(1): 93–107.

Wankel LM and Kreisel PSJ (1985) Factors underlying enjoyment of youth sports: Sport and age group comparisons. *J Sports Psyc* **7**: 51–64.

World Health Organization (1997) *Obesity: Preventing and managing the global epidemic. Report of a WHO consultation on obesity*. WHO, Geneva, Switzerland.

9

Diabetes, Obesity and Cardiovascular Disease – Therapeutic Implications

Jayadave Shakher and **Anthony H. Barnett**

Introduction

Obesity and overweight are independent risk factors for cardiovascular morbidity and mortality (Sjostrom, 1992a,b; Allison *et al.* 1999). These figures are mainly based on the epidemiological studies in a white population. There may be gender and ethnic differences, as for example, coronary heart disease risk is proportionately increased at a lower body mass index (BMI) in the Asian population. Risk of morbidity and mortality begins to rise at BMI $> 25\,\mathrm{kg/m^2}$ and the risk increases sharply at BMI $> 30\,\mathrm{kg/m^2}$. Although BMI is used as a surrogate indicator of cardiovascular risks, central or abdominal obesity is considered to be a better predictor.

The mechanism by which obesity causes increased cardiovascular morbidity and mortality is attributed to associated co-morbidities and risk factors such as hypertension, dyslipidaemia, type 2 diabetes and insulin resistance. The co-occurrence of some or all of these risk factors along with obesity is termed the cardiometabolic syndrome.

Until recently the mechanism of atherosclerosis in obesity was not well understood. The recognition of adipose tissue as a metabolically active endocrine organ, capable of synthesizing and secreting mediators like tumour necrosis factor-α (TNF-α), interleukin-6 (IL-6), plasminogen activator inhibitor-1 (PAI-1)

Obesity and Diabetes. Edited by Anthony H. Barnett and Sudhesh Kumar
© 2004 John Wiley & Sons, Ltd ISBN: 0-470-84898-7

and angiotensin II (AII) may help explain the process of accelerated atherosclerosis. Endothelial dysfunction, which is a recognized complication of obesity and type 2 diabetes mellitus, plays an important role in thrombus formation. The secretion of adipocytokines like adiponectin may be implicated in the pathogenesis of type 2 diabetes mellitus. Thus, favourably modifying lipids, decreasing blood pressure, achieving near normoglycaemia, and reducing pro-inflammatory cytokines and adhesion molecules through weight loss and pharmocotherapy, may prevent progression of atherosclerosis or occurrence of acute coronary syndrome events in obese high risk populations with type 2 diabetes.

Obesity and mortality

The association between excess body weight and death is confirmed by the Nurses' Health Study, with mortality rising progressively in woman with BMI > 29 kg/m^2 (Manson *et al.* 1995). The increased mortality was also noted in the American Cancer Society's Cancer Prevention Study I and II. Cancer Prevention Study II involved 457 785 men and 588 369 women followed for 14 years. The lowest mortality for men was within BMI 23.5–24.9 kg/m^2 and for women 22.0–23.4 kg/m^2. For BMI > 40 kg/m^2, the relative risk of death was 2.6 times higher for men and 2 times higher for women compared with BMI between 23.5 and 24.9. There was an ethnic difference with the relative risk of death – 1.4 for black men and 1.2 black women with a BMI > 40 kg/m^2 (Calle *et al.*, 1999).

Obesity and cardiovascular disease

Obesity is a major contributor to the risk of cardiovascular disease. In the Framingham Heart Study, the 26-year incidence of coronary heart disease (CHD) was increased by a factor of 2.4 in obese women and 2 in obese men under age of 50 years (Hubert *et al.*, 1983). Excess weight was an independent predictor of coronary artery disease, coronary death and congestive heart failure after adjusting for other known recognized risk factors.

In the Nurses' Health Study from the United States, the risk of developing CHD increased 3.3-fold with BMI > 29 kg/m^2 and 1.8-fold between 25 and 29 kg/m^2, compared to those women with BMI < 21 kg/m^2 (Manson *et al.*, 1990, 1995). Each kg of weight gained from the age of 18 years was associated with 3.1% higher risk of cardiovascular disease (Willett *et al.*, 1995).

This increased risk extends to overweight children and adolescents, who are at risk of premature cardiovascular morbidity and death. Excess weight in adolescence was a better predictor of these risks than excessive weight in adulthood (Gunnell *et al.*, 1998).

Along with an increased risk of CHD, obese populations experience a higher recurrence of cardiac event rates after acute myocardial infarction. The relative risk of recurrent infarction or death was 1.5 with BMI 30–34.5 kg/m^2 and 1.8 with BMI $>$ 35 kg/m^2 compared to BMI 16–24 kg/m^2 as seen in a population based study of 2541 patients (Rea *et al.*, 2001).

The increased CHD risk is better correlated with abdominal or central obesity than simple BMI (Rich-Edwards *et al.*, 1995). In the Nurses' Health Study, a waist–hip ratio (WHR) of $\geq$0.88 versus WHR $<$ 0.72 was associated with an increased relative risk of CHD of 3.25 (Rexrode *et al.*, 1998).

The increased CHD morbidity and mortality could be related to traditional risk factors like hypertension and dyslipidaemia or due to the effect of obesity *per se* on the cardiovasculature. Obesity is associated with disturbances in cardiac function and structural changes in the absence of hypertension and underlying organic heart disease. There is an increase in total blood volume in proportion to body weight resulting in higher cardiac output. Volume overload of the left ventricle results in increased left ventricular stress which stimulates eccentric hypertrophy of the ventricle with resultant diastolic dysfunction. Over time, excessive wall stress causes ventricular dilatation resulting in systolic dysfunction, termed obesity cardiomyopathy. The presence of hypertension in obesity exacerbates left ventricular wall changes, which can increase progression towards heart failure (Albert and Hashini, 1993).

Left ventricular wall abnormality is implicated in the propensity for sudden death seen in obesity. The reason for sudden death from cardiomyopathy may be due to complex ventricular arrhythmias. Prolonged Q-T interval which predisposes to cardiac arrhythmias, occurs in up to one third of obese subjects (Frank *et al.*, 1986). Other ECG changes observed in a study of 100 obese subjects compared with 100 normal subjects, without any evidence of cardiac disease included more leftward shift of P, QRS and T axes, evidence of left ventricular hypertrophy and left atrial abnormality and T-wave flattening seen in the inferior and lateral leads (Alpert *et al.*, 2000). Autonomic dysfunction due to alteration in parasympathetic and sympathetic cardiac innervation may also contribute towards arrhythmias.

The structural and functional changes are also seen in the right side of the heart in obesity. Right ventricular dysfunction could be secondary to left ventricular dysfunction or due to obstructive sleep apnoea and/or obesity hyperventilation syndrome which occurs in 5 per cent of morbidly obese individuals (Alpert and Hashini, 1993).

Obesity and hypertension

A rise in blood pressure is associated with increased body weight. Epidemiological studies indicate that obesity is a strong independent risk factor for hypertension (Modan *et al.*, 1985; Stamler *et al.*, 1993). In the Framingham Study, for example, the prevalence of hypertension among obese individuals was twice that of those individuals with normal weight irrespective of sex and age (Hubert *et al.*, 1983). The INTERSALT Study involving 10 000 men and women showed that a 10-kg increase in weight was associated with 3-mmHg rise in systolic and 2.3-mmHg rise in diastolic blood pressure (Dyer and Elliott, 1989). This level of blood pressure elevation is associated with a 12 per cent increase risk for CHD and 24 per cent increase for stroke. In the Nurses' Health Study, the relative risk of hypertension in those women who gained 5.0 to 9.9 kg and greater than 25.0 kg was 1.7 and 5.2, respectively (Huang *et al.*, 1998). The risk of hypertension was even higher with abdominal obesity (WHR $\geq$ 0.9 in men and $\geq$ 0.85 in women) (Blair *et al.*, 1984).

The exact mechanism of the association of central obesity and hypertension is not fully defined. Insulin resistance may provide a metabolic link perhaps through hyperinsulinaemia. Hyperinsulinaemia enhances sodium reabsorption directly through its effects on distal renal tubules (De Fronzo *et al.*, 1975) and indirectly through the stimulation of central sympathetic nervous system (Moan *et al.*, 1995; Rearen *et al.*, 1996). It also augments angiotensin-II-mediated aldosterone secretion (Landsberg, 1992). The resultant hypervolaemia causes an increase in cardiac output, yet the total peripheral resistance remains near normal with failure of vasodilatation of the systemic vasculature. Vasodilation is thought to be mediated by nitric oxide (NO) and this vasodilatory effect is blunted in obese and hypertensive subjects (Baron *et al.*, 1995; Steinberg *et al.*, 1996).

Another mechanism which may cause increased vascular tone is through alterations in cation transport. Insulin has been shown to stimulate NA/K ATPase activity with accumulation of intracellular sodium along with increase in intracellular calcium leading to vascular resistance and hypertension (Sowers and Draznin, 1998).

This link between hyperinsulinaemia and hypertension is not seen in Pima Indians despite commonly having hyperinsulinaemia, insulin resistance and obesity (Saad *et al.*, 1991). These discrepancies might be explained by difference in genetic susceptibility to the development of hypertension or to the effects of insulin on blood pressure. Another explanation is that there might be 'selective insulin resistance' with impaired ability of insulin to cause glucose uptake, but preservation of some actions such as renal sodium retention, activation of the renin–angiotensin system, alteration in cation flux and stimulation of the sympathetic nervous system.

Obesity and dyslipidaemia

Obesity is associated with alteration in lipoprotein metabolism resulting in increase in total cholesterol (TC), triglycerides (TG), low-density lipoprotein cholesterol (LDLc), very-low-density lipoprotein cholesterol (VLDL) and reduced level of high-density cholesterol (HDLc) (Hubert *et al.*, 1983; Grundy and Barnett, 1990). Epidemiological studies such as the Framingham Heart

Study and the Multiple Risk Factor Intervention Trial (MRFIT) showed a significant positive correlation between plasma cholesterol levels and increased risk of death due to CHD (Stamler *et al.*, 1993).

In the PROCAM study, involving 4407 German men aged between 40 and 65 years, without cardiac disease at the start of the study, the combination of high TG, TC and low HDL levels for example was associated with the increased risk of coronary heart disease. In men with plasma cholesterol levels above 6.5 mmol/l with HDLc less than 0.9 mmol/l, the risk of myocardial infarction over 6 years was as high as 20–30 per cent (Assmann and Schulte, 1992).

Indeed, epidemiological studies confirm that low plasma HDL cholesterol is a better predictor of risk of CHD. The univariate analysis of the data from PROCAM indicates a significant association between CHD and HDL ($P <$ 0.001), which remained after adjustment for other risk factors (Assmann and Schulte, 1992). The Framingham Study also shows a clear correlation between low HDLc and increased risk of CHD mortality and morbidity, regardless of LDL cholesterol levels (Hubert *et al.*, 1983).

Although there is an inverse relationship between low HDL and elevated triglyceride levels, triglyceride concentration as an independent risk factor of coronary heart disease remains controversial. Studies such as the PROCAM, the Stockholm Prospective Study and the Paris Prospective Study showed positive correlations between TG and CHD risks (Carlson *et al.*, 1979; Cambien *et al.*, 1986; Assmann *et al.*, 1998).

The meta-analyses of 16 population-based studies showed that after adjusting for HDLc, every 1 mmol/l increase in TG was associated with relative risk increase in CHD by 14 per cent in men and 37 per cent in women (Austin *et al.*, 1998).

Despite the controversy, there is a growing consensus that TG directly causes atherosclerotic cardiovascular disease, or at least acts as a marker for CHD risk factors. The pathogenesis of atherosclerosis is believed to be related to TG-rich lipoproteins (TGRLPs) which include VLDL, chylomicrons, and their remnants and IDL, all of which contain more cholesterol than LDLc (NIH Consensus Panel, 1993; Krauss, 1998; Hodis, 1999). These small TGRLPs appear to possess atherogenic potential similar to small dense LDLc, with ability to infiltrate arterial wall and leads to atherosclerosis (Ross, 1999).

The role of LDLc in the pathogenesis of CHD has been well established and indeed the predominance of small, dense LDL particles are reported to be more prevalent in CHD patients than in healthy controls (Fisher, 1983). This was confirmed in the Quebec Cardiovascular Study, which showed dense LDL particles are associated with increase risk of CHD over 5 years and the combination of small dense LDLc and elevated apolipoprotein B (ApoB) concentration resulted in a six-fold increase in risk of CHD (Lamarche *et al.*, 1996, 1997). Plasma insulin levels were found to be 18 per cent higher in men who develop CHD compared to men who remain healthy and fasting plasma insulin concentration was found to be an independent CHD risk factor after taking into account lipid and lipoprotein concentration (Despres *et al.*, 1996).

Though ApoB and LDLc are considered as good predictors of CHD, the use of ApoB in clinical practice is limited by lack of standardization and calculation of LDLc using the Friedewald equation (LDLc = TC − HDLc − TG/2.2 mmol/l) is less accurate with increasing TG levels and inapplicable at TG > 4.52 mmol/l (Friedewald *et al.*, 1972).

Recently, non-HDLc was considered to be a better predictor of CHD risk as it encompasses all cholesterol present in atherogenic lipoprotein particles (VLDL, IDL, LDL, lipoprotein a) and there appears to be a correlation between non-HDLc and ApoB. The measurement of non-HDLc (total cholesterol minus HDLc) required only TC and HDLc, which can be measured in non-fasting samples (Frost and Harel, 1998).

Obesity, type 2 diabetes and insulin resistance

Insulin resistance is a common feature of obesity and its incidence rises with increasing BMI. Visceral obesity is an even better predictor than BMI of hyperinsulinaemia, insulin resistance and type 2 diabetes (Despres, 1998; Ferrannini and Camastra, 1998). The clustering of cardiovascular risk factors with insulin resistance was first described as syndrome X by Reaven in 1988 and included central obesity, hypertension, glucose intolerance and dyslipidaemia (the 'deadly quartet') (De Fronzo and Ferrannini, 1991; Reaven, 1993; Williams, 1994). Other features of the syndrome have since been added to include a pro-coagulant state and accelerated atherosclerosis, appropriately called the 'cardiometabolic syndrome'. Recent guidelines from the National Cholesterol Education Programme (Adult Treatment Panel III, ATP III) suggests that clinical criteria for definition of insulin resistance or metabolic syndrome should be based upon any three of the following (Executive Summary, 2002; Figure 9.1).

1. Abdominal obesity defined as waist circumference in men of > 102 cm (40 in) and in woman more than 88 cm (35 in)

2. Fasting triglyceride level > 150 mg/dl (1.7 mmol/l).

3. HDL cholesterol < 40 mg/dl (< 1 mmol in men)
   < 50 mg/dl (< 1.3 mmol in women)

4. Blood pressure ≥ 130/85 mmHg

5. Fasting glucose > 110 mg/dl (> 6.1 mmol/l)

Based on these criteria, the Third National Health and Nutrition Examinations Survey (NHANES), found an overall prevalence of metabolic syndrome at 22 per cent and the prevalence increasing steadily with age. African-American women

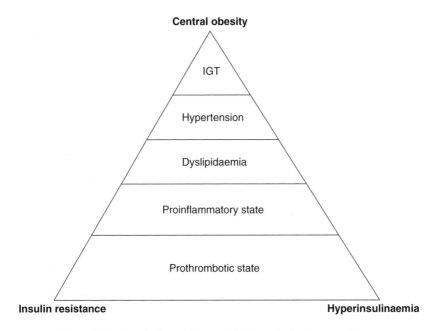

Figure 9.1   Metabolic syndrome. IGT, impaired glucose tolerance.

have approximately 57 per cent higher prevalence and Hispanic women have approximately 26 per cent higher prevalence than their male counterparts. Ford and colleagues found that in men and women with metabolic syndrome from NHANES, approximately 50 per cent showed evidence of insulin resistance suggesting that the link between obesity and IGT or type 2 diabetes may be through this mechanism (Ford *et al.*, 2002).

There are a variety of factors that contribute to insulin resistance, including the distribution of body fat, the role of free fatty acids (FFA), adipocytokines, proinflammatory mediators and genetic factors.

In obese individuals, there is increased release of FFA from the visceral fat which is more resistant to the metabolic effect of insulin and more sensitive to lipolytic hormones. An increased delivery of FFA to the liver may reduce insulin binding to hepatocytes, and impair insulin action with increased hepatic glucose production. Along with increased production of FFA, there is decreased utilization with defects in uptake and oxidation of FFA by the skeletal muscle in obesity and type 2 diabetes (Jensen *et al.*, 1989; Wiesenthal *et al.*, 1999). Regular exercise induces an increase in type 1 (aerobic, red) muscle fibres with enhanced insulin sensitivity by utilizing FFA, whereas type 2 (anaerobic, white) fibres predominate in sedentary subjects contributing to insulin resistance (McFarlane *et al.*, 2001).

Fat cells produce adiponectin and resistin, which may play a role in development of insulin resistance and type 2 diabetes. A low concentration of adiponectin is related to insulin resistance and hyperinsulinaemia and has an increased risk of type 2 diabetes in human subjects. The administration of thiazolidine-diones in insulin-resistant subjects increases serum adiponectin levels without affecting body weight (Weyer *et al.*, 2001; Lindsay *et al.*, 2002). There is a debate about the physiological role of resistin in human subjects, but in mice administration of resistin reduces insulin-stimulated glucose uptake (Steppan *et al.*, 2001).

TNF-α, an inflammatory cytokine, also secreted by adipocytes, is elevated in animal models of obesity and insulin resistance and neutralization of TNF-α ameliorates insulin resistance in obese rats. TNF-α mRNA expression is increased in obesity and levels of TNF-α correlate with serum insulin and BMI.

TNF-α is implicated in causing insulin resistance by different mechanisms. It increases hormone sensitive lipase activity with resultant FFA release from adipose tissue stores to the liver. At the post-receptor level, TNF-α interferes with insulin signalling and insulin receptor substrate (IRS) protein formation. This impairs insulin-mediated glucose uptake by adipocytes through down regulation of GLUT 4, the insulin-responsive glucose transporter. It also down-regulates peroxisome proliferator-actived receptor expression (Hauner *et al.*, 1995; Kern *et al.*, 1995).

There may be genetic factors which contribute to developing insulin resistance. Disruption of the IRS gene (*IRS-2*) in mice, results in insulin resistance and hyperglycaemia. A β 3 adrenergic receptor mutation in humans is associated with high risks of obesity and early onset of type 2 diabetes (Walston *et al.*, 1995; Withers *et al.*, 1998). The β 3 adrenergic receptor regulates lipolysis in visceral fat and increases thermogenesis. CD36 deficiency is also associated with higher serum TG, raised fasting plasma glucose, lower serum HDLc and increased blood pressure. CD36 is a fatty acid transporter and one of the macrophage scavenger receptors. The exact mechanism by which it causes the insulin resistance syndrome is not yet established (Miyaoka *et al.*, 2001).

Obesity and type 2 diabetes

Obesity is a powerful risk factor for the development of type 2 diabetes and more than two-thirds of patients with type 2 diabetes are obese. The risk of type 2 diabetes correlates positively with increasing obesity (Larsson *et al.*, 1981; Harris, 1989). In the Nurses Health Study, the risk of developing diabetes increased five-fold in women with BMI of $25 \, \text{kg/m}^2$ compared with those with BMI of $22 \, \text{kg/m}^2$ The risk becomes higher reaching 28-fold with BMI of $30 \, \text{kg/m}^2$ and 93-fold with BMI $> 35 \, \text{kg/m}^2$ (Colditz *et al.*, 1996).

The risk of obesity and type 2 diabetes was better defined by a high WHR and waist circumference (Larsson *et al.*, 1984). Additionally, the duration of obesity was directly related to the risk of diabetes (Everhart *et al.*, 1992). The risk of type 2 diabetes from obesity is more prevalent across certain ethnic groups such as South Asians and Afro-Caribbeans (Bhopal, 2002).

The increasing prevalence of type 2 diabetes is paralleled by the rise in the level of obesity in the general population. This process occurred over too short a period to implicate genetic factors *per se*. It is most likely that environmental factors interact with genetic susceptibility in the pathogenesis of type 2 diabetes. The 'thrifty genotype hypothesis' has been proposed as an explanation for the increased prevalence of type 2 diabetes. This hypothesis suggests that during times of famine alternating with times of plenty, the ability to store fat efficiently leads to a survival advantage. In western society, when there is permanent 'plenty', this genetic 'advantage' has become a liability with increased risk of development of obesity and diabetes (Neel, 1962).

Insulin resistance and cardiovascular disease

Various studies have shown that hyperinsulinaemia is a predictor of cardio-vascular disease. The Quebec Study showed that fasting insulin concentrations are independent predictors of CHD. Haffner and colleagues found that people who developed diabetes had higher fasting glucose and insulin concentrations along with elevated blood pressure, lower HDLc and higher TG than in those whose glucose metabolism remained normal. Thus, for the macrovascular complications of type 2 diabetes like stroke or myocardial infarction, the period of increased risk begins or 'the clock starts ticking' even before the onset of hyperglycaemia (Haffner *et al.*, 1990).

Evidence is emerging that inflammation and endothelial dysfunction are likely to be the important contributors to the accelerated atherosclerosis seen in people with insulin resistance, obesity and type 2 diabetes. Atherosclerosis precedes the development of type 2 diabetes and the inflammation may be involved in the underlying process (Pradhan and Ridker, 2002).

Yudkin *et al.* (1999) showed that inflammatory markers like C-reactive protein (CRP), pro-inflammatory cytokines, IL-6 and TNF-α correlate with obesity and IR. In a prospective study, Pradhan *et al.* (2001) followed 27 628 women free of diagnosis of diabetes and cardiovascular disease for 4 years and found that baseline elevated markers of systemic inflammation like CRP and IL-6 powerfully predict the development of type 2 diabetes. Ridker *et al.* found that elevated level of CRP in the previously healthy women predicted the development of type 2 diabetes as well as likelihood of developing myocardial infarction (Pradhan and Ridker, 2002).

Increased levels of circulating inflammatory markers are also found in groups at risk of developing type 2 diabetes such as obese children, women with poly-cystic ovary syndrome, women with a family history of type 2 diabetes and people of South Asian origin and Pima Indians, independently of total BMI (Cook *et al.*, 2000; Forouhi *et al.*, 2001; Kelly *et al.*, 2001; Pannacciulli *et al.*, 2002). These studies showed that inflammatory markers which are related to atherosclerosis also predicted the onset of cardiovascular disease and type 2 diabetes ('common soil hypothesis') (Stern, 1995; Pradhan and Ridker, 2002).

Loss of normal endothelial cell (EC) function is thought to be an early marker of development of atherosclerosis. In type 2 diabetes, there is early endothelial injury probably as a result of hyperglycaemia, hypertension, dyslipidaemia and insulin resistance. Impaired EC dysfunction is also seen in the early stages of diabetes, IGT and in first degree relatives of type 2 diabetes (Figures 9.2 and 9.3).

EC serve as a metabolically active barrier between the lumen and the vessel wall and play a pivotal role in vascular homeostasis. Normal endothelial function includes regulation of vasomotor tone, homeostasis, leucocyte trafficking and vascular smooth muscle cell proliferation and migration. Endothelial cells elaborates Nitric oxide (NO) which mediates vasodilation, antagonizes thrombosis, and has anti-inflammatory properties and inhibits growth of vascular smooth muscle cells (VSMC) (McVeigh *et al.*, 1992; Williams *et al.*, 1996; Stehouwer *et al.*, 1997; Loscalzo, 2001; Storey *et al.*, 2001). In a dysfunctional state, apart from the loss of NO secretion, EC release substances such as AII and endothelin. They mediate vasoconstriction, aggravate thrombosis and activate platelets. These substances are proinflammatory and in the absence of NO, promote growth of VSMC and stimulate adhesion molecules like ICAM and VCAM (intracellular and vascular cell adhesion molecules) (Lim *et al.*, 1999; Figure 9.3).

The mechanisms of EC dysfunction are secondary to hyperglycaemia and resistance to insulin. Hyperglycaemia contributes to EC dysfunction in several ways (glucose hypothesis). Exposure to a high glucose level results in intracellular hyperglycaemia that damages the cells by several mechanisms. These

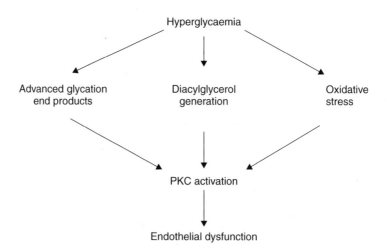

Figure 9.2 Mechanisms of hyperglycaemia – induced endothelial dysfunction. PKC, protein kinase C.

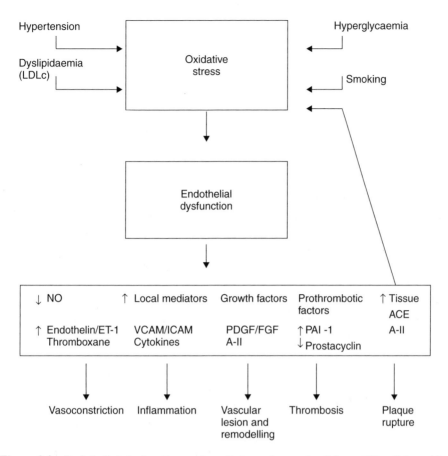

Figure 9.3 Endothelial dysfunction and mediators of vascular injury. NO, nitric oxide; VCAM, vascular cell adhesion molecule; ICAM intracellular adhesion molecule; PDGF, platelet-derived growth factor; FGF, fibroblast growth factor; AII, angiotensin II; PAI-1, plasminogen activator inhibitor-1.

include increased activity of the aldose reductase/sorbitol pathway, increased formation of advanced glycation end products (AGE) and increased synthesis of diacylglycerol (DAG) with generation of protein kinase C (PKC). All these mechanisms reflect a single upstream process which is the overproduction of superoxide by the mitochondrial electron transport chain. Generation of super-oxide O_2 reduces the availability of NO (Hawthorne *et al.*, 1989; Bucala *et al.*, 1991; Wolf *et al.*, 1991; Tesfamariam *et al.*, 1993; Figure 9.2).

Insulin resistance has shown to be associated with EC dysfunction even in the absence of hyperglycaemia (insulin hypothesis). Insulin resistance is implicated in the development of cardiovascular disease. Postreceptor pathway involving phosphatidylinositol-3 (PI-3) kinase activity is implicated in insulin resistance. Insulin normally binds to its receptors and phosphorylates IRS-1, which in turn activates the PI-3 kinase. PI-3 kinase plays a major role in both insulin mediated glucose disposal in adipose tissue and also in NO production by the EC.

The insulin stimulation of PI-3 kinase is reduced in obese subjects and almost absent in type 2 diabetes (Nolan *et al.*, 1997), whereas, insulin action on the mitogen-activated protein kinase (MAPK) is unaffected. This 'selective insulin resistance' results in enhancement of the mitogenic pathway with increased VSMC growth and migration and increase in plasminogen activator inhibitor-1 (PAI-1) and endothelin. This pathway is present in vasculature, heart and kidneys (Begum *et al.*, 1998).

Adipocytes also contribute towards endothelial dysfunction. Adipocyte releases IL-6 and TNF-α. IL-6 is one of the key promoter of hepatic CRP synthesis. CRP in turn has been shown to down-regulates ENOS *in vitro* and also regulates PAI-1 synthesis and secretion. TNF-α may have a direct effect on EC (Hotamisligil *et al.* (1993).

Endothelial dysfunction predisposes to atherosclerosis in the presence of increased prothrombotic factors like coagulation abnormalities, increased platelet activation, inflammatory mediators and the presence of oxidized lipoproteins.

Visceral obesity and insulin resistance are associated with an increased level of PAI-1, increased plasma level of fibrinogen, factor VII, and factor VIII C coagulant activities. High levels of PAI-1 predisposes to CHD. Hyperinsulinaemia, hyperglycaemia and A II are all important simulators of PAI-1 gene expression and PAI-1 production (Meigs *et al.*, 1997; McFarlane *et al.*, 2001). Elevated PAI-1 levels have been found in non-diabetic first degree relatives of type 2 diabetic probands and in patients with established cardiovascular disease. Hyperfibrinogenaemia is a strong independent risk factor for CHD and acts synergistically with dyslipidaemia and hypertension to promote atherosclerosis (Thompson *et al.*, 1995).

Type 2 diabetes and dyslipidaemia

Dyslipidaemia is common in type 2 diabetes and contributes significantly to the increased risk of CHD. The characteristic dyslipidaemia consists of elevated TG and low HDLc (Syvanne and Taskinen, 1997; Haffner, 1998). The Framingham Heart Study reported no difference with regards to total and LDL cholesterol levels between diabetic men and women compared with their non-diabetic counterparts. People with diabetes, however, have an increased proportion of small dense atherogenic LDL particles and twice the prevalence of low HDLc with high TG compared with non-diabetics (Tchernof *et al.*, 1996; Laakso, 1997).

Low HDL levels are independent predictors of CHD and have a strong inverse relationship with TG levels. The risk weakens as the HDLc concentration rises above 1 mmol/l. In the UKPDS there is a significant association between the risk of CHD and elevated levels of LDLc and TG and decreased concentration of HDLc. For each 1 mmol/l increase in LDL concentration, there was 1.57-fold increase in the risk of CHD and for each increase in 0.1 mmol/l of HDL cholesterol the risk was decreased by 0.15-fold (Turner *et al.*, 1998).

Some studies have reported that TG are better predictors of CHD risks than LDLc. The Diabetes Intervention Study and the PARIS prospective study demonstrated that TG levels were significantly higher in people who died from CHD than who survived (Fontbonne *et al.*, 1989; Hanefeld *et al.*, 1996). The mechanism by which raised TG cause atherosclerosis is attributed to the presence of TG-rich lipoproteins (TGRLPs), as described above.

There are also changes to apolipoprotein composition in diabetic patients with increased susceptibility of apolipoproteins A1 and B to glycation which results in decreased affinity for HDL receptors and increased susceptibility to oxidative modification (Hedrick *et al.*, 2000).

Type 2 diabetes and hypertension

The prevalence of hypertension in the diabetic population is 1.5 to 3 times higher than that of the non-diabetic age-matched population (Wingard, 1995). In type 2 diabetes, hypertension may be present at the time of the diagnosis or precedes the development of hyperglycaemia (HDS, 1993) and is implicated in development of both micro- and macrovascular complications. Epidemiological studies indicate that diabetic individuals with hypertension have greatly increased risks of cardiovascular disease, renal inefficiency and retinopathy. In UKPDS, every 10-mm rise in systolic blood pressure was associated with a 15 per cent increase in risk of coronary artery disease. Both systolic and diastolic hypertension markedly accentuate the progression of diabetic nephropathy and aggressive antihypertensive management will decrease the rate of fall of glomerular filtration rate (UKPDS, 1998).

Hypertension is also implicated as a risk factor for diabetic retinopathy resulting in increasing hard exudate, hemorrhage and progression of diabetic retinopathy. Studies in the diabetic population have shown a markedly higher frequency of progression of diabetic retinopathy when diastolic blood pressure is in excess of 70 mm (Janka *et al.*, 1989).

The pathophysiology of hypertension in diabetes is postulated to be related to hyperinsulinaemia. (for mechanisms, see Obesity and hypertension) (De Fronzo *et al.*, 1975; Moan *et al.*, 1995; Reaven *et al.*, 1996). Apart from the functional changes, diabetes can cause arterial wall structural changes. This may be due to non-enzymatic glycation of proteins including collagen and other matrix proteins to form AGEs (Bucala *et al.*, 1991).

Type 2 diabetes and CHD

Type 2 diabetes predisposes to macrovascular complications such as myocardial infarction, peripheral vascular disease and stroke. Epidemiological studies have shown that the risk of CHD is increased two- to six-fold in patients with type 2 diabetes compared with non-diabetic subjects (Pyörälä *et al.*, 1987; Stamler *et al.*, 1993). Indeed, in the non-diabetic subjects, there has been a substantial decline in mortality from coronary heart disease in many parts of the world in recent years. The effect was considerably less in adults with diabetes with perhaps even an increase in women with diabetes (Gu *et al.*, 1999).

More than 50 per cent of diabetic patients have evidence of CHD at diagnosis, which does not take into account the high prevalence of sub-clinical CHD in the diabetic population (Kuller *et al.*, 2000). Conversely, among people with established CHD, there is a high prevalence of diabetes. In fact, one-quarter of patients who had myocardial infarction in the PROCAM Study have diabetes (Assmann *et al.*, 1997).

CHD is responsible for more than three quarters of deaths in type 2 diabetic patients and mortality from CHD is approximately three times higher in diabetic patients than in the general population (Kannel and McGee, 1979; Jarrett and Shipley, 1985). In the PROCAM study, there were 419 diabetic patients among the cohort of 4849 men and overall mortality was twice as high in diabetic group compared with non-diabetic subjects. The excess mortality was largely explained by cardiovascular mortality. (Assmann *et al.*, 1997). The cardioprotective effect in females is lost in diabetes and the proportionate increase in CHD mortality is significantly greater in women than in men (Smith *et al.*, 1984).

There is also an ethnic variation in the prevalence CHD, with lower rate of prevalence in the Japanese population in both diabetic and non-diabetic persons (Sabaki *et al.*, 1989). This is in contrast to the high risk of CHD among south Asian migrants to the UK and elsewhere (Bhopal, 2002). This population has increased susceptibility to insulin resistance and type 2 diabetes with a tendency to abdominal fat deposition and abnormal lipid profile. Pima Indians who are obese with a high prevalence of diabetes, however, have a lower risk of dying from CHD compared with the non-diabetic population in the Framingham study (Nelson *et al.*, 1990). This may be due to genetic susceptibility and/or a better lipid profile with low concentration of LDLc and TC.

CHD is also more severe in patients with diabetes and tends to occur at a younger age, with higher rates of diffuse multivessel disease, low ejection fraction, and increased tendency to develop congestive cardiac failure. It has a poorer outcome following myocardial infarction with higher rates of cardiac failure and death in the early postinfarction period (Smith *et al.*, 1984; Singer *et al.*, 1989; Aconson *et al.*, 1997). In the Bypass Angioplasty Revascularization Investigation (BARI), the diabetic subgroup awaiting revascularization, showed a higher incidence of triple vessel disease, greater left ventricular dysfunction and a lower 5-year survival rate. The BARI Study also showed that 5-year survival was significantly higher in diabetic patients undergoing coronary artery bypass graft compared to percutaneous transluminal coronary angioplasty. Coronary artery bypass graft CABG may therefore be the preferred procedure in diabetic patients with diffuse atherosclerosis (Bypass Angioplasty Revascularization Investigation Investigators, 2000).

The increased risk of CHD in type 2 diabetes is not entirely explained by traditional risk factors, though the diabetic population tends to have lower HDLc, higher total cholesterol/HDLc ratio and more hypertension. In the Multiple Risk Factor Intervention Trial (MRFIT), increasing the number of traditional risk factors like hypercholesterolaemia, smoking or hypertension increased the cardiovascular mortality, but the diabetic patients had approximately three times the risk compared with non-diabetic subjects for the same given number of risk factors (Stamler *et al.*, 1993). The CHD mortality of diabetic patients without a history of myocardial infarction was found to be similar to that of patients without diabetes who had a previous myocardial infarction (Haffner *et al.*, 1998).

Several mechanisms may be involved which explain this increased risk of CHD in type 2 diabetes. These include increased inflammatory and prothrombotic mediators, endothelial dysfunction, increased oxidative stress, AGE, platelet hyperactivity, reduced fibrinolytic capacity, as well as autonomic neuropathy, predisposing patients to ventricular arrhythmia.

Hyperglycaemia is a well-established risk factor for small vessel disease in diabetes, and improving glycaemic control reduces the risk of severe microvascular complications (The Diabetes Control and Complication Trial, 1993). The link between hyperglycaemia and the risk of CHD is unclear in type 2 diabetes. In the UKPDS study, a reduction of 0.9 per cent in glycated haemoglobin did not demonstrate significant benefit with regards to macrovascular disease, although a reduction of 16 per cent in myocardial infarction in the intensive treated group was almost significant ($P = 0.052$) (Turner *et al.*, 1998). The group of patients treated intensively with metformin, however, had a 39 per cent reduction in incidence of myocardial infarction compared with the conventionally treated group and those in the intensively treated group who received insulin or sulphonylurea. From an 'epidemiological updated HbA1c model', the rate of myocardial infarction doubled comparing HbA1c 5.5 per cent with 11 per cent, but there was a 10-fold increase in microvascular events.

The reasons for the relatively poor correlation between glycaemia and CHD have been debated. It has been suggested that post-prandial hyperglycaemia measured by 2-h glucose concentration after an oral glucose tolerance test may be more strongly related to CHD morbidity and mortality than fasting blood glucose concentration or HbA1c (Barzilay *et al.*, 1999). It is also believed that the risk factor for cardiovascular disease appear even before diabetes becomes recognizable ('ticking clock hypothesis').

Apart from chronic hyperglycaemia, acute hyperglycaemia influences CHD outcome in people with myocardial infarction as seen in the DIGAMI Study. In this trial, people who were intensively treated with insulin therapy (insulin glucose infusion for 24 h followed by intensive insulin treatment), compared with a controlled group managed by conventional therapy, showed a reduction in mortality to 33 per cent compared with 44 per cent in the conventionally treated group. The exact mechanism may not be related to improvement in hyperglycaemia and could be through indirect effects on improving platelet function, lipoprotein abnormalities and prothrombotic factors etc. (Malmberg, 1997).

Benefits of weight loss

Overweight and obesity are the results of interaction between social behaviour, cultural, physiological, metabolic and genetic factors in association with sedentary lifestyle and consumption of high energy dense diets. A weight loss programme would need to address the lifestyle modification involving changes in dietary intake, physical activity and behavioural therapy.

Even modest weight reduction in the ranges of 5 to 10 per cent of initial body weight are associated with a significant clinical improvement in a wide range of co-morbid conditions. The benefits include reduction in blood pressure, improved lipid profile, reduced left ventricular mass and an overall improvement in the CV risk profile. Weight loss as little 5 per cent of initial weight is associated with significant improvement haemoglobin A1c levels (Wing *et al.*, 1987; Goldstein, 1992; Bosello *et al.*, 1997).

New therapeutic lifestyle change (TLC) treatment programmes involve prescription diet and exercise based on an individual patient's eating habits and activity profile, combined with behavioural care provided through telephone, mail or attending a clinic (Perri *et al.* 1988; Perri, 1992). TLCs have been shown to improve the risks factors involved in the metabolic syndrome and to treat associated co-morbidities. Behavioural therapy was found to be an important part of the programme. The longer the duration of the behavioural therapy, the better the long-term weight loss outcome compared with standard treatment (Wadden *et al.*, 1994, 1997). The basic dietary therapy in TLC is reduction in saturated fat with an increase in the polyunsaturated and monounsaturated fats. The total percentage of fat is less than 30 per cent of total calories.

The structured meal plans and/or meal replacements, as opposed to traditional diets, give greater freedom and flexibility to substitute different types of meals and have been shown to be more effective in weight management. The success of structured meal plans over traditional diets was thought to be due to increased patients' empowerment with improved self monitoring and meal planning skills (Wing and Jeffery, 2001).

The clinical trials demonstrating diet and exercise delay or preventing the development of type 2 diabetes are discussed elsewhere.

Exercise

Although physical activity and exercise are key factors in weight reduction programmes, the effects of exercise alone on weight loss are considerably less dramatic than those of calorie restriction alone (Wood *et al.*, 1988; Anderssen *et al.*, 1995). Exercise is a key determinant, however, of successful long-term maintenance of weight loss (Schoeller *et al.*, 1997; Wyatt, 2002). The US Surgeon General recommends a regular programme of moderate to vigorous intense physical activity for a minimum of 30 min per day (US Surgeon General, 1996). Recent recommendation have favoured 60 min of physical activity daily.

Pharmacotherapy

The role of anti-obesity drugs is discussed in detail in the text.

Management of hypertension

Weight reduction has been shown to be an effective non-pharmacological approach to improve blood pressure in several studies (Schotte and Stunkard, 1990; Krzesinski *et al.*, 1993). Loss of 1 kg body weight is associated with a mean decrease in blood pressure of 1 mmHg (Staessen *et al.*, 1989). The reduction in blood pressure is related to the amount of weight loss rather than to the various treatment modalities employed such as different caloric restrictions or behaviour therapy. Weight reduction can also reduce the number of antihypertensive medications prescribed (Fagerberg *et al.*, 1984).

The role of sodium restriction is controversial. The INTERSALT Study showed that dietary sodium restriction can independently lower blood pressure and is additive with weight loss (Fagerberg *et al.*, 1984). Studies have shown that moderate sodium restriction to 100 mmol (2300 mg) per day can reduce systolic pressure by 5 mmHg and diastolic pressure by 2–3 mmHg (Cutler *et al.*, 1997). In addition, the response to antihypertensive therapy appears to be more effective in salt-restricted subjects. Physical activity, involving 30–45 min of brisk walking has been shown to lower blood pressure, as well as smoking cessation, and reduction of alcohol intake (Joint National Committee, 1997; Haire-Joshu *et al.*, 1999; American Diabetes Association, 2002).

A number of large studies in diabetic patients with hypertension have shown important benefits in CHD outcomes from lowering blood pressure (UKPDS, 1998; Heart Outcomes Prevention Evaluation Study, 2000). The UKPDS showed that tight blood pressure group was associated with significant reduction in macrovascular complications compared to the less intensively treated group (10/5 mmHg difference between the groups) (UKPDS, 1998).

Proteinuria is considered as a harbinger for CHD as well as renal disease and it is postulated that angiotensin-converting enzyme (ACE) inhibitors may offer some unique benefit in preventing CHD as well as nephropathy in type 2 diabetes. Indeed, in the Heart Outcomes Prevention Evaluation substudy, (MICRO-HOPE) and in the Captopril Prevention Project (CAPPP) Trial, the

Table 9.1   Major hypertension trials in subjects with diabetes

Study	n randomized	n diabetes	Follow up (years)	Main comparison	Endpoint reduction (diabetes)
UKPD	1148	1148	9	Captopril versus atenolol	Diabetes related death 32% Stroke 44%
SHEP	4736	583	5	Chlorthalidone versus placebo	All cardiovascular events (46–66%)
CAPPP	10985	572	6	Captopril versus β blocker or thiazide	Captopril group fatal/non-fatal 34%
SYS-Euro	4695	492	2	Nitrendipine versus Placebo	All major cardiovascular events (41–70%)
HOT	18790	1501	4	Felodipine	All cause mortality 39%
MICRO-HOPE		3577	4.5	Ramipril versus Placebo	Total mortality 29% CV deaths 37% MI 22%
ALLHAT	24335	8633	4.9	Amlodipine, doxazosin, lisinopril, chlorthalidone	Total mortality -39%
LIFE	9193	1195	4.8	Losartan versus atenolol	Losartan group all cause mortality 39%
ABCD	470	470	5	Nisoldipine versus enalapril	Discontinuation of study

CV, cardiovascular; MI, myocardial infarction; UKPD, UK Prospective Diabetes; HOPE, heart outcomes Prevention Evaluation; HOT, hypertension optimal treatment; SHEP, systolic Hypertension Elderly Program; CAPPP, Captopril Prevention Project Trial; SYST-EURO, Systolic Hypertension Europe; MICRO, Microalbuminuria Cardiovascular and Renal Outcomes; ALLHAT, Antihypertensive and Lipid Lowering Treatment to Prevent Heart Attack Trial; LIFE, Losartan Intervention For Endpoint Reduction Study; ABCD, Appropriate Blood Pressure Control in Diabetes.

diabetic subgroup on ACE inhibitors had better cardiovascular outcome events (Table 9.1) (HOPES, 2000).

Further studies involving ACE inhibitors, the FACET (Fosinopril vs Amlodipine Cardiovascular Randomized Events Trial) and the ABCD trial (Appropriate Blood Pressure Control in Diabetes) appeared to suggest that calcium channel blockers might be inferior to ACE-I in the context of cardiovascular disease and/or the beneficial outcome observed is a reflection of the cardioprotective effect of an ACE inhibitor. These studies should be interpreted with caution as the trials were not designed and powered to assess a difference between two treatment groups with regard to cardiovascular events (Tatti et al., 1998; Estacio et al., 2000).

The controversy surrounding the calcium antagonist therapy with regard to adverse cardiovascular events was not demonstrated in the Systolic Hypertension

Europe (SYS-Eur) Trial and the Hypertension Optimal Treatment Study (HOT) (see Table 9.1; Hansson *et al.*, 1998; Tuomilehto *et al.*, 1999).

The HOT Study also looked at the optimal diastolic target blood pressure. Felodipine was used as an initial treatment with other agents introduced in a five step regime to achieve the diastolic target value <90 mmHg, <85 mmHg or <80 mmHg. Among the diabetic group, aggressive diastolic blood pressure lowering to less than 80 mmHg was associated with the 51 per cent reduction in the risk of major cardiovascular events and 43 per cent reduction in the risk of cardiovascular mortality (Hansson *et al.*, 1999).

Similarly, much has been debated about the adverse effects of diuretic therapy especially in diabetic subjects. The beneficial effect of chlorthalidone as an antihypertensive agent was seen in the Systolic Hypertension in the Elderly Program (SHEP), which demonstrated reduction in major cardiovascular events in older type 2 diabetics and non-diabetics who had isolated systolic hypertension (ISH). (Table 9.1; Curb *et al.*, 1996).

Recently published data from the largest hypertensive trial, ALLHAT (33 357 subjects), compared the effect on cardiovascular endpoints of three newer agents (amlodipine, lisinopril or doxazosin) with a diuretic (chlorthalidone). After a mean follow up of 4.9 years, there was no difference in the relative risk of the primary outcome (combined fatal CHD or non-fatal myocardial infarction) or all cause mortality between amlodipine, lisinopril and chlorthalidone (Table 9.1; ALLHAT Collaborative Group, 2002).

These studies have not shown particular benefits of the newer drug classes compared with long established agents. The recent understanding of the role of A II in the pathogenesis of atherosclerosis and it's effect on myocardial tissues might suggest that A II type 1 receptor blockers (ARB) may prove to have genuine drug class differences in relation to cardiovascular outcomes.

Indeed, the LIFE (Losartan Intervention For Endpoint Reduction) Study looked at the effect of losartan or atenolol on 9193 hypertensive patients with left ventricular hypertrophy. Losartan not only reduced the cardiovascular outcomes, but there was approximately a two-fold greater ECG-left ventricular hypertrophy regression compared with the atenolol group. More impressive results were seen in sub-set of 1195 patients with diabetes, with a 39 per cent risk reduction in all cause mortality compared with the atenolol group. These benefits were above and beyond those attributable to blood pressure reduction alone (Table 9.1; Dahlof *et al.*, 2002).

Recently, three large placebo-controlled trials involving ARBs have demonstrated reduction of progression of albuminuria and the development and progression of nephropathy in hypertensive patients with type 2 diabetes. These differences were not explained by the blood pressure reduction achieved. It is postulated that ARBs have renal protective effects over and above blood pressure lowering in patients with type 2 diabetes (Brenner *et al.*, 2001; Lewis *et al.*, 2001; Parving *et al.* 2001).

Management of dyslipidaemia

Sedentary lifestyle is a major risk factor for CHD which increases lipid and non-lipid risk factors seen in obesity, metabolic syndrome and type 2 diabetes. Weight loss and exercise can reduce TG, increase HDLc and, in some persons, lower LDLc levels (Wood *et al.*, 1988; Goldstein, 1992). Regular physical activity should be a standard part on any lipid management programme. The American Diabetes Association (ADA) suggests a reduction in the proportion of dietary saturated fats with increase in carbohydrate or monounsaturated fat or both. The ATP III recommends therapeutic lifestyle changes including dietary changes combined with regular exercise and weight management as the first line treatment for all risk factors associated with metabolic syndrome (National Cholesterol Education Program, 2002). Diets high in *trans* fatty acids, like margarine, biscuits and white bread, that can raise LDLc as well as lower HDLc should be avoided. National Cholesterol Education Program and ADA recommend drug therapy only after lifestyle interventions has been tried except for those patients with clinical evidence of CHD or with very high LDLc levels. Several studies have shown that aggressive dietary therapy alone or in combination with exercise has beneficial effects on lipid levels and CHD.

The St. Thomas' Atherosclerosis Regression Study (STARS) randomized men with CHD and TC above 6.0 mmol/l to conventional care or a low-fat diet. Weight reduction measures and exercise programmes were provided for overweight subjects. After 3 years, the progression rate of coronary atherosclerosis slowed in the diet-treated group (Watts *et al.*, 1992). The clinical trials involving omega 3 fatty acids also showed significant benefit on cardiovascular end points. In the Diet and Reinfarction Trial (DART), men recovering from myocardial infarction, who were randomized to dietary advice consisting of increased fatty fish consumption had a 29 per cent reduction on all cause mortality at 2-year follow up (Burr *et al.*, 1989).

In the GISSI Prevention Trial, patients randomized to receive omega 3 fatty acid supplementation (1 g/day) had a significant 10–15 per cent reduction in combined primary endpoints of death, and fatal/non-fatal stroke (GISSI Prevenzione Investigators, 1999). In the Lyon Diet Heart Study, patients on a Mediterranean diet instead of a western diet had a reduction in death from cardiovascular causes; non-fatal acute myocardial infarction of 73 per cent, cardiovascular mortality of 76 per cent and all cause mortality of 70 per cent (De Lorgeril *et al.*, 1996, 1999).

Several large-scale, controlled, randomized clinical trials have established that intervention with statins reduces CHD risks. This is seen in both the primary and secondary prevention settings and it is mediated mainly by reducing the LDL cholesterol (Table 9.2).

The landmark Scandinavian Simvastatin Survival Study (4S) convincingly demonstrated that coronary events and total mortality were decreased by 30

Table 9.2 CHD prevention trials with statins in patients with diabetes – subgroup analysis

Study	Drug	N	Baseline LDLc (mmol/l)	LDLc lowering (%)	CHD risk reduction (%) Overall	CHD risk reduction (%) Diabetes
Primary prevention						
AF CAPS/TexCAPS	Lovastatin	155	3.9	25	37	43 (NS)
HPS	Simvastatin	2982	3.4	29	24	22
Secondary prevention						
CARE	Pravastatin	586	3.6	27	23	25
4S	Simvastatin	202	4.8	36	32	55
LIPID	Pravastatin	782	3.9	25	24	19 (NS)
HPS	Simvastatin	1978	3.3	30	24	18

NS, not significant.

per cent with LDLc reduction of 36 per cent. The Cholesterol and Recurrent Events (CARE) and Long Term Intervention with Pravastatin in Ischemic Disease (LIPID) demonstrated similar benefits in patients with relatively average TC and LDLc (Sacks *et al.*, 1996; LIPID, 1998).

The link between increasing LDL and CHD is well established in statin trials. There is a roughly linear relationship between CHD events rates and LDLc levels on treatment with statins. Those at the highest CHD risk experience the greatest benefit from the decrease in LDLc and tends to plateau at lower LDLc level. The lowest event rate is in the CARE pravastatin group, who achieved a mean LDLc of less than 2.6 mmol/l, which is in accordance with the NCEP guideline of LDLc target ≤2.6 mmol/l. The baseline LDLc level in 4S was 4.88 mmol/l, in CARE 3.6 mmol/l, and 3.88 mmol/l in LIPID. In all these trials, statins approximately reduced LDLc level by about one third. In the recent Heart Protection Study, (HPS) 33 per cent of the total 20 536 subjects had baseline LDLc <3 mmol/l, 25 per cent between 3 and 3.5 mmol/l and 42 per cent had levels >3.5 mmol/l. The simvastatin (40 mg) group, when compared to placebo, had significant reduction in all cause mortality, CHD deaths and major cardiovascular events. The benefit in reduction of events was similar in all the three tertiles of baseline LDLc (MRC/BHF, 2002).

The benefit of aggressive lipid lowering is also extended to the Regression Growth Evaluation Statin Study (REGRESS) where pravastatin delayed the progression of atherosclerosis on angiography and reduction in clinical events at 24 months in the 885 men who took part. These benefits occurred at all lipid levels, including those in the lowest quintile with LDLc concentration between 2.2 and 3.8 mmol/l (Jukema *et al.*, 1995) The Atorvastatin Versus Revascularisation Treatment Study (AVERT) compared the outcome of aggressive lipid lowering with atorvastatin (80 mg/day) to that of angioplasty in 341 stable CHD patients with coronary vessel disease. The atorvastatin group (*n* = 164) achieved a greater reduction of LDLc to 2.0 mmol/l, as opposed to 3.0 mmol/l in angioplasty group followed by usual care. The incidence of ischaemic events was 36 per cent lower in the atorvastatin group over 18 months, although not statistically significant, there was lower rate of coronary artery bypass graft and percutaneous transluminal coronary angioplasty as well as hospitalization for worsening angina (Pitt *et al.*, 1999).

This raises the point 'the lower the LDLc, the better?' and the issue as to whether there is a threshold LDLc below which no benefit occurs. It has been postulated that the cardiovascular benefits of lowering LDLc may be due, at least in part, to improvement in endothelial dysfunction and the anti-inflammatory properties of statins rather than lipid lowering. In the substudy of CARE, it was shown that pravastatin was associated with improved endothelium dependent vasodilatation and reduction of CRP. Studies in 4S and WOSCOP demonstrated benefit within 6 months of randomization, too soon for the benefit to be explained by regression of atherosclerosis. Acute coronary syndromes arise as a result of rupture of unstable plaque which poses a greater threat than the plaque size or severity of stenosis. The vulnerability of the atherogenic plaque is related to the size of the lipid-rich core, foam cells, inflammatory cells and the thickness of the fibrous cap which is contributed by the vascular smooth muscle cells. Statins reduce the lipid rich core and inflammatory cells especially macrophages and T lymphocytes and directly inhibits metalloproteinase secretion by macrophages that digest collagen in the plaque (Jukema *et al.*, 1995; Aronow *et al.*, 2001; Corti *et al.*, 2001).

The clinical equivalent to this effect was shown in the Myocardial Ischaemia Reduction with Aggressive Cholesterol Lowering study (MIRACL) in which 3086 patients with unstable angina or non-Q wave myocardial infarction received either atorvastatin 80 mg/day or placebo within 4 days of hospital admission. The primary endpoint (recurring infarction, cardiac arrest with resuscitation, worsening angina requiring hospitalization) was less frequent with atorvastatin at 16 weeks compared to placebo with a relative risk reduction of 16 per cent, but the benefit was primarily due to a 26 per cent reduction in hospitalization for worsening angina (Schwartz *et al.*, 2001).

The beneficial effect of statins was not seen in the recent lipid arm of ALL-HAT study. One possible explanation is that a relatively large proportion of patients taking pravastatin (22.6 per cent) stopped the medication and around 26 per cent of people in the 'usual care' have been started on a statin (ALLHAT Collaborative Group, 2002).

The role of statins in diabetic dyslipidaemia is based on subgroup analyses from the major statin studies. Patients with diabetes benefit as much or more than non-diabetics from statin treatment, but the majority of the outcomes did not reach statistical significance due to the small number of diabetic patients compared to non-diabetic subjects (Table 9.2).

Table 9.3 CHD prevention trials with fibrates in patient with diabetes

Secondary prevention	Drug	N	CHD risk reduction (%)
VA-HIT	Gemfibrozil	309	24
DIAS	Fenofibrate	207	23 (NS)

NS, not significant; VA-HIT, Veterans Affairs HDL Intervention Trial; DIAS, Diabetes Atherosclerosis Intervention Study.

In fact, statins reduce CHD events by only approximately 30 per cent with a residual risk of 70 per cent, which may be related to suboptimal LDLc lowering or due to the presence of other untreated lipid abnormalities. In a retrospective analysis, low baseline HDLc was found to be a strong inverse risk factor for both placebo and pravastatin groups in the CARE and LIPID trials. The conclusion was that low HDLc is a powerful negative risk factor for coronary events despite treatment with statin and the risks associated with a low HDLc is not altered by statin therapy. There is evidence that fibrates which increases HDLc may be effective for secondary prevention of CHD as observed in the Veterans Affairs HDL Intervention Trial (VA-HIT) (Table 9.3; Rubins *et al.*, 1999; Bloomfield *et al.*, 2001). The DIAS (the Diabetes Atherosclerosis Intervention Study) demonstrated that the progression of focal, localized atherosclerosis was reduced by 40 per cent on two measurements in the fenofibrate group compared with the control group. There was a non significant trend towards reduction in combined coronary events, fewer deaths, MI and coronary intervention in the treatment arm (Table 9.3; DIAS, 2001).

Antiplatelet therapy

Patients with insulin resistance have high levels of circulating PAI-1, a protein that inhibits fibrinolysis. Diabetic platelets show a greater number of GP IIb/IIIa receptors and increased tendency to adhesion and aggregation. Endothelial dysfunction results in reduced NO and prostaglandin I2 production with well known antiplatelet aggregation properties and increase level of the pro-aggregatory substances adenosine diphosphate and thromboxane A2 (Tschoepe *et al.*, 1990; Aronson *et al.*, 1996).

Antiplatelet therapy has been shown in numerous multicentre intervention trials to reduce the rate of cardiovascular events in both non-diabetic and diabetic patients. The HOT trial demonstrated that aspirin 75 mg/day significantly reduced cardiovascular events by 15 per cent and myocardial infarction by 36 per cent in both diabetic and non-diabetic subjects compared to placebo (Hansson *et al.*, 1998).

The recent meta-analysis of the Antithrombotic Trialists' Collaboration confirmed that antiplatelet therapy reduced the combined outcome of any serious vascular event by approximately one quarter, non-fatal myocardial infarction by one-third, non-fatal stroke by one-quarter and vascular mortality by one-sixth. In all of the high-risk categories, coronary heart disease, non-haemorraghic cerebrovascular disease, and peripheral vascular disease, the absolute benefits substantially outweighed the absolute risks of major cranial and extracranial bleeding (Collaborative meta-analysis, 2002).

The addition of dipyradimole to aspirin did not produce a significant further reduction in vascular events compared with aspirin alone. Clopidrogel was found to be slightly more effective than aspirin with reduction in vascular events by 10 per cent compared with 4 per cent for aspirin and with lower risk of gastrointestinal bleeding as it does not reduce the synthesis of cytoprotective prostaglandins in the gastrointestinal tract (Peters *et al.*, 2002).

The evaluation of platelet GbIIb/IIIa inhibition for stenting (EPISTENT) showed that among diabetic patients, the combination of abixicam and stenting was associated with a lower rate of repeat target vessel revascularization at 6 months (8.1 per cent) than stenting and placebo (11.6 per cent) or angioplasty and abixicam (18.4 per cent). There was also a significant reduction in death and myocardial infarction rate at 6 months in abixicam and stent compared to other two groups (Marso *et al.*, 1999).

A recent meta-analysis of six randomized trials that enrolled 6485 diabetic patients showed that GbIIb/IIIa inhibition was associated with a significant reduction in mortality in acute coronary syndrome as well as in those undergoing revascularization regardless of procedures (Roffi *et al.*, 2001).

Conclusion

Obesity and type 2 diabetes are major risk factors for cardiovascular disease. There are a number of evidence-based treatments available to reduce cardiovascular complications in diabesity. Clinicians should adopt multifactorial therapeutic approach to address cardiovascular risk factors by achieving good glycaemic control, reducing lipid levels, lowering blood pressure and improving prothrombotic milieu. As obesity is the underlying problem in these patients, treatment of obesity itself would be a logical addition to above therapies and can lead to significant reduction in risk factors.

References

ALLHAT Collaborative Group (2002) Major outcomes in high risk hypertensive patients randomized to ACE inhibitor or calcium channel blocker vs diuretic. *JAMA* **287**:2981–97.
American Diabetes Association (2002) *Smoking and Diabetes* (Position Statement). *Diabetes Care* **25**(Suppl. 1):S80–S81.
Allison BD, Fontaine KR, Manson JE *et al.* (1999) Annual deaths attributable to obesity in the United States. *JAMA* **282**:1530.
Alpert MA and Hashini MW (1993) Obesity and the heart. *Am J Med Sci* **306**:117.

Alpert MA, Terry BE, Cohen MV *et al.* (2000) The electrocardiogram in morbid obesity. *Am J Cardiol* **85**:908.

Anderssen S, Holme I, Urdae P and Hjermann I (1995) Diet and exercise intervention have favourable effects on blood pressure in mild hypertensives: the Oslo Diet and Exercise Study (ODES). *Blood Press* **4**:343–9.

Aronow HD, Topol EJ, Roe MT *et al.* (2001) Effect of lipid-lowering therapy on early mortality after acute coronary syndromes: an observational study. *Lancet* **357**:1063.

Aronson D, Bloomgarden Z and Rayfield EJ (1996) Potential mechanism for promoting restenosis in diabetic patients (Review). *J Am Coll Cardiol* **27**:528–35.

Aronson D, Rayfield EJ and Chesebro JH (1997) Mechanisms of determining course and outcome of diabetic patients who have had acute myocardial infarction. *Ann Intern Med* **126**:296–306.

Assmann G and Schulte H (1992) Relation of high density lipoprotein cholesterol and triglycerides to incidence of atherosclerotic coronary artery disease (The PROCAM Experience). *Am J Cardiol* **70**:733–7.

Assmann G, Schulte H and Cullen P (1997) New and classical risk factors – the Munster heart study (PROCAM). *Eur J Med Res* **2**:237–42.

Assmann G, Schulte H, Funke H and von Eckardstein A (1998) The emergence of triglycerides as a significant independent risk factor in coronary artery disease. *Eur Heart J* **19**(suppl M) 8–14.

Austin MA, Hokanson JE and Edwards KL (1998) Hypertriglyceridaemia as a cardiovascular risk factor. *Am J Cardiol* **81**(suppl 4A):7B–12B.

Bypass Angioplasty Revascularization Investigation Investigators (2000) Seven-year outcome in the Bypass Angioplasty Revascularization Investigation (BARI) by treatment and diabetic status. *J Am Coll Cardiol* **35**:1122–9.

Baron AD, Steinberg HO, Chaker H *et al.* (1995) Insulin mediated skeletal muscle vasodilation contributes to both insulin sensitivity and responsiveness in lean humans. *J Clin Invest* **96**:786.

Barzilay JI, Spiekerman CF, Wahl PW *et al.* (1999) Cardiovascular disease in older adults with glucose disorders: comparison of ADA criteria for diabetes mellitus with WHO criteria. *Lancet* **354**:622–5.

Begum N, Ragolia L, Rienzie J *et al.* (1998) Regulation of mitogen activated protein kinase induction by insulin in vascular smooth muscle cells. *J Biol Chem* **273**:25164–70.

Bhopal R (2002) Epidemic of cardiovascular disease in South Asians. *Br Med J* **324**:625–6.

Blair D, Habicht JP, Sins EA *et al.* (1984) Evidence for increased risk for hypertension with centrally located body fat and the effect of race and sex. *Am J Epidemiol* **119**:526–40.

Bloomfield Rubins H, Davenport J, Babikian V *et al.* (2001) Reduction in stroke with gemfibrozil in men with coronary heart disease and low HDL cholesterol: the Veterans Affairs HDL Intervention Trial (VA-HIT). *Circulation* **103**:2828.

Bosello O, Armellini F, Zamboni M and Fitchet M (1997) The benefits of modest weight loss in type II diabetes. *Int J Obes Relat Metab Disord* **21**(suppl 1):S10–S13.

Brenner BM, Cooper MG, de Zeeuw D *et al.* (2001) Effects of losartan on renal and cardiovascular outcomes in patients with type 2 diabetes and nephropathy. *N Engl J Med* **345**:861–9.

Bucala R, Tracey KJ and Cerami A (1991) Advanced glycosylation endproducts – quench nitric oxide and mediate defective endothelium-dependent vasodilatation, in experimental diabetes. *J Clin Invest* **87**:432–8.

Burr ML, Fehily AM, Gilbert JF *et al.* (1989) Effects of changes in fat, fish and fibre intakes on death and myocardial infarction: Diet and Reinfarction Trial(DART). *Lancet* **2**:757–61.

Collaborative meta-analysis of randomised trials of antiplatelet therapy for prevention of death, myocardial infarction, and stroke in high risk patients. *Br Med J* **324**:71.

Calle EE, Thun MJ, Petrelli JM *et al.* (1999) Body mass index and mortality in a prospective cohort of US adults. *N Engl J Med* **341**:1097.

Cambien F, Jacqueson A, Richard JL *et al.* (1986) Is the level of serum triglyceride a significant predictor of coronary death in 'normocholesterolemic' subjects? The Paris Prospective Study. *Am J Epidemiol* **124**:624–32.

Carlson LA, Bottiger LE and Ahfeldt PE (1979) Risk factors for myocardial infarction in the Stockholm prospective study (role of plasma TG and TC) *Acta Medica Scand* **206**:351–60.

Colditz GA, Willett WC, Stampfer MJ *et al.* (1990) Weight as a risk factor for clinical diabetes in women. *Am J Epidemiol* **132**:501–13.

Cook DG, Mendall MA, Whincup PH *et al.* (2000) C-reactive protein concentration in children. Relationship to adiposity and other cardiovascular risk factors. *Atherosclerosis* **149**:139–50.

Corti R, Fayad ZA, Fuster V *et al.* (2001) Effects of lipid-lowering by simvastatin on human atherosclerotic lesions: a longitudinal study by high-resolution, noninvasive magnetic resonance imaging. *Circulation* **104**:249.

Curb JD, Piessel SL, Cutler JA *et al.* (1996) Effect of diuretic-based antihypertensive treatment on cardiovascular disease risk in older diabetic patients with isolated systolic hypertension: Systolic Hypertension in the Elderly Program Cooperative Research Group. *JAMA* **276**:1886–92.

Cutler JA, Follmann D and Allender PS (1997) Randomized trials of sodium reduction: an overview. *Am J Clin Nutr* **65** (Suppl. 2):643S–651S.

Diabetes Atherosclerosis Intervention Study Investigators (2001) *Lancet* **357**:905–10.

Dahlof B, Devereux RB, Kjeldson *et al.* (2002) Cardiovascular morbidity and mortality in the Losartan for Endpoint Reduction in Hypertensive Study. *Lancet* **359**:995–1003.

De Fronzo RA, Cooke CR, Andres R *et al.* (1975) The effect of insulin on renal handling of sodium, potassium, calcium, and phosphate in man. *J Clin Invest* **55**:845–55.

De Lorgeril M, Salen P, Bontemps L *et al.* (1999) Mediterranean diet, traditional risk factors, and the rate of cardiovascular complications after myocardial infarction. Final report of the Lyon Diet Heart Study. *Circulation* **99**:779.

De Lorgeril M, Salen P, Martin JL *et al.* (1996) Effect of a Mediterranean type of diet on the rate of cardiovascular complications in patients with coronary heart disease. Insights into the cardioprotective effect of certain nutriments. *J Am Coll Cardiol* **28**:1103.

DeFronzo RA and Ferrannini E (1991) Insulin resistance. A multifaceted syndrome responsible for NIDDM, obesity, hypertension, dyslipidemia, and atherosclerotic cardiovascular disease. *Diabetes Care* **14**:173.

Despres JP (1998) The insulin resistance–dyslipidemic syndrome of visceral obesity: effect on patients' risk. *Obes Res* **6**(suppl 1):8S–17S.

Despres JP, Lamarche B, Mauriege P *et al.* (1996) Hyperinsulinaemia as an independent risk factor for ischemic heart disease. *NEJM* **334**:952–7.

Dyer AR and Elliott P (1989) The INTERSALT Study: relations of body mass index to blood pressure. *J Hum Hypertens* **3**:299–308.

Executive Summary of the Third Report of National Cholesterol Education Programme. *JAMA* **285**:2486, 2002.

Estacio R, Jeffers BW, Gifford N and Schrier RW (2000) Effect of blood pressure control on diabetic microvascular complications in patients with hypertension and type 2 diabetes. *Diabetes Care* **23**(Suppl. 2):B54–B64.

Everhart JE, Pettitt DJ, Bennett PH and Knowler WC (1992) Duration of obesity increases the incidence of NIDDM. *Diabetes* **41**:235–40.

Fagerberg B, Andersson OK, Isaksson B and Bjorntorp P (1984) Blood pressure control during weight reduction in obese hypertensive men. *Br Med J* **119**:11–14.

Ferrannini E and Camastra S (1998) Relationship between IGT, NIDDM and obesity. *Eur J Clin Invest* **28**(suppl2):3–6; discussion 6–7.

Fisher WR (1983) Heterogeneity of plasma low density lipoprotein. *Metabolism* **32**:283–91.

Fontbonne A, Eschwege E, Cambien F *et al.* (1989) Hypertriglyceridaemia as a risk factor for coronary heart disease, 11 yr follow up, of the Paris Prospective Study. *Diabetologia* **32**:300–4.

Ford ES, Giles WH and Dietz WH (2002) Prevalence of the metabolic syndrome among US adults: Findings from the Third National Health and Nutrition Examination Survey. *JAMA* **287**:356.

Forouhi NG, Sattar N and McKeigue PM (2001) Relation of CRP to cardiovascular risks in European and South Asians. *Int J Obes* **25**:1327–31.

Frank S, Colliver JA and Frank A (1986) The electrocardiogram in obesity. *Am J Coll Cardiol* **7**:295–9.

Friedewald WT, Levy RI and Fredrickson DS (1972) Estimation of the concentration of LDLc in plasma, without the use of the preparative ultracentrifuge. *Clin Chem* **18**:499–552.

Frost PH and Harel RJ (1998) Rationale for use of non-high-density lipoprotein cholesterol rather than low-density lipoprotein cholesterol as a tool for lipoprotein cholesterol screening and assessment of risk and therapy. *Am J Cardiol* **81**(4A):26B–31B.

GISSI Prevenzione Investigators: Dietary supplementation with n-3 polyunsaturated fatty acids and vitamin E after myocardial infarction. *Lancet* **354**:447–55.

Goldstein DJ (1992) Beneficial health effects of a modest weight loss. *Int J Obes* **16**:397–415.

Grundy SM and Barnett JP (1990) Metabolic and health complications of obesity. *Dis Mon* **36**:641.

Gunnell DJ, Frankel SJ, Nanchahal K *et al.* (1998) Childhood obesity and adult cardiovascular mortality. *Am J Clin Nutr* **67**:1111–18.

Gu K, Cowie CC and Harris MI (1999) Diabetes and decline in heart disease mortality in US adults. *JAMA* **282**:1291–7.

Hypertension in Diabetic Study (HDS): I prevalence of hypertension in newly presenting type 2 diabetic patients and the association with risk factors for cardiovascular and diabetic complications. *J Hypertens* **11**:309–17, 1993.

Heart Outcomes Prevention Evaluation Study Investigators (2000) Effects of ramipril on cardiovascular and microvascular outcomes in people with diabetes mellitus: results of the HOPE study and MICRO-HOPE substudy. *Lancet* **355**:253–9.

Haffner SM (1998) Management of dyslipidemia in adults with diabetes. *Diabetes Care* **21**(1):160–78.

Haffner SM, Lehto S, Ronnemaa T *et al.* (1998) Mortality from coronary heart disease in subjects with type 2 diabetes and in nondiabetic subjects with and without prior myocardial infarction. *N Engl J Med* **339**(4):229–34.

Haffner SM, Stern MP, Hazuda JP *et al.* (1990) Cardiovascular risk factors in prediabetic individuals. *JAMA* **263**:2893–8.

Haire-Joshu D, Glasgow RE and Tibbs TL (1999) Smoking and diabetes (Technical Review). *Diabetes Care* **22**:1887–9.

Hanefeld M, Fischer S, Julius U *et al.* (1996) Risk factors for myocardial infarction and death in newly detected NIDDM: the Diabetes Intervention Study, 11 year follow up. *Diabetologia* **39**:1577–83.

Hansson L, Zanchetti A, Carruthers SG *et al.* (1998) Effects of intensive blood-pressure lowering and low-dose aspirin on patients with hypertension: principal results of the Hypertension Optimal Treatment (HOT) randomised trial. *Lancet* **351**:1755–62.

Harris MI (1989) Impaired glucose tolerance in the US population. *Diabetes Care* **12**:464.

Hauner H, Petiuschke T, Russ M *et al.* (1995) Effects of TNF-α on glucose transport and lipid metabolism of newly-differentiated human fat cells in cell culture. *Diabetologia* **38**:764–71.

Hawthorne GC, Bartlett K, Hetherington CS and Albertic KG (1989) The effect of high glucose on polyol pathway activity in cultured human endothelial cells. *Diabetologia* **32**:196–9.

Hedrick CC, Thorpe SR, Fu MX *et al.* (2000) Glycation impairs HDLc function. *Diabetologia* **43**:312–20.

Hodis HN (1999) Triglyceride-rich lipoprotein remnant particles and risk of atherosclerosis. *Circulation* **99**:2852–2854.

Hotamisligil GS, Shargill NS and Spiegelman BM (1993) Adipose expression of TNF-α: direct role in obesity linked insulin resistance. *Science* **259**:87–91.

Huang Z, Willett WC, Manson JE *et al.* (1998) Body weight, weight change and risk for hypertension in women. *Ann Intern Med* **128**:81.

Hubert HB, Feinleib M, McNamara PM and Castelli WP (1983) Obesity as an independent risk factor for cardiovascular disease: a 26 year follow-up of participants in the Framingham Heart Study. *Circulation* **67**:968–77.

Joint National Committee on Prevention, Detection, Evaluation and Treatment of High Blood Pressure (1997) The Sixth Report of the Joint National Committee on Prevention, Detection, Evaluation and Treatment of High Blood Pressure (JNC VI). *Arch Int Med* **157**:2413–2446.

Janka HU, Warram JH, Rand LI and Krolewski AS (1989) Risk factors for progression of background retinopathy in long-standing IDDM. *Diabetes* **38**:460–4.

Jarrett RJ and Shipley MJ (1985) Mortality and associated risk factors in Diabetes. *Acta Endocrinol (Suppl)* **272**:21–6.

Jensen MD, Haymond MW, Rizza RA *et al.* (1989) Influence of body fat distribution on free fatty acid metabolism in obesity. *J Clin Invest* **83**:1168–73.

Jukema JW, Bruschke AV, van Boren AJ *et al.* (1995) Effects of lipid lowering by pravastatin on progression and regression of coronary artery disease in men with normal to moderately elevated serum cholesterol levels: The Regression Growth Evaluation Statin Study (REGRESS). *Circulation* **91**:2528.

Kannel WB and McGee DL (1979) Diabetes and cardiovascular risk factors: the Framingham study. *Circulation* **59**:8–13.

Kelly CC, Lyall H, Petric JR *et al.* (2001) Low-grade chronic inflammation in women with polycystic ovarian syndrome. *J Clin Endocrinol Metab* **86**:2453–5.

Kern PA, Saghizadeh M, Ong JM *et al.* (1995) The expression of tumour necrosis factor in human adipose tissue. Regulation by obesity, weight loss, and relationship to lipoprotein lipase. *J Clin Invest* **95**:2111–19.

Krauss RM (1998) Atherogenicity of triglyceride-rich lipoproteins *Am J Cardiol* **81**:13B–17B.

Krzesinski JM, Janssens M, Vanderspeeten F and Rorive G (1993) Importance of weight loss and sodium restriction in the treatment of mild and moderate essential hypertension. *Acta Clin Belg* **48**:234–245.

Kuller LH, Velentgas P, Barzilay J *et al.* (2000) Diabetes mellitus: subclinical cardiovascular disease. *Arterioscler Thromb Vasc Biol* **20**:823–9.

Long-Term Intervention with Pravastatin in Ischaemic Disease (LIPID) Study Group. Prevention of cardiovascular events and death with pravastatin in patients with coronary heart disease and a broad range of initial cholesterol levels. *N Engl J Med* **339**:1349.

Laakso M (1997) Dyslipidemia, morbidity, and mortality in non-insulin-dependent diabetes mellitus. Lipoproteins and coronary heart disease in non-insulin-dependent diabetes mellitus. *J Diabetes Complications* **11**(2):137–41.

Lamarche B, Moorjani S, Lupien PJ *et al.* (1996) Apo A1 and B levels and the risk of ischemic heart disease – five year follow-up of men in Quebec Cardiovascular Study. *Circulation* **94**:273–8.

Lamarche B, Tchernof A, Moorjani *et al.* (1997) Small dense LDLc as a predictor of ischaemic heart disease in men – Quebec Cardiovascular Study. *Circulation* **95**:69–75.

Landsberg L (1992) Hyperinsulinaemia: a possible role in obesity – induced hypertension. *Hypertension* **19**(suppl 1):161–5.

Larsson B, Bjorntorp P and Tibblin G (1981) The health consequences of obesity. *Int J Obes* **5**:97–116.

Larsson B, Svardsudd K, Welin L *et al.* (1984) Abdominal obesity and risk of cardiovascular disease and death. *Br Med J (Clin Res Ed)* **288**:1401–4.

Lewis EJ, Hunsicker LG, Clarke WR *et al.* (2001) Renoprotective effect of the angiotensin-receptor antagonist irbesartan in patients with nephropathy due to type 2 diabetes. *N Engl J Med* **345**:851–60.

Lim SC, Caballero AE, Smakowski *et al.* (1999) Soluble intercellular adhesion molecule, vascular cell adhesion molecule, and impaired microvascular reactivity are early markers of vasculopathy in type 2 diabetic individuals without microalbuminuria. *Diabetes Care* **22**:1865–70.

Lindsay, RS, Funahashi T, Hanson RL *et al.* (2002) Adiponectin and development of type 2 diabetes in the Pima Indian population. *Lancet* **360**:57.

Loscalzo J (2001) Nitric oxide insufficiency, platelet activation and arterial thrombosis. *Circ Res* **88**:756–62.

MRC/BHF Heart Protection Study of cholesterol lowering with Simvastatin in 20536 high-risk individuals: a randomised placebo-controlled trial. *Lancet* **360**:7.

Malmberg K (1997) Prospective randomised study of intensive insulin treatment on long term survival after acute myocardial infarction in patients with diabetes mellitus. Diabetes Mellitus, Insulin-Glucose Infusion in Acute Myocardial Infarction (DIGAMI) Study Group. *Br Med J* **314**:1512–15.

Manson JE, Colditz GA, Stampfer MJ *et al.* (1990) A prospective study of obesity and risk of coronary heart disease in women. *NEJM* **322**:882.

Manson JE, Willett WC, Stampfer MJ *et al.* (1995) Body weight and mortality among women. *N Engl J Med* **333**:677.

Marso SP, Lincott AM, Ellis SG *et al.* (1999) Optimizing the percutaneous interventional outcomes for patients with diabetes mellitus: results of EPISTENT. *Circulation* **100**:2477–84.

McFarlane SI, Banerji M and Sowers JR (2001) Insulin resistance and cardiovascular disease. *J Clin Endocrinol Metab* **86**(2):713–8.

McVeigh GE, Brennan GM, Johnston GD *et al.* (1992) Impaired endothelium dependent/independent vasodilation in patients with NIDDM. *Diabetologia* **35**:771–6.

Meigs JB, D'Agostino RB Sr, Wilson PW *et al.* (1997) Risk variable clustering in insulin resistance syndrome. The Framingham Offspring Study. *Diabetes* **46**:1594–600.

Miyaoka K, Kiwasako T, Hisano K *et al.* (2001) CD36 deficiency associated insulin resistance. *Lancet* **357**:686.

Moan A, Nordby G, Rostrup M *et al.* (1995) Insulin sensitivity, sympathetic activity and cardiovascular reactivity in young men. *Am J Hypertens* **8**:268.

Modan M, Halkin H, Almog S *et al.* (1985) Hyperinsulinaemia. A link between hypertension obesity and glucose intolerance. *J Clin Invest* **75**:809–17.

NIH Consensus Development Panel on Triglyceride, High Density Lipoprotein and Coronary Heart Disease (1993) *JAMA* **269**:505–10.

National Cholesterol Education Program (NCEP) Expert Panel on detection, evaluation, and treatment of high blood cholesterol in adults (Adult Treatment Panel III) (2002) Final report. US Department of Health and Human Services; Public Health Service; National Institutes of Health; National Heart, Lung, and Blood Institute. [NIH Publication No. 02–5215. September 2002.] *Circulation* **106**:3143.

Neel JV (1962) Diabetes mellitus: a 'thrifty' genotype rendered detrimental by process. *Am J Hum Genet* **14**:353–62.

Nelson RG, Sievers ML, Knowler WC *et al.* (1990) Low incidence of fatal coronary heart disease in Pima Indians. *Circulation* **81**:987–95.

Nolan JJ, Ludvik B, Baloga J *et al.* (1997) Mechanisms of the kinetic defect in insulin action in obesity and NIDDM. *Diabetes* **46**:494–500.

Perri MG (1992) *Improving the Long-term Management of Obesity: Theory Research and Clinical Guidelines.* Wiley, New York, NY.

Pannacciulli N, De Pergola G, Giorgino F and Giorgino R (2002) A family history of type 2 diabetes is associated with increased plasma levels of C-reactive protein in non-smoking healthy adult women. *Diabet Med* **19**:689–92.

Parving HH, Lehnert H, Brodiner-Mortensen J *et al.* (2001) The effect of irbesartan on the development of diabetic nephropathy in patients with type 2 diabetes. *N Engl J Med* **345**:870–8.

Perri MG, McAllister DA, Gange JJ *et al.* (1988) Effects of four maintenance programs on the long-term management of obesity. *J Consult Clin Psychol* **56**:529–34.

Peters RJ, Zao F, Lewis BS *et al.* for the CURE Investigators (2001) Aspirin dose and bleeding events in the CURE study (abstract). *Eur Heart J* Suppl, p. 510.

Pitt B, Waters D, Brown WV *et al.* (1999) Atorvastatin Versus Revascularization Treatment Investigators. Aggressive lipid-lowering therapy compared with angioplasty in stable coronary artery disease. *N Engl J Med* **341**:70.

Pradhan AD and Ridker PM (2002) Do atherosclerosis and type 2 diabetes share a common inflammatory basis? *Eur Heart J* **23**:831–4.

Pradhan AD, Manson JE, Rifai N *et al.* (2001) C-reactive protein, interleukin-6 and risk of developing type diabetes. *JAMA* **286**:327–34.

Pyörälä K, Laakso M, Uusitupa M (1987) Diabetes and atherosclerosis: an epidemiologic view. *Diabetes Metab Rev* **3**(2):463–524.

Randomised trial of cholesterol lowering in 4444 patients with coronary heart disease: the Scandinavian Simvastatin Survival Study (4S). *Lancet* **344**:1383.

Reaven GM (1993) Role of insulin resistance in human disease (syndrome X): *Annu Rev Med* **44**:121.

Reaven GM, Lithell H and Landsberg L (1996) The role of insulin resistance and the sympathoadrenal system. *N Engl J Med* **334**:374.

Rea TD, Hechbert SR, Kaplan RC *et al.* (2001) Body mass index and the risk of recurrent coronary events following acute myocardial infarction. *Am J Cardiol* **88**:467.

Rexrode KM, Carey VJ, Hennekens CH *et al.* (1998) Abdominal obesity and coronary heart disease in women. *JAMA* **280**:1843.

Rich-Edwards JW, Manson JE, Hennekens CH and Buring JE (1995) The primary prevention of coronary heart disease in women. *N Engl J Med* **332**:1758.

Roffi M, Chew DP, Mukherjee D *et al.* (2001) Platelet glycoprotein llb/llla inhibitors reduce mortality in diabetic patients with non-ST segment elevation acute coronary syndromes *Circulation* **104**:2767–71.

Ross R (1999) Atherosclerosis – an inflammatory disease. *N Engl J Med* **340**:115–26.

Rubins HB, Robins SJ, Collins D *et al.* (1999) Gemfibrozil for the secondary prevention of coronary heart disease in men with low levels of high-density lipoprotein cholesterol. Veterans Affairs High-Density Lipoprotein Cholesterol Intervention Trial Study Group. *N Engl J Med* **341**:410.

Saad MF, Lillioja S, Nyomba BL *et al.* (1991) Racial differences in the relation between blood pressure and insulin resistance. *N Engl J Med* **324**:733.

Sacks, FM, Pfeffer MA, Moye LA *et al.* (1996) The effect of pravastatin on coronary events after myocardial infarction in patients with average cholesterol levels. Cholesterol and Recurrent Events Trial investigators. *N Engl J Med* **335**:1001.

Sasaki A, Horiuchi N, Hasegawa R and Uehara M (1989) Mortality in type 2 diabetic patients. A long term follow up study in Osaka District, Japan. *Diab Res Clin Pract* **7**:33–40.

Schoeller DA, Shay K and Kushner RF (1997) How much physical activity is needed to minimise weight gain in previously obese women? *Am J Clin Nutr* **66**:551–6.

Schotte DE and Stunkard AJ (1990) The effects of weight reduction on blood pressure in 301 obese patients. *Arch Int Med* **150**:1701–4.

Schwartz, GG, Olsson AG, Ezekowitz MD *et al.* (2001) Effects of atorvastatin on early recurrent ischaemic events in acute coronary syndromes. The MIRACL Study: A randomized controlled trial. *JAMA* **285**:1711.

Singer DE, Moulton AW and Nathan DM (1989) Diabetic myocardial infarction. Interaction of diabetes with other preinfarction risk factors. *Diabetes* **38**:350–7.

Sjostrom LV (1992a) Mortality of severely obese subjects. *Am J Clin Nutr* **55**:516S.

Sjostrom LV (1992b) Morbidity of severely obese subjects. *Am J Clin Nutr* **55**(suppl 2).

Smith JW, Marcus FI and Serokman R (1984) Prognosis of patients with diabetes mellitus after myocardial infarction. *Am J Cardiol* **54**:718–21.

Sowers JR and Draznin B (1998) Insulin, cation metabolism and insulin resistance. *J Basic Clin Physiol Pharmacol* **9**:223–33.

Staessen J, Fagard R, Lijnen P and Amery A (1989) Body weight, sodium intake and blood pressure. *J Hypertens* **7**(Suppl. 1):S19–S23.

Stamler J, Vaccaso O, Neaton JD and Wentworth D (1993) Diabetes, other risk factors and 12 yr cardiovascular mortality for men – the Multiple Risk Factor Intervention Trial. *Diabetes Care* **16**:434–44.

Stehouwer CD, Lambert J, Donker AJ and van Hinsbergh VW (1997) Endothelial dysfunction and pathogenesis of diabetic angiopathy. *Cardiovasc Res* **34**:55–68.

Steinberg HO, Chaker H, Leaming R *et al.* (1996) Obesity/insulin resistance-endothelial dysfunction. *J Clin Invest* **97**:2601.

Steppan, CM, Bailey ST, Bhat S *et al.* (2001) The hormone resistin links obesity to diabetes. *Nature* **409**:307.

Stern MP (1995) Diabetes and cardiovascular disease. 'the common soil' hypothesis *Diabetes* **44**:369–74.

Storey AM, Perry CJ and Petric JR (2001) Endothelial dysfunction in type 2 diabetes. *Br J Diabetes Vasc Dis* **1**:22–7.

Syvanne M and Taskinen MR (1997) Lipids and lipoproteins as coronary risk factors in NIDDM. *Lancet* **350**(Suppl I):20–3.

The Diabetes Control and Complication Trial. *N Engl J Med* **329**:977–86, 1993.

Tatti P, Pahor M, Byington RP *et al.* (1998) Outcome results of fosinopril versus amlodipine cardiovascular events randomised trial (FACET) in patients with hypertension and NIDDM. *Diabetes Care* **21**:597–603.

Tchernof A, Lamarche B, Prud'Homme D *et al.* (1996) The dense LDL phenotype: association with plasma lipoprotein levels, visceral obesity, and hyperinsulinemia in men. *Diabetes Care* **19**:629–37.

Tesfamariam B, Palacino JJ, Weisbrod RM and Cohen RA (1993) Aldose reductase inhibition restores endothelial cell function in diabetic rabbit aorta. *J Cardiovasc Pharm* **21**:205–11.

Thompson SG, Kienast J, Pyke SD *et al.* (1995) Hemostatic factors and the risk of myocardial infarction or sudden death in patients with angina pectoris. *N Engl J Med* **332**:635–41.

Tschoepe D, Rosen P, Kaufmann L *et al.* (1990) Evidence for abnormal platelet glycoprotein expression in diabetes mellitus. *Eur J Clin Invest* **20**:166–70.

Tuomilehto J, Raotenyte D, Birkenhager WH *et al.* (1999) Effects of calcium channel blockade in older patients with diabetes and systolic hypertension. *N Engl J Med* **340**:677–84.

Turner RC, Millns H, Neil HA *et al.* (1998) Risk factors for coronary artery disease in non-insulin dependent diabetes mellitus. United Kingdom Prospective Diabetes Study. (UKPDS-23). *Br Med J* **316**:823–8.

US Surgeon General (1996) *Physical Activity and Health: A Report of the Surgeon General.* US Department of Health and Human Services, Washington, DC.

UK Prospective Diabetes Study Group (1998) Tight blood pressure control and risk of macrovascular and microvascular complications in type 2 diabetes: UKPDS 38. *Br Med J* **317**:703–13.

Wingard DL (1995) Heart disease and diabetes. In *Diabetes in America.* US Govt. Printing Office, Washington, DC, pp. 429–48 (NIH publ. no. 95–1468).

Wyatt HR (2002) The National Weight Control Registry. In Bessesen DH and Kushner RF, (eds). *Evaluation and Management of Obesity.* Hanley & Belfus Inc, Philadelphia, pp. 119–124.

Wadden TA, Foster GD and Letizia KA (1994) One-year behavioural treatment of obesity: comparison of moderate and severe caloric restriction and the effects of weight maintenance therapy. *J Consult Clin Psychol* **62**:165–71.

Wadden TA, Vogt RA, Andersen RE *et al.* (1997) Exercise in the treatment of obesity: effects of four interventions on body composition, resting energy expenditure, appetite, and mood. *J Consult Clin Psychol* **65**:269–77.

Walston J, Silver K, Bogardus C *et al.* (1995) Time of onset of non-insulin-dependent diabetes mellitus and genetic variation in the ß3-adrenergic-receptor gene. *N Engl J Med* **333**:343.

Watts GF, Lewis B, Brunt JN *et al.* (1992) Effects on coronary artery disease of lipid-lowering diet or diet plus cholestyramine in the St. Thomas' Atherosclerosis Regression Study (STARS). *Lancet* **339**:563.

Weyer C, Funahashi T, Tanaka S *et al.* (2001) Hypoadiponectinemia in obesity and type 2 diabetes: close association with insulin resistance and hyperinsulinemia. *J Clin Endocrinol Metab* **86**:1930.

Weyer C, Yudkin JS, Stehouwer CD *et al.* (2002) Humoral markers of inflammation and endothelial dysfunction in relation to adiposity in Pima Indians. *Atherosclerosis* **161**:233–42.

Wiesenthal SR, Sandhu H, McCall RH *et al.* (1999) Free fatty acid impair hepatic insulin extraction *in vivo. Diabetes* **48**:766–74.

Willett WC, Manson JE, Stampfer MJ *et al.* (1995) Weight, weight change and coronary heart disease in women. *JAMA* **273**:461–5.

Williams B (1994) Insulin resistance: the shape of things to come. *Lancet* **344**:521.

Williams SB, Cusco JA, Roddy MA *et al.* (1996) Impaired nitric oxide-mediated vasodilation in patients with NIDDM. *J Am Coll Cardiol* **27**:567–74.

Wing RR and Jeffery RW (2001) Food provision as a strategy to promote weight loss. *Obes Res* **9**(suppl 4):271S–275S.

Wing RR, Koeske R, Epstein LH *et al.* (1987) Long-term effects of modest weight loss in type II diabetic patients. *Arch Intern Med* **147**:1749–53.

Withers DJ, Gutierrez JS, Towery H *et al.* (1998) Disruption of IRS-2 causes type 2 diabetes in mice. *Nature* **391**:900.

Wolf BA, Williamson JR, Easan RA *et al.* (1991) Diacylglycerol accumulation and microvascular abnormalities induced by elevated glucose levels. *J Clin Invest* **87**:31–8.

Wood PD, Stefanick ML, Dieon DM *et al.* (1988) Changes in plasma lipids and lipoproteins in overweight men during weight loss through dieting as compared with exercise. *N Engl J Med* **319**:1173–9.

Yudkin JS, Stehouwer CD, Emeis JJ and Coppack SW (1999) C-reactive protein in healthy subjects: association with obesity, insulin resistance and endothelial dysfunction. *Arterioscler Thromb Vasc Biol* **19**:972–8.

10

Drug Therapy for the Obese Diabetic Patient

John P. H. Wilding

Introduction

Type 2 diabetes is strongly associated with obesity and overweight, such that the majority of patients (at least 80 per cent in Caucasian populations) will have a body mass index of at least $25 \, kg/m^2$, and well over 50 per cent will be clinically obese (WHO Study Group, 1997). Hence, any discussion of drug therapy in patients with type 2 diabetes must give serious consideration to the special problems encountered when treating obese subjects. This is particularly important as polypharmacy is now the norm for patients with type 2 diabetes, given the evidence that an aggressive, multifactorial approach to risk factor reduction is of benefit when attempting to reduce the risk of micro- and macrovascular complications (Gaede et al., 2003). More specifically, there is good evidence that weight loss can be an effective treatment for type 2 diabetes, resulting in improved control and reducing risk from cardiovascular disease (Wing et al., 1987; Lean et al., 1990; Pories et al., 1995; Figure 10.1). In this chapter I will discuss those aspects of pharmacotherapy in patients with type 2 diabetes that are relevant to obesity; namely the effects of drugs used to treat hyperglycaemia on body weight, the choice of drugs used to treat other risk factors such as hypertension, drugs used to treat complications and consider the role of specific therapy for weight reduction and weight maintenance in the treatment and prevention of type 2 diabetes.

Drugs for hyperglycaemia

Treatment of hyperglycaemia is arguably the most difficult task when treating obese patients with type 2 diabetes. For example in the United Kingdom

Obesity and Diabetes. Edited by Anthony H. Barnett and Sudhesh Kumar
© 2004 John Wiley & Sons, Ltd   ISBN: 0-470-84898-7

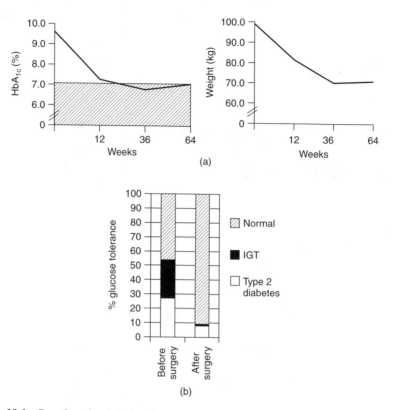

Figure 10.1 Benefits of weight loss in type 2 diabetes. (a) Changes in weight and HbA$_{1c}$ in subjects who succeeded in losing at least 13.6 kg during a behavioural weight loss programme (redrawn using data from Wing *et al.*, 1987). (b) Change in glucose tolerance status after gastric bypass surgery (data from Pories *et al.*, 1995). IGT, impaired glucose tolerance.

Prospective Diabetes Study (UKPDS), the progressive worsening of glycaemic control over time, despite regular stepwise increases in therapy in an attempt to maintain predetermined levels of fasting glycaemia (Turner, 1999) was particularly apparent in obese patients (Turner *et al.*, 1999). Furthermore, with the exception of metformin and acarbose, drugs used to treat hyperglycaemia often lead to further weight gain in patients with diabetes, which will tend to increase insulin resistance, sometimes creating a vicious cycle of increasing weight and drug dose, and adversely affecting risk factors such as blood pressure and low-density lipoprotein (LDL)-cholesterol (Yki-Jarvinen *et al.*, 1997). Newer strategies, either combining drugs to minimize weight gain, or treating obesity itself with drugs may eventually result in more effective strategies than those used in the UKPDS study.

Metformin

There is now good evidence that whenever possible, metformin should be used as first line therapy in overweight and obese patients with type 2 diabetes, when hyperglycaemia cannot be adequately controlled by lifestyle changes alone. In the UKPDS, early treatment of obese patients with metformin, both improved hyperglycaemia, resulting in average HbA_{1c} values 0.6 per cent lower compared to patients predominantly treated with diet alone, and prevented most of the weight gain that occurred in subjects treated with insulin or sulphonylureas (Turner et al., 1998, 1999). Overweight or obese subjects randomized to metformin had a 32 per cent reduction in the composite endpoints for both micro- and macrovascular complications, including retinopathy, nephropathy, peripheral neuropathy, myocardial infarction, and stroke, compared to lifestyle change alone (Turner et al., 1998). This is in contrast to other treatments, which only significantly reduced microvascular complications. It is tempting to speculate that the apparent additional protective effect of metformin on the incidence of macrovascular disease was due to its effects on body weight, although it is not possible to determine this from the UKPDS data. Some studies have suggested that metformin causes modest weight loss, and this may be the case in some patients; however its potency as a weight loss agent is not sufficient for it to be classed as such. The mechanism whereby metformin influences body weight is not known; many patients report nausea and gastrointestinal disturbance as a side effect, and this leads to withdrawal of the drug in about 5 per cent of patients. This suggests that metformin may act predominantly by reducing energy intake, and there is evidence that this is the case (Makimattila et al., 1999). There has been some concern about lactic acidosis as a side effect of metformin therapy; this precludes its use in many patients due to contraindications that include renal impairment, cardiac and hepatic failure, that are common in the obese diabetic population. Despite this, there is evidence that it is widely used in patients with contraindications, without much evidence of adverse effects (lactic acidosis remains very rare) and there have been recent calls for these to be reviewed in the light of this experience (Jones et al., 2003). Metformin also has a potential role in the prevention of diabetes, with a 30 per cent reduction seen over 4 years in the recently reported US diabetes prevention programme, although this was less than with an intensive diet and exercise programme (that reduced diabetes incidence by 58 per cent, it may be a suitable choice for people unable or unwilling to undertake such an approach, particularly in younger patients (Diabetes Prevention Program Research Group, 2002).

Sulphonylureas

Weight gain, in the range of 3–4 kg over the first 6–12 months of therapy is usual with drugs such as glibenclamide and chlorpropamide, as was seen in the UKPDS. Similar effects are usually seen with newer agents, such as glipizide and gliclazide, although some studies report no weight gain with glipizide, this may be because these studies were of short duration (Simonson et al., 1997; Cefalu et al., 1998). Such drugs should therefore be considered as second-line agents in obese patients with type 2 diabetes, usually as add-on therapy to metformin, and only used as monotherapy only if metformin is contraindicated or poorly tolerated. The mechanisms whereby sulphonylureas cause weight gain are not fully understood, and have not been studied in detail. Improved metabolic control, with reduction of glycosuria has been suggested as one possible mechanism, but weight gain also occurs in patients without glycosuria. Studies of energy intake and metabolic rate in diabetic patients on sulphonylureas versus metformin show little difference in energy expenditure, but this is slightly lower in those on sulphonylureas after adjusting for fat free mass (Chong *et al.*, 1995). Hyperglycaemia itself is correlated with basal metabolic rate, perhaps due to the energy costs of increased gluconeogenesis and futile glucose cycling; so part of the weight gain could be due to a reduction in metabolic rate related to improvements in hyperglycaemia during therapy (Efendic *et al.*, 1985; Franssilakallunki and Groop, 1992). Hyperinsulinaemia, leading to increased deposition of lipid in adipose tissue might also increase metabolic efficiency. Hypoglycaemia is said to increase hunger, and is a known side-effect of sulphonylureas, but hypoglycaemia is uncommon in poorly controlled obese patients with type 2 diabetes. A recent report suggesting that the sulphonylurea receptor is expressed in adipocytes and increases expression of lipogenic enzymes such as fatty acid synthase could be of relevance, but the clinical significance of this *in-vitro* observation remains uncertain (Shi *et al.*, 1999). Receptors for sulphonylureas are also present in the hypothalamus and other appetite-regulating areas of the central nervous system, but the possibility of direct effects on appetite and/or central nervous system (CNS) modulation of energy expenditure by sulphonylureas and related compounds has not been systematically investigated (Treherne and Ashford, 1991).

Non-sulphonylurea insulin secretagogues

Newer insulin secretagogues, acting on the K-ATP channel, glitinides, such as nateglinide and repaglinide have recently become available for clinical use. They are very short-acting, and are therefore given prior to meals to control post-prandial hyperglycaemia. They appear to be equivalent to sulphonylureas in terms of their effects on overall glycaemic control as measured by HbA_{1c}. There have been some claims that these newer agents cause less weight gain than sulphonylureas, but these have been in relatively short-term studies, or from observational data and there are no definitive data from comparative long-term randomized trials to substantiate claims of superiority in this respect (Landgraf *et al.*, 2000).

Acarbose

Acarbose is an α-glucosidase inhibitor that inhibits the breakdown of some complex sugars to glucose within the intestinal lumen, thus reducing the rise in glucose seen after a carbohydrate meal. This undigested carbohydrate is eventually broken down by bacterial fermentation in the large bowel, and most of the sugars are therefore eventually absorbed. Acarbose therefore does not usually cause weight loss, although this has been reported in some studies (Wolever *et al.*, 1997), but it does reduce HbA$_{1c}$ by about 0.6 per cent on average, without weight gain (Holman *et al.*, 1999). It can therefore be helpful in obese patients with type 2 diabetes, but its use is frequently limited by gastrointestinal side effects.

Thiazolidinediones

Thiazolidinediones are a relatively new addition to the range of drugs used to treat hyperglycaemia in type 2 diabetes. They are agonists at the peroxisome proliferator activated receptor-γ (PPARγ), a nuclear receptor found predominantly in adipose tissue, the function of which is thought to be regulation of aspects of adipocyte differentiation and adipocyte function (Spiegelman, 1998). These drugs act to sensitize tissues such as adipose tissue and muscle to insulin, via a range of effects that include a reduction in circulating non-esterified fatty acids, and alterations in expression of adipocytokines such as tumour necrosis factor-α (TNF-α), leptin and adiponectin that may influence insulin sensitivity (Nolan *et al.*, 1999; Wang *et al.*, 1997). Weight gain and redistribution of body fat appear to be closely linked to the therapeutic effects of this class of drugs. In animal models weight gain is dose dependent, and occurs in all animal models of obesity studied to date, including the fatty Zucker rat, which lacks functional leptin receptors (thus dispelling the notion that weight gain is secondary to the reduction in leptin synthesis seen with thiazolidinedione treatment) (Wang *et al.*, 1997). The effect is also dependent on diet, with greater effects seen when rats are provided with a highly palatable diet (Pickavance *et al.*, 1999). Part of the weight gain may be due to increased energetic efficiency as weight gain still occurs when animals are pair-fed with controls (Pickavance *et al.*, 2001). Thiazolidinediones also cause some fluid retention through an unknown mechanism, but the majority of weight gain is due to an increase in adipose tissue rather than body water. In humans, the average weight gain over 12 months of treatment is in the range of 3–4 kg, which is similar to that observed with sulphonylureas (Raskin *et al.*, 2001). The changes in fat distribution are of some interest, and been claimed to be beneficial, as investigation using magnetic resonance imaging or computerized tomography has shown decreases in visceral adipose tissue whilst subcutaneous adipose tissue mass increases (Kelly *et al.*, 1999). Animal and human studies have also demonstrated the synergistic effect of drug treatment plus lifestyle changes – thus avoidance of weight gain enhances the therapeutic effect (Pickavance *et al.*, 2001; Reynolds *et al.*, 2002).

Insulin

The natural history of type 2 diabetes is that of declining β-cell function, such that insulin therapy is often required, either as a substitute or as add-on therapy to oral agents. In the UKPDS 53 per cent of sulphonylurea-treated patients required insulin during the course of the study. Insulin treatment is frequently, but not invariably associated with significant weight gain; in the UKPDS the average weight gain in subjects randomized to insulin was 7.5 kg over 10 years (compared to 2.5 kg in those randomized to diet alone; Turner, 1999). In one study in the US of intensive insulin therapy in type 2 diabetes, good control (average glucose fell from 17.5 to 7.7 mmol/l) was only achieved at the expense of weight gain of nearly 9 kg in just 6 months. Weight gain with insulin treatment can be attenuated by up to 80 per cent with the addition or continuation of metformin, and where possible this should be considered standard treatment of obese patients with type 2 diabetes when insulin therapy is required.

The role of anti-obesity drugs in diabetic management

Given the overwhelming evidence that obesity is of fundamental importance in the aetiology of type 2 diabetes, as well as many of its co-morbid conditions such as hypertension, dyslipidaemia and other aspects of the metabolic syndrome, it is surprising how little attention has been given to weight management, compared to the extensive studies that have been conducted with drugs to control hyperglycaemia, hypertension and dyslipidaemia. There is little doubt that reduction of excess body weight can be very effective treatment. Dietary intervention studies suggest that a weight loss of approximately 10 per cent is required to significantly improve HbA_{1c} in subjects with established type 2 diabetes, although some subjects may respond dramatically to lesser degrees of weight loss (Wing et al., 1987). Modest weight loss early in the course of the disease, combined with other changes to diet and lifestyle can also be extremely effective, as was shown during the first 3 months of dietary treatment in the UKPDS (Manley et al., 2000). Prevention studies, conducted in obese and overweight subjects with impaired glucose tolerance, have shown that weight loss of only 3 or 4 kg can have dramatic effects to prevent or delay the onset of type 2 diabetes (Tuomilheto et al., 2001; DPPRG, 2002). Thus there is heterogeneity of response to weight loss in type 2 diabetes that may be in part related to the duration of the disease with weight loss becoming less effective as β-cell dysfunction develops. Nevertheless, even in insulin-requiring patients, weight loss can be beneficial, and on occasion can result in normalization of blood glucose, especially after surgical intervention, such as gastric bypass (Pories et al., 1995).

What then, is the role of anti-obesity drugs? The fenfluramines have now been withdrawn on grounds of safety, following reports of development of carcinoid-like valvular heart lesions in some patients in the United States. Phentermine and diethylpropion, somewhat controversially, remain available for short-term use (up to 3 months), despite of lack of long-term trial data of sufficient quality to support their continued use. Two newer agents, orlistat and sibutramine, are now in widespread use, and data is available regarding their role in the management of patients with type 2 diabetes.

Orlistat

Orlistat is an inhibitor of pancreatic and intestinal lipases, and therefore prevents the breakdown of dietary fat into fatty acids and glycerol within the gut lumen, resulting in approximately 30 per cent malabsorption of dietary fat. For individuals on a Western diet, this typically results in a daily caloric deficit of about 200–300 kcal; without dietary restraint, this should result in a weight loss of about 0.2–0.3 kg per week, or 5–7.5 kg over 6 months. This will of course be somewhat attenuated by the fall in metabolic rate that occurs with weight loss, so weight loss tends to gradually reach a plateau after 6–9 months of treatment. Clinical trials with orlistat have usually included dietary advice to help weight loss, and recommendations about increasing physical activity, hence the average weight loss achieved in non-diabetic subjects is on average about 10 kg (compared to 6 kg with diet and exercise alone). There is some evidence that the early response to treatment is a good predictor of future weight loss (Sjostrom *et al.*, 1998). Once weight loss has stopped, the role of continued drug use is to promote weight maintenance, as weight is soon regained if the drug is stopped. Side-effects of orlistat are confined to the gastrointestinal tract, as the drug is not systemically absorbed and include loose fatty stools, oily spotting and rarely faecal incontinence. These side-effects tend to reduce with time, as patients learn to avoid foods that are high in fat. Circulating concentrations of fat-soluble vitamins and β-carotene fall by about 10 per cent but clinical vitamin deficiency is very rare, and can be prevented by use of a multivitamin supplement.

Several studies have been conducted using orlistat in diabetic patients, either treated with diet or with a variety of oral agents and insulin. Typically, subjects with type 2 diabetes find it more difficult to lose weight than those without diabetes (Wing *et al.*, 1987), and in general the weight loss observed is less; for example in sulphonylurea-treated patients with type 2 diabetes, weight loss over 12 months was 6 kg with orlistat compared to 3 kg with placebo, so that twice as many patients achieved 5 and 10 per cent weight loss with orlistat. This modest weight loss did, however, result in improvements in glycaemic control that were proportional to weight loss, and moreover, there were also favourable changes in the lipid profile (Hollander *et al.*, 1998). Similar results have been shown in metformin and insulin-treated patients, but these trials have yet to be reported in full (Bray *et al.*, 2001; Miles *et al.*, 2001). The Xendos trial, a trial of diabetes prevention with orlistat has also recently reported, and supports the use of orlistat as an adjunct to diet and exercise in subjects at high risk of developing type 2 diabetes, as well as demonstrating efficacy at weight maintenance for up to 4 years (Anon, 2002).

Sibutramine

Sibutramine is a centrally acting drug that is an inhibitor of serotonin and norepinephrine (noradrenaline) reuptake. As a reuptake inhibitor, it is in some ways pharmacologically similar to reuptake inhibitors used as antidepressants, but sibutramine does not have antidepressant or euphoric properties. It is pharmacologically distinct from serotonin releasing agents, such as dexfenfluramine, that have been reported to cause cardiac valvular lesions similar to those seen in carcinoid syndrome (Connolly et al., 1997; Gundlah et al., 1997; Bach et al., 1999). Sibutramine is thought to act by both increasing post-prandial satiety (the feeling of fullness after a meal), and by increasing thermogenesis, particularly by attenuating the usual fall in energy expenditure that occurs with weight loss (Halford et al., 1994; Hansen et al., 1998). CNS-mediated side effects include dry mouth, insomnia and constipation; there is also a modest increase in sympathetic nervous system activity, which is responsible for the change in thermogenesis, but also can result in increases in heart rate and blood pressure in some patients, although the average changes seen in clinical trials are of 2–4 bpm in heart rate, and 1–2 mmHg of systolic and diastolic blood pressure, although no significant changes are seen in obese hypertensive patients whose blood pressure is well controlled (Hazenberg, 2000). The efficacy of sibutramine for both weight loss and weight maintenance has been tested in clinical trials of up to two years duration. For example in the Sibutramine Trial of Weight Reduction and Maintenance (STORM) study, conducted in non-diabetic patients, mean weight loss of 12 per cent occurred over the first 6 months of the study; this was largely maintained for a further 18 months in those subjects in whom the active drug was continued, whereas significant weight regain occurred in subjects switched to placebo, despite continuing dietary and lifestyle advice. Nearly 50 per cent of patients maintained weight loss of at least 10 per cent for the duration of the study. As well as inducing weight loss, there were significant improvements in the lipid profile with weight loss in this study, with reduction in LDL, very low-density lipoprotein cholesterol, triglycerides and an increase in high-density lipoprotein (HDL) cholesterol, such that the cholesterol HDL ratio fell by 13.3 per cent (James et al., 2000). These beneficial effects may have been offset to some extent by increases in blood pressure, although a meta-analysis of such changes suggests an overall decrease in cardiovascular risk, as assessed using the Framingham risk equation (Lauterbach, 2000). Sibutramine has also been evaluated in diabetic patients treated with diet, metformin, and sulphonylureas (Serrano-Rios et al., 2002). As with orlistat, weight loss proved more elusive in trials in diabetic patients, but, for example, in metformin-treated patients, an average weight loss of about 5 per cent was achieved and maintained for 12 months, compared to virtually no weight loss in placebo-treated subjects, despite intensified dietary advice. This was associated with improvements in HbA_{1c}, lipid profile and little change in blood pressure in subjects who lost weight, although there was an increase in heart rate, and more sibutramine-treated patients experienced a rise in blood pressure (McNulty et al., 2003). These encouraging results, together with legitimate concerns regarding the cardiovascular effects of sibutramine, has led to the design of the Sibutramine

Cardiovascular Outcomes Trial (SCOUT), that will investigate the effects of weight loss with sibutramine on cardiovascular endpoints in high risk patients, including many with type 2 diabetes.

In summary, there is now good evidence that use of drugs for weight loss can be a useful adjunct to improve glycaemic, lipid and possibly blood pressure control in patients with type 2 diabetes. However at present, careful selection of motivated patients is important, as with any weight loss programme, and definitive trials examining hard endpoints are yet to be conducted.

Drugs in development

Given the high level of recent interest in developing drugs for weight loss, it seems likely that newer, perhaps more effective agents will eventually become available. Agents currently under evaluation include new lipase inhibitors, β_3-receptor agonists, cholecystokinin receptor agonists, cannabinoid receptor-1 receptor antagonists, the anticonvulsant topiramate, and leptin analogues. Diabetes management would be transformed if a safe, highly effective weight loss agent became available, but this seems unlikely in the near future.

Antihypertensive treatment

Although many intervention trials have been conducted using different anti-hypertensive agents in diabetic and non-diabetic subjects, few studies have been conducted exclusively in obese subjects, and some studies have specifically excluded very obese patients. The average body mass index (BMI) in the UKPDS study was approximately $29 \, \text{kg/m}^2$, but no sub-group analysis based on BMI has been reported. There is clear evidence from the literature that obese hypertensive patients have higher circulating catecholamine concentrations and greater activity of the renin–angiotensin system than non-obese patients, but it is unknown whether this is also the case in diabetic patients. It is therefore difficult to draw firm conclusions about the optimal antihypertensive strategy for obese patients with type 2 diabetes. Angiotensin-converting enzyme (ACE) inhibitors are certainly effective, and may have other advantages in subjects with cardiovascular disease, nephropathy and retinopathy; they have been shown to reduce complication rates in the UKPDS study (Stearne et al., 1998); angiotensin II receptor blockers have similar effects, and can be used if patients are intolerant of ACE inhibitors, combination with ACE inhibitors may be indicated in patients with microalbuminuria. Low dose thiazide diuretics are safe, but slightly less efficacious than ACE inhibitors – they are a reasonable first-line choice in patients without microalbuminuria. β-blockers are certainly effective antihypertensive drugs, but they can cause weight gain, and were less well tolerated than ACE inhibitors in the UKPDS, so should perhaps be considered as second-line agents, although they may be specifically indicated in patients with

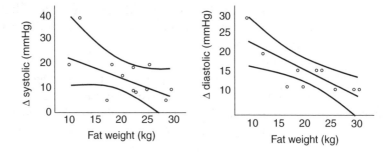

Figure 10.2 Obese patients respond less well to nifedipine as antihypertensive treatment. Data redrawn from Stoabirketvedt *et al.* (1995).

angina, some dysrhythmias, and in heart failure. Calcium channel blockers seem to be less effective in patients with obesity-related hypertension (Stoabirketvedt *et al.*, 1995), but are useful as add-on therapy (Sharma *et al.*, 2001; Figure 10.2). Other drugs such as α-blockers, methyldopa and clonidine and may have a role as adjunctive therapy where blood pressure is difficult to control.

Lipid-lowering treatment

Although weight loss may have beneficial effects on lipids, particularly on HDL cholesterol and triglycerides, the evidence for use of lipid-lowering agents in subjects at high risk of cardiovascular disease is now very strong, and it would therefore be difficult to justify withholding such treatment on the grounds of expected effects of weight loss. Clearly, if substantial weight loss is achieved, then the continuing need for lipid-lowering drugs should be reviewed.

Use of other drugs that may cause weight gain

There is a long list of drugs, mainly centrally acting, that can cause weight gain (Table 10.1), and these are often prescribed to patients with diabetes. Of particular note are tricyclic antidepressants and anticonvulsants such as carbamazepine and gabapentin used for symptom control in painful neuropathy. Other drugs include antipsychotic drugs, notably the newer atypical antipsychotic agents, such as clozapine and olanzapine, that can cause substantial weight gain, and have been suggested to independently worsen insulin resistance and perhaps increase diabetes risk in non-diabetic subjects (Hedenmalm *et al.*, 2002). Pizotifen, a serotonin antagonist used in the management of migraine, may cause increased appetite and therefore weight gain (Galanopoulou *et al.*, 1990). Corticosteroids and some progesterone preparations, such as medroxyprogesterone acetate may also cause substantial weight gain, and in the case of corticosteroids, worsen insulin resistance and impair β-cell function. Finally, antiretroviral therapy, used in the management of HIV infection, may cause lipodystrophy with

Table 10.1 Drugs causing weight gain

Class	Examples	Mechanism of effect
Anticonvulsants	Sodium valproate	Unknown
	Phenytoin	
	Gabapentin	
Antidepressants	Citalopram	Serotonin
	Mirtazepine	
Antipsychotics	Chlorpromazine	? Dopamine agonism
	Risperidone	
	Olanzepine	
β-Blockers	Atenolol	? Inhibition of thermogenesis
Corticosteroids	Prednisolone	Promote fat deposition
	Dexamethasone	Increase appetite
Insulin	All formulations	
Sex steroids	Medroxyprogesterone acetate	Increase appetite
	Progesterone	
	Combined oral contraceptives	
Insulin secretagogues	Glibenclamide	Changes in metabolic rate, and increased appetite implicated
	Gliclazide	
	Repaglinide	
Thiazolidinediones	Rosiglitazone	Changes in metabolic rate, and increased appetite implicated
	Pioglitazone	
Drugs for migraine	Pizotifen	Serotonin antagonist
Protease inhibitors	Indinavir	Promote site-specific fat deposition
	Ritonavir	

increased central adiposity and thus either predispose to diabetes, or exacerbate existing glucose intolerance (Carr *et al.*, 1998). Whilst it may not be possible to avoid the use of many of these drugs, it is important to be aware of their potential effects on body weight, keep doses to the minimum, and give appropriate advice to patients, with regard to dietary restraint when they are taking drugs that may result in weight gain.

References

Anon (2002) Xendos study: Orlistat plus diet prevents, delays diabetes onset in obese patients. *Formulary* **37**:504.

Bach DS, Rissanen AM, Mendel CM *et al.* (1999) Absence of cardiac valve dysfunction in obese patients treated with sibutramine. *Obes Res* **7**:363–9.

Bray GA, Pi-Sunyer FX, Hollander P and Kelley DE (2001) Effect of orlistat in overweight patients with type 2 diabetes receiving insulin therapy. *Diabetes* **50**:A107.

Carr A, Samaras K, Chisholm DJ and Cooper DA (1998) Pathogenesis of HIV-1-protease inhibitor-associated peripheral lipodystrophy, hyperlipidaemia, and insulin resistance. *Lancet* **351**:1881–3.

Cefalu WT, Bell-Farrow A, Wang ZQ et al. (1998) Effect of glipizide GITS on insulin sensitivity, glycemic indices, and abdominal fat composition in NIDDM. *Drug Devel Res* **44**:1–7.

Chong PKK, Jung RT, Rennie MJ and Scrimgeour CM (1995) Energy-expenditure in type-2 diabetic-patients on metformin and sulfonylurea therapy. *Diabet Med* **12**:401–8.

Connolly HM, Crary JL, McGoon MD et al. (1997) Valvular heart disease associated with fenfluramine-phentermine. *N Engl J Med* **337**:581–8.

Diabetes Prevention Program Research Group (2002) Reduction in the incidence of type 2 diabetes with lifestyle intervention or metformin. *N Engl J Med* **346**:393–403.

Efendic S, Wajngot A and Vranic M (1985) Increased activity of the glucose cycle in the liver – early characteristic of type-2 diabetes. *Proc Natl Acad Sci USA* **82**:2965–9.

Franssilakallunki A and Groop L (1992) Factors associated with basal metabolic-rate in patients with type-2 (non-insulin-dependent) diabetes-mellitus. *Diabetologia* **35**:962–6.

Gaede P, Vedel P, Larsen N et al. (2003) Multifactorial Intervention and Cardiovascular Disease in Patients with Type 2 Diabetes. *N Engl J Med* **348**:383–93.

Galanopoulou P, Giannacopoulos G, Theophanopoulos C et al. (1990) Behavioural changes on diet selection and serotonin (5-HT) turnover in rats under pizotifen treatment. *Pharmacol Biochem Behav* **37**:461–4.

Gundlah C, Martin KF, Heal DJ and Auerbach SB (1997) *In vivo* criteria to differentiate monoamine reuptake inhibitors from releasing agents: Sibutramine is a reuptake inhibitor. *J Pharmacol Exp Ther* **283**:581–91.

Halford JCG, Heal DJ and Blundell JE (1994) Investigation of a new potential antiobesity drug, sibutramine, using the behavioral satiety sequence. *Appetite* **23**:306–7.

Hansen DL, Toubro S, Stock MJ et al. (1998) Thermogenic effects of sibutramine in humans. *Am J Clin Nutr* **68**:1180–6.

Hazenberg BP (2000) Randomized, double-blind, placebo-controlled, multicenter study of sibutramine in obese hypertensive patients. *Cardiology* **94**:152–8.

Hedenmalm K, Hagg S, Stahl M et al. (2002) Glucose intolerance with atypical antipsychotics. *Drug Saf* **25**:1107–16.

Hollander PA, Elbein SC, Hirsch IB et al. (1998) Role of orlistat in the treatment of obese patients with type 2 diabetes – A 1-year randomized double-blind study. *Diabetes Care* **21**:1288–94.

Holman RR, Cull CA and Turner RC (1999) A randomized double-blind trial of acarbose in type 2 diabetes shows improved glycemic control over 3 years (UK Prospective Diabetes Study 44). *Diabetes Care* **22**:960–4.

James WPT, Astrup A, Finer N et al. (2000) Effect of sibutramine on weight maintenance after weight loss: a randomised trial. *Lancet* **356**:2119–25.

Jones GC Alexander WM and Macklin JP (2003) Contraindications to the use of metformin. *Br Med J* **326**:4–5.

Kelly IE, Han TS, Walsh K and Lean MEJ (1999) Effects of a thiazolidinedione compound on body fat and fat distribution of patients with type 2 diabetes. *Diabetes Care* **22**:288–93.

Landgraf R, Frank M, Bauer C and Dieken ML (2000) Prandial glucose regulation with repaglinide: its clinical and lifestyle impact in a large cohort of patients with Type 2 diabetes. *Int J Obes* **24**:S38–S44.

Lauterbach K (2000) Framingham analysis: Coronary heart disease risk reduction with weight loss in obesity on sibutramine treatment. *Obes Res* **8**:B83.

Lean ME, Powrie JK, Anderson AS and Garthwaite PH (1990) Obesity, weight loss and prognosis in type 2 diabetes. *Diabet Med* **7**:228–33.

Makimattila S, Nikkila K and Yki-Jarvinen H (1999) Causes of weight gain during insulin therapy with and without metformin in patients with Type II diabetes mellitus. *Diabetologia* **42**:406–12.

Manley SE, Stratton IM, Cull CA *et al.* (2000) Effects of three months' diet after diagnosis of Type 2 diabetes on plasma lipids and lipoproteins (UKPDS 45). UK Prospective Diabetes Study Group. *Diabet Med* **17**:518–23.

McNulty SJ, Ur E and Williams G (2003) A randomized trial of sibutramine in the management of obese type 2 diabetic patients treated with metformin. *Diabetes Care* **26**:125–31.

Miles J, Aronne L, Hollander P and Klein S. Effect of orlistat in overweight and obese type 2 diabetes patients treated with metformin. *Diabetologia* **44**:890.

Nolan JJ, Olefsky JM, Nyce MR *et al.* (1996) Effect of troglitazone on leptin production – studies in-vitro and in human-subjects. *Diabetes* **45**:1276–8.

Pickavance LC, Buckingham RE and Wilding JPH (2001) Insulin-sensitizing action of rosiglitazone is enhanced by preventing hyperphagia. *Diabetes Obes Metab* **3**:171–80.

Pickavance LC, Tadayyon M, Widdowson PS *et al.* (1999) Therapeutic index for rosiglitazone in dietary obese rats: separation of efficacy and haemodilution. *Br J Pharmacol* **128**:1570–6.

Pories WJ, Swanson MS, MacDonald KG *et al.* (1995) Who would have thought it – an operation proves to be the most effective therapy for adult-onset diabetes-mellitus. *Ann Surg* **222**:339–52.

Raskin P, Rendell M, Riddle MC *et al.* (2001) A randomized trial of rosiglitazone therapy in patients with inadequately controlled insulin-treated type 2 diabetes. *Diabetes Care* **24**:1226–32.

Reynolds LR, Konz EC, Frederich RC and Anderson JW (2002) Rosiglitazone amplifies the benefits of lifestyle intervention measures in long-standing type 2 diabetes mellitus. *Diabetes Obes Metab* **4**:270–5.

Serrano-Rios M, Meichionda N and Moreno-Carretero E (2002) Role of sibutramine in the treatment of obese Type 2 diabetic patients receiving sulphonylurea therapy. *Diabet Med* **19**:119–24.

Sewter CP, Digby JE, Blows F *et al.* (1999) Regulation of tumour necrosis factor-alpha release from human adipose tissue *in vitro*. *J Endocrinol* **163**:33–8.

Sharma AM, Pischon T, Engeli S and Scholze J. (2001) Choice of drug treatment for obesity-related hypertension: where is the evidence? *J Hypertens* **19**:667–74.

Shi H, Moustaid-Moussa N, Wilkison WO and Zemel MB (1999) Role of the sulfonylurea receptor in regulating human adipocyte metabolism. *FASEB J* **13**:1833–8.

Simonson DC, Kourides IA, Feinglos M *et al.* (1997) Efficacy, safety, and dose-response characteristics of glipizide gastrointestinal therapeutic system on glycemic control and insulin secretion in NIDDM – Results of two multicenter, randomized, placebo-controlled clinical trials. *Diabetes Care* **20**:597–606.

Sjostrom L, Rissanen A, Andersen T *et al.* (1998) Weight loss and prevention of weight regain in obese patients: a 2-year, European, randomised trial of orlistat. *Lancet* **352**:167–72.

Spiegelman BM (1998) PPAR-gamma: Adipogenic regulator and thiazolidinedione receptor. *Diabetes* **47**:507–14.

Stearne MR, Palmer SL, Hammersley MS *et al.* (1998) Tight blood pressure control and risk of macrovascular and microvascular complications in type 2 diabetes: UKPDS 38. *Br Med J* **317**:703–13.

Stoabirketvedt G, Thom E, Aarbakke J and Florholmen J (1995) Body-fat as a predictor of the antihypertensive effect of nifedipine. *J Intern Med* **237**:169–73.

Treherne JM and Ashford ML (1991) The regional distribution of sulphonylurea binding sites in rat brain. *Neuroscience* **40**:523–31.

Tuomilheto J, Lindstrom J, Erickson JG *et al.* (2001) Prevention of type 2 diabetes mellitus by changes in lifestyle amongst subjects with impaired glucose tolerance. *N Engl J Med* **344**:1343–50.

Turner RC (1999) Intensive blood-glucose control with sulphonylureas or insulin compared with conventional treatment and risk of complications in patients with type 2 diabetes (UKPDS 33) (vol 352, pg 837, 1998). *Lancet* **354**:602.

Turner RC, Cull CA, Frighi V and Holman RR (1999) Glycemic control with diet, sulfonylurea, metformin, or insulin in patients with type 2 diabetes mellitus – Progressive requirement for multiple therapies (UKPDS 49). *JAMA* **281**:2005–12.

Turner RC, Holman RR, Stratton IM *et al.* (1998) Effect of intensive blood-glucose control with metformin on complications in overweight patients with type 2 diabetes (UKPDS 34). *Lancet* **352**:854–65.

Wang Q, Dryden S, Frankish HM *et al.* (1997) Increased feeding in fatty Zucker rats by the thiazolidinedione BRL 49653 (rosiglitazone) and the possible involvement of leptin and hypothalamic neuropeptide Y. *Br J Pharmacol* **122**:1405–10.

WHO Study Group (1997) *Prevention of Diabetes Mellitus.* WHO, Geneva, p. 844.

Wing RR, Koeske R, Epstein LH *et al.* (1987) Long-term effects of modest weight-loss in type-II diabetic- patients. *Arch Intern Med* **147**:1749–53.

Wing RR, Marcus MD, Epstein LH and Salata R (1987) Type-II diabetic subjects lose less weight than their overweight nondiabetic spouses. *Diabetes Care* **10**:563–6.

Wolever TMS, Chiasson JL, Josse RG *et al.* (1997) Small weight loss on long-term acarbose therapy with no change in dietary pattern or nutrient intake of individuals with non-insulin-dependent diabetes. *Int J Obes* **21**:756–63.

Yki-Jarvinen H, Ryysy L, Kauppila M *et al.* (1997) Effect of obesity on the response to insulin therapy in noninsulin-dependent diabetes mellitus. *J Clin Endocrinol Metab* **82**:4037–43.

11

The Role of Bariatric Surgery in the Management of Type 2 Diabetes

David D. Kerrigan, James Evans and **John Pinkney**

Introduction

The epidemic of obesity afflicting the USA and much of the developed world represents one of the most serious threats to the health of our species. Bariatric surgery (Gk *baros* weight, *iatrikos* the art of healing) is a rapidly evolving branch of surgical science, which aims to induce substantial weight loss in those whose obesity places them at significant risk of developing serious health problems. For most diseases, this risk does not become acute until individuals are more than 50 per cent overweight (corresponding to a body mass index (BMI) of $40 \, \mathrm{kg/m^{-2}}$; Kral, 1985), a condition known as *morbid* obesity. In an attempt to balance the risks of surgery against the benefits of weight loss, bariatric operations are currently only performed in the morbidly obese, or those with a $\mathrm{BMI} > 35 \, \mathrm{kg/m^{-2}}$ who have already developed co morbidity such as diabetes or hypertension (IFSO, 1997).

Obesity and type 2 diabetes:

Obesity is the most significant risk factor for type 2 diabetes, which is three times more common in overweight individuals ($\mathrm{BMI} > 25 \, \mathrm{kg/m^{-2}}$) than in those of normal body weight (Pi-Sunyer, 1993; Perry *et al.*, 1995; Colditz *et al.*, 1995). In the morbidly obese, the relative risk of type 2 diabetes is at least 5 per cent

Obesity and Diabetes. Edited by Anthony H. Barnett and Sudhesh Kumar
© 2004 John Wiley & Sons, Ltd ISBN: 0-470-84898-7

for men and 8–20 per cent in women (Mason *et al.*, 1992; Sjostrom *et al.*, 1999; Kral, 2001). Approximately 30 per cent of those considered for weight reduction surgery have type 2 diabetes (Gleysteen *et al.*, 1990; Pories *et al.*, 1995; Wittgrove *et al.*, 1996; Cowan and Buffington, 1998; Noya *et al.*, 1998), and a further 5–27 per cent have impaired glucose tolerance (Pories *et al.*, 1995; Wittgrove *et al.*, 1996; Cowan *et al.*, 1998).

Even allowing for a degree of selection bias in these surgical reports, obesity is clearly a major problem for a significant proportion of type 2 diabetics, particularly as treatment of the diabetes with oral hypoglycaemics can often exacerbate further weight gain.

It has been suggested that modest weight loss in type 2 diabetics may prolong survival (Lean *et al.*, 1990) and reduces the incidence of new diabetes by 58 per cent within 4 years in overweight populations with impaired glucose tolerance (Tuomilehto *et al.*, 2001; Knowler *et al.*, 2002). Several short-term studies of diet and exercise programmes in obese type 2 diabetics have also shown significant improvements in glycaemic control with weight loss (Di Base *et al.*, 1981; Hanefeld and Weck, 1989; Fukuda *et al.*, 1989; Wing *et al.*, 1988, 1991, 1994; Rotella *et al.*, 1994; Capstick *et al.*, 1997; Williams *et al.*, 1998). However, in clinical practice, it is far more difficult to reproduce these encouraging results in an unselected group of diabetics. Even those who do lose weight usually relapse because maintenance of weight loss using low calorie diets and lifestyle changes is beyond most patients (Zilli *et al.*, 2000).

Although diabetic patients may struggle to maintain a beneficial degree of weight loss with non-surgical treatment, there is an increasing body of evidence to suggest that surgically induced weight loss can ameliorate many of the pathophysiological abnormalities found in type 2 diabetes, or even offer the prospect of a 'surgical cure' for the condition. This chapter explores the evidence behind these claims.

Surgical techniques

Broadly speaking, weight reduction operations fall into one of two groups, *restrictive* procedures, and those that combine restriction of gastric size with a degree of *malabsorption*. In experienced hands, these are all safe procedures with an operative mortality of 0.5–1 per cent, and an acceptably low risk of serious long-term complications.

Restrictive procedures

Purely restrictive procedures limit the patients' capacity for food intake by creating a very small pouch from the proximal stomach, just beneath the gastro-oesophageal junction (Figures 11.1 and 11.2). The pouch is constructed in such a way that it must drain via a narrow opening, which effects a degree of resistance

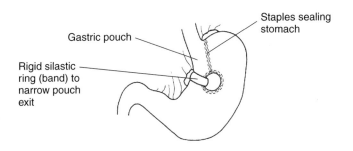

Figure 11.1   Vertical banded gastroplasty (VBG).

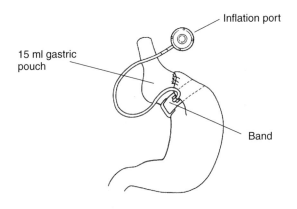

Figure 11.2   Laparoscopic gastric band.

to the emptying of solid food (although liquids empty normally). The aim is to produce enough resistance to retain food in the gastric pouch so that the patient feels full after a relatively small meal. Ingested food drains through into the more distal stomach, but this happens gradually, and so the sensation of satiety lasts for longer than usual. In this way, calorie intake is dramatically reduced.

The most widely practised restrictive operation in the 1980s and early 1990s was the vertical banded gastroplasty (VBG; Figure 11.1). Although VBG is an effective means of inducing sustained weight loss, it is associated with a fairly high risk (4–48 per cent) of disruption of the stapled gastric partition and weight regain (MacLean *et al.*, 1990; Capella and Capella, 1996; Dietel, 1997; Sven-heden *et al.*, 1997; Toppino *et al.*, 1999; Balsiger *et al.*, 2000). Consequently, the VBG has largely been superseded by laparoscopic adjustable gastric banding as the restrictive operation of choice.

Laparoscopic banding (Figure 11.2) is a 'keyhole' technique in which the upper stomach is encircled by an inflatable silicone cuff, or 'band'. Postopera-tively, the band is progressively inflated with small volumes of fluid (utilizing an injection port hidden under the patient's skin), until the desired degree of compression of the stomach beneath the food pouch is obtained and an adequate rate of weight loss commences.

Both VBG and laparoscopic banding produce similar degrees of weight loss, with a typical patient losing 50–60 per cent of their excess body weight over the first 2 years postoperatively (Dietel *et al.*, 1986; Fobi and Fleming, 1986; MacLean *et al.*, 1987; Favretti *et al.*, 1995; Belachew *et al.*, 1998; Fielding *et al.*, 1999; O'Brien *et al.*, 1999; Hell and Miller, 2000).

Restrictive/malabsorptive procedures

There are two types of operation that utilize a combination of restricted gastric size and a variable degree of small intestinal bypass to achieve superior weight loss.

The Roux en Y gastric bypass (Figure 11.3) is the most widely performed operation for weight reduction in the USA. Creating a 15-ml gastric pouch beneath the gastro-oesophageal junction induces a similar degree of gastric restriction to the VBG and laparoscopic band. However, after gastric bypass, food is separated from digestive juices by surgically diverting it away from the duodenum and proximal jejunum. The amount of bowel bypassed is varied according to the patient's BMI, but in general the total length of small bowel available for calorie absorption is reduced by about 150–300 cm. Nevertheless, gastric bypass is still thought to work largely by reducing stomach capacity.

Biliopancreatic diversion (BPD) involves a much more extensive intestinal bypass, with diverted food rejoining bile and pancreatic secretions in the terminal

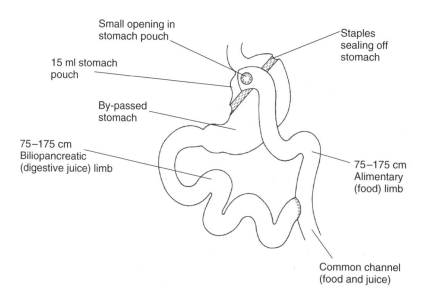

Figure 11.3   Roux-en-Y gastric bypass.

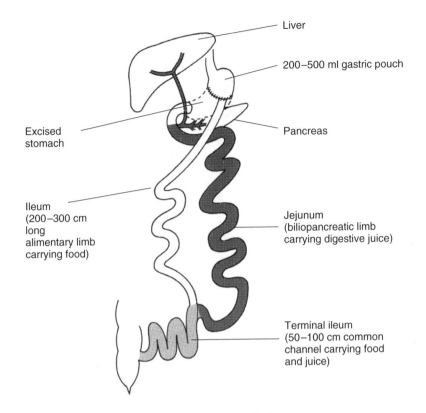

Figure 11.4   Biliopancreatic diversion.

ileum, just 50–100 cm from the ileocaecal valve (Figure 11.4). This situation leads to a greater degree of malabsorption, which, after compensatory bowel hypertrophy, means only 60 per cent of ingested calories are absorbed (Scopinaro *et al.*, 2000). Unlike the obsolete jejunoileal bypass operations performed in the 1970s, BPD is not associated with excessive diarrhoea and malnutrition, as it does not create a 'blind loop' of unused, excluded small bowel prone to toxic bacterial overgrowth (although a milder degree over bacterial overgrowth still occurs). BPD patients malabsorb proportionately more fat and starch, with relative sparing of protein absorption. However, protein loss from the gut is still increased by five times the normal rate (Scopinaro *et al.*, 1998) (approximately 30 g/day), and so it essential that the patient resumes a fairly normal eating pattern quickly to achieve a protein intake of 70–100 g daily. For this reason, a much larger 200–500 ml stomach remnant is preserved, although some gastric restriction is still required to initiate weight loss and reduce the risk of peptic ulceration.

The duodenal switch procedure (Figure 11.5) is a modification of the BPD in which the vagus nerves, antrum, pylorus and proximal duodenum are preserved (Marceau *et al.*, 1999), thereby reducing the incidence of postoperative diarrhoea and dumping syndrome to less than 10 per cent (Marceau *et al.*, 1998).

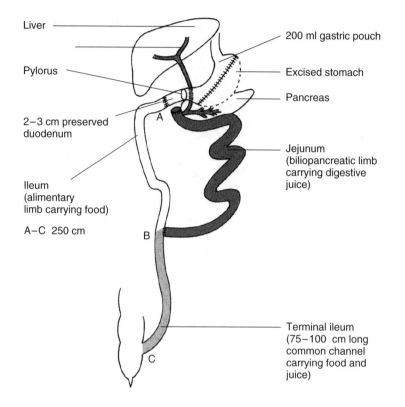

Figure 11.5   Duodenal switch.

All malabsorptive operations bypass the duodenum and proximal jejunum and thus carry a risk of trace element deficiency (particularly calcium, iron and zinc). Reduction in gastric size can also result in reduced vitamin B12 absorption in up to a third of patients. Vitamin and mineral deficiencies are equally prevalent after gastric bypass and BPD, but generally tend to be minor as long as a daily multivitamin supplements are taken (Skroubis *et al.*, 2002).

Although they were developed as open surgical procedures, both BPD/duodenal switch (Baltasar *et al.*, 2002; Paiva *et al.*, 2002; Scopinaro *et al.*, 2002; Rabkin *et al.*, 2003) and Roux-en-Y gastric bypass (Wittgrove *et al.*, 1996; Champion *et al.*, 1999; Gagner *et al.*, 1999; Wittgrove and Clark, 1999; Higa *et al.*, 2000; DeMaria *et al.*, 2002) can now be performed using laparoscopic minimally invasive techniques. All of these operations reduce excess weight by 70–80 per cent, although there is some evidence that gastric bypass may be somewhat less effective than BPD/duodenal switch in those with a BMI > 55 (Hess and Hess, 1998; MacLean *et al.*, 2000; Feng and Gagner, 2002). Furthermore, it would appear that long-term maintenance of weight loss is better after BPD/duodenal switch (Pories *et al.*, 1992, 1995; Hess and Hess, 1998; Scopinaro *et al.*, 2000; Baltasar *et al.*, 2001).

Resolution of diabetes after bariatric surgery

The best known report of diabetes remission after weight reduction surgery came from Walter Pories and his team in Greenville, USA, not least because of its provocative title 'Who would have thought it? An operation proves to be the most effective therapy for adult-onset diabetes mellitus' (Pories *et al.*, 1995). In an uncontrolled observational series, Pories studied 165 patients with type 2 diabetes (and a further 165 with impaired glucose tolerance) after gastric bypass surgery. A remarkable 83 per cent of the diabetic patients (and 99 per cent of those with impaired glucose tolerance) were rendered euglycaemic. Furthermore, 10 of the 27 patients who remained diabetic were found to have technical failures due to disruption of the gastric staple line, leaving just 17 true non-responders. Analysis of this sub-group showed them to be older than euglycaemic patients (by about 7 years) and to have been diagnosed with diabetes for significantly longer. Retrospectively, Pories also noted that 9-year mortality in a group of diabetics who had not undergone surgery (because of personal preference or their insurance company's refusal to pay) was 28 per cent compared to 9 per cent in the surgical group (including perioperative deaths). The percentage of control subjects treated with oral hypoglycaemics or insulin increased from 56 to 87 per cent during the period of review, but fell from 32 to 9 per cent after gastric bypass (McDonald *et al.*, 1997). These two groups were not particularly well matched, but the results are intriguing.

The second major study with important data on this issue is the Swedish Obese Subjects (SOS) study. This is a well-designed prospective, but non-randomized comparison of patients who had undergone a variety of bariatric operations and those who had been treated with best medical therapy (which at the time, did not include orlistat or sibutramine). Within the study group were 156 patients with type 2 diabetes. After 2 years of follow-up, the requirement for on-going drug treatment to control hyperglycaemia in the surgical arm was half that in the non-surgical group (Sjostrom *et al.*, 1999). Furthermore, in a matched population of non-diabetic patients observed for 8 years, surgically treated patients with (by surgical standards) a reasonably poor degree of maintained weight loss (16 per cent) showed a dramatic reduction in the incidence of newly diagnosed diabetes. No weight loss was observed in the non-surgical control group over the 8 years of study (Sjostrom *et al.*, 2000).

The surgical literature is littered with other enthusiastic, personal and largely uncontrolled series which appear to confirm the widely held view that most diabetics can be 'cured' by surgically induced weight loss (Scopinaro *et al.*, 1996; Smith *et al.*, 1996; Cowan and Buffington, 1998; Hess and Hess, 1998; Noya *et al.*, 1998; Dhabuwala *et al.*, 2000; Dietel, 2000; Schauer *et al.*, 2000; Abu-Abeid *et al.*, 2001; Haciyanli *et al.*, 2001; Angrisani *et al.*, 2002; Bacci *et al.*, 2002; DeMaria *et al.*, 2002; Dixon and O'Brien, 2002; O'Brien *et al.*, 2002; Rubino *et al.*, 2002; Dolan *et al.*, 2003; Mittermair *et al.*, 2003). A problem that is frequently overlooked when assessing these reports is that none of these studies were specifically designed to test the efficacy of bariatric surgery as a treatment for diabetes. The recruitment of diabetics into these studies was haphazard and unintentional. Furthermore, many patients were only diagnosed with diabetes at baseline screening, and may not therefore represent a typical type 2 diabetic clinic population with emerging microvascular disease. It is essential that any diabetes study looks at the progression of microvascular complications; unfortunately, we have no data on how bariatric surgery affects this important endpoint.

How does surgery 'cure' diabetes?

The simplistic explanation for observed improvements in glycaemic control after bariatric surgery is the rapid weight loss induced by decreased food intake and postoperative malabsorption. However, although our understanding is far from complete, there is increasing evidence that weight loss is simply a surrogate marker for improved diabetes control, but not the direct cause of any observed benefit.

Modification of dietary intake

Bariatric surgery results in a substantial reduction in nutrient intake which may account for the normalization of plasma glucose reported. In a recent study, a sham operated individual who followed the same strict postoperative diet recommended to Roux-en-Y gastric bypass patients showed similar improvements in insulin and glucose levels. This suggests that calorific restriction is a major factor in promoting glycaemic control after weight loss surgery (Pories *et al.*, 1995). Furthermore, there are some indications that gastric bypass may alter the type of food patients ingest. Induction of the 'dumping syndrome' or postoperative changes in taste and food preference result in a preferential reduction in carbohydrate ingestion (Sugarman *et al.*, 1992). This may enhance diabetic control because it is known that obese individuals with a high carbohydrate intake (especially simple sugars), have increased insulin secretion. Hyperinsulinaemia favours anabolic metabolism (Woods *et al.*, 1974; Wiener, 1980) and stimulates hyperphagia with carbohydrate craving, producing yet further increases in insulin secretion. Consequently, insulin-induced receptor downregulation occurs, followed by insulin resistance, and a vicious cycle of increasing carbohydrate consumption and weight gain. Successful weight loss is almost impossible by conventional means under these circumstances, but bariatric surgery may allow the cycle to be broken.

Although this evidence provides a cogent argument for the role of reduced calorie intake mediating improved diabetes control, other observations indicate that this can not be the sole explanation. Whilst energy intake is drastically reduced immediately after surgery, over the ensuing months it progressively increases without adversely affecting glucose and insulin levels. This is particularly true in the case of patients undergoing BPD/duodenal switch, who achieve excellent long-term glycaemic control, even though their eating capacity is usually fully restored within 12 months of surgery (Scopinaro et al., 1998). This point is illustrated by a fascinating case report of a young *non-obese* diabetic woman who underwent BPD to treat chylomicronaemia. Due to an unrestricted high fat and carbohydrate post-operative diet, she actually put on weight, but her plasma insulin and blood glucose returned to normal within 3 months (Mingrove et al., 1997).

If reduced food intake was the sole explanation for improved diabetes control, purely restrictive procedures such as laparoscopic gastric banding and VBG should be as effective as Roux-en-Y gastric bypass. There is no doubt that laparoscopic banding and VBG do indeed appear to ameliorate diabetes, but unfortunately there are no randomized trials comparing these techniques with gastric bypass. The few small observational studies available report resolution of diabetes in about two-thirds of patients undergoing banding (Dixon et al., 2002; O'Brien et al., 2002; Dolan et al., 2003), a somewhat less impressive outcome than that reported after gastric bypass and BPD/duodenal switch. Gastric bypass has been reported to abolish the requirement for medical treatment in 82–95 per cent of type 2 diabetic patients (Pories et al., 1995; Smith et al., 1996; Dhabuwala et al., 2000; Schauer et al., 2000; DeMaria et al., 2002), and (within the limitations outlined earlier) results after BPD/duodenal switch are even more spectacular (100 per cent diabetes remission) (Scopinaro et al., 1996; Hess and Hess, 1998).

Perhaps the most striking argument against weight loss being the most important factor in promoting diabetes control is the rapidity with which serum glucose returns to normal after gastric bypass, BPD and duodenal switch. This dramatic onset of euglycaemia sometimes occurs within days of surgery, and long before there is any significant weight loss (Pories et al., 1995; Hess and Hess, 1998; Scopinaro et al., 1998; Pies et al., 2001). In contrast, resolution of diabetes is not usually seen until about 6 months after purely restrictive operations such as laparoscopic banding (Dolan et al., 2003). A common feature of gastric bypass, BPD and duodenal switch operations is that food is diverted away from the hormonally active proximal small bowel. This has led to the concept that these operations disturb a complex neurohumoral signalling mechanism within the antrum, duodenum and proximal jejunum, which modulates the production and metabolism of insulin. The implication is that type 2 diabetes may, in fact, be a disease of the foregut rather than the pancreas.

Diabetes as a foregut disease

The gut secretes insulinotropic hormones called incretins which stimulate β-cell production of insulin in response to food, especially carbohydrate, entering the foregut. The principle incretins are glucagons, glucagon-like peptide-1

(GLP-1) and glucose-dependant insulinotropic peptide (GIP) (Kellum *et al.*, 1990; Creutzfeldt and Nauck, 1992; Gutnaik *et al.*, 1992; Holst, 1994). Any disturbance of this 'enteroinsular axis' following surgical diversion of food into the more distal small intestine could therefore affect glucose homeostasis and possibly lead to changes in insulin resistance.

Pories and colleagues proposed that hyperinsulinaemia in type 2 diabetes is the result of over stimulation of the islet cells by an abnormal incretin signal from the gut, a stimulus which is abolished by re-routing food away from the duodenum and upper jejunum (Pories and Albrecht, 2001). Although plausible, Rubino and Gagner (2002) have extended this argument and proposed the presence of as-yet unidentified 'anti-incretin' factors secreted by the duodenum, which would act as a homeostatic counterbalance to the effect of incretins (Figure 11.6). They speculate that type 2 diabetes occurs when there is an imbalance due to a relative excess of anti-incretin activity, leading to a delayed insulin response to ingested carbohydrate and thus glucose intolerance. If anti-incretins also blocked the actions of insulin at a receptor or post-receptor level, insulin resistance with secondary hyperinsulinaemia would result.

By diverting food away from the duodenum, both gastric bypass and BPD may avoid excessive stimulation of incretins (as proposed by Pories) or anti-incretins (as proposed by Rubino and Gagner), which would have the effect lowering plasma insulin and/or glucose. These hypotheses do not fully explain the excellent resolution of type 2 diabetes seen after the duodenal switch procedure, in which at least 2–5 cm of proximal duodenum is retained (Figure 11.5),

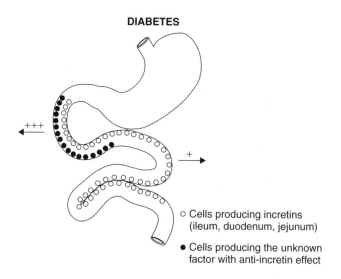

DIABETES

○ Cells producing incretins
(ileum, duodenum, jejunum)

● Cells producing the unknown
factor with anti-incretin effect

Figure 11.6 Hypothesis 1. Type 2 diabetes results from over production of duodenal anti-incretins causing imbalance with secretion of incretins by the foregut. This would lead to delayed insulin response to food and impaired insulin action. With permission from Lippincott Williams & Wilkins.

but all three operations (particularly BPD and duodenal switch) result in chyme entering the distal small bowel at a much earlier phase of digestion than normal. Stimulation of the terminal ileum by nutrients releases GLP-1, a powerful incretin, which could improve the action of insulin, promoting euglycaemia (Figure 11.7). GLP-1 also delays gastric emptying, and probably explains the marked early satiety noted after BPD and duodenal switch.

There is certainly some experimental evidence to substantiate aspects of the hypothesis that surgery improves diabetes via modulation of the enteroinsular axis, as jejuno-ileal bypass (an operation abandoned in the early 1980s) and BPD have both been associated with raised levels of the incretins enteroglucagon (an old name for what is almost certainly GLP-1) and GIP, which can persist for over 20 years after surgery (Sarson *et al.*, 1981; Naslund *et al.*, 1998). Exogenous GLP-1 infusion in type 2 diabetics has been shown to have an anti-diabetogenic effect, by stimulating insulin release and increasing glucose utilization, resulting in reduced post-prandial insulin requirements and plasma free insulin concentrations (Gutnaik *et al.*, 1992). The suggestion is that long-term control of diabetes after gastric bypass and malabsorptive surgery is the result of increased endogenous GLP-1 production. This has led to the suggestion that ileal transposition into a more proximal position in the small intestine would be an ideal operation for treatment of type 2 diabetes, as it would maximize GLP-1 release, without the need for extensive malabsorption. However, before this experimental approach could be recommended, well-planned studies of ileal transposition in

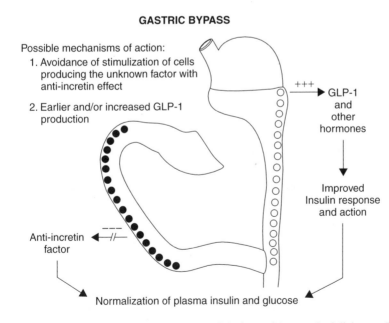

GASTRIC BYPASS

Possible mechanisms of action:
1. Avoidance of stimulization of cells producing the unknown factor with anti-incretin effect

2. Earlier and/or increased GLP-1 production

+++ → GLP-1 and other hormones

↓

Improved Insulin response and action

Anti-incretin factor ←//—

Normalization of plasma insulin and glucose

Figure 11.7 Hypothesis 2. Mechanisms responsible for rapid control of diabetes after gastric bypass. With permission from Lippincott Williams & Wilkins.

type 2 diabetes and obesity are required to evaluate safety and clinical efficacy (Mason, 1999).

Changes in serum lipids

In obese diabetics undergoing BPD and duodenal switch, enhancement of insulin sensitivity and glucose tolerance occurs before any major effect on body weight is noted. It has been suggested that the lipid malabsorption and subsequent reduction in plasma lipids these operations induce may play a major role in reversal of insulin resistance (Mingrove *et al.*, 1997). Abnormal fat deposition in skeletal muscle has been identified as a mechanism for obesity-related insulin resistance and it is proposed that lipid deprivation may deplete intramyocellular fat, thereby reversing insulin resistance. Greco and colleagues (2002) studied quadriceps muscle biopsies in morbidly obese patients before and after BPD or a low calorie diet. After BPD, insulin resistance was fully reversed within 6 months. Even though most patients were still obese at this stage, intramyocellular lipids had decreased, whereas after non-surgical weight loss, only very modest changes in insulin sensitivity and myocellular lipids were noted.

An alternative suggestion implicates decreased hepatic clearance of insulin (causing hyperinsulinaemia) as a cause of insulin resistance. It is proposed that increased free fatty acids in portal blood (Stromblad and Bjorntorp, 1986) and/or increased free fatty acid oxidation (Randle *et al.*, 1965) (which in turn inhibits glucose oxidation), prevent effective handling of glucose and insulin by the liver, an effect which is reversed by the decrease in lipid absorption and reduced intra-abdominal adipose tissue seen after BPD/duodenal switch.

Conclusions

Is surgery helpful in controlling type 2 diabetes?

There is a wealth of non-randomized clinical evidence to support the view that the majority of patients with type 2 diabetes experience greatly improved glycaemic control and reduced insulin resistance after bariatric surgery. This effect appears to be independent of weight loss, and probably results from a combination of reduced calorie intake, increased intestinal secretion of GLP-1, and lipid malabsorption.

Which is the best operation for diabetes control?

Due to a lack of published randomized trials, it is not possible to recommend any particular surgical procedure as the optimum choice for diabetic patients, but it would appear that gastric bypass, BPD and duodenal switch produce more complete and rapid resolution of type 2 diabetes compared with simple restrictive procedures such as laparoscopic banding and VBG.

Which type 2 diabetics should be offered bariatric surgery?

Pories and Albrecht (2001) have demonstrated that over a 10-year period gastric bypass reduced mortality in a population of diabetic patients to 1 per cent for every year of follow-up, compared to 4.5 per cent per year in a matched group of diabetics who did not undergo bariatric surgery. In observational studies, gastric bypass, BPD and duodenal switch are associated with diabetes remission in 80–100 per cent of patients, although randomized studies looking at diabetes-specific endpoints are awaited.

Pories *et al.* (1995) reported a small number of patients whose diabetes appeared to be resistant to bariatric surgery. Some of these were due to failures in operative technique, but most were older patients who had suffered with diabetes for longer and others whose type 2 diabetes was sufficiently severe to require insulin, presumably as a result of well-established islet secretory failure. It follows that it may be advisable to offer weight reduction surgery to younger diabetics and those at an earlier stage in their disease, before insulin secretory failure becomes irreversible.

Should non-obese type 2 diabetics be offered bariatric surgery?

The current recommendation is that only diabetics with a BMI > 35 should be offered surgery. However, there is published evidence of 90 per cent diabetes remission in a group of patients with only moderate obesity (mean BMI 33) (Noya *et al.*, 1998). As earlier intervention may be more likely to successfully control plasma glucose and insulin, there is an argument for lowering the BMI threshold for surgical intervention in type 2 diabetes. This is supported by the observation that insulin resistance only increases with increasing obesity up to a BMI of 30, after which it plateaus (Elton *et al.*, 1994); thus patients with a BMI of 30 are likely to have a similar degree of insulin resistance to heavier individuals. Unfortunately, at the present time, we have no randomized evidence with which to challenge the hypothesis that surgical intervention at a BMI of 30 will prove as cost-effective as intervention at a BMI of 35 or greater.

The advent of minimally invasive laparoscopic surgical approaches to banding, gastric bypass, BPD and even duodenal switch operations will almost certainly increase the acceptability of surgery, but it should be remembered that enthusiasm for a more aggressive surgical approach needs to be tempered by an awareness of the small but not insignificant risks of death (1 per cent) and complications (2–10 per cent).

References

Abu-Abeid S, Keidar A and Szold A (2001) Resolution of chronic medical conditions after laparoscopic adjustable silicone gastric banding for the treatment of morbid obesity in the elderly. *Surg Endosc* **15**:132–4.

Angrisani L, Furbetta F, Doldi SB *et al.* (2002) Results of the Italian multicenter study on 239 super-obese patients treated by adjustable gastric banding. *Obes Surg* **12**:846–50.

Bacci V, Basso MS, Greco F *et al.* (2002) Modifications of metabolic and cardiovascular risk factors after weight loss induced by laparoscopic gastric banding. *Obes Surg* **12**:77–82.

Balsiger BM, Poggio JL, Mai J *et al.* (2000) Ten and more years after vertical banded gastroplasty as primary operation for morbid obesity. *J Gastrointest Surg* **4**:598–605.

Baltasar A, Bou R, Bengochea M *et al.* (2001) Duodenal switch: an effective therapy for morbid obesity – intermediate results. *Obes Surg* **11**:54–8.

Baltasar A, Bou R, Miro J *et al.* (2002) Laparoscopic biliopancreatic diversion with duodenal switch: technique and initial experience. *Obes Surg* **12**:245–8.

Belachew M, Legrand M, Vincent V *et al.* (1998) Laparoscopic adjustable gastric banding. *World J Surg* **22**:955–63.

Capella JF and Capella RF (1996) The weight reduction operation of choice: Vertical banded gastroplasty or gastric bypass? *Am J Surg* **171**:74–9.

Capstick F, Brokks BA, Burns CM *et al.* (1997) Very low calorie diet (VLCD): a useful alternative in the treatment of the obese NIDDM patient. *Diabetes Res Clin Pract* **36**:105–11.

Champion JK, Hunt T and DeLisle N (1999) Laparoscopic vertical banded gastroplasty and Roux-en-Y gastric bypass in morbid obesity. *Obes Surg* **9**:123.

Colditz GA, Willett WC, Ronitzky A *et al.* (1995) Weight gain as a risk factor for clinical diabetes mellitus in women. *Ann Intern Med* **122**:481–6.

Cowan GSM Jr and Buffington CK (1998) Significant changes in blood pressure, glucose and lipids with gastric bypass surgery. *World J Surg* **22**:987–92.

Creutzfeldt W and Nauck M (1992) Gut hormones and diabetes mellitus. *Diabetes Metab Rev* **8**:149–77.

DeMaria EJ, Sugarman HJ, Kellum JM *et al.* (2002) Results of 281 consecutive total laparoscopic Roux-en-Y gastric bypasses to treat morbid obesity. *Ann Surg* **235**:640–5.

Dhabuwala A, Cannan RJ and Stubbs RS (2000) Improvement in comorbidities following weight loss from gastric bypass surgery. *Obes Surg* **10**:428–35.

Di Biase G, Mattioli PL, Contaldo F and Mancini M (1981) A very low calorie formula diet (Cambridge Diet) for the treatment of diabetic-obese patients. *Int J Obes* **5**:319–24.

Dietel M (1997) Staple disruption in vertical banded gastroplasty (commentary). *Obes Surg* **7**:139–41.

Dietel M (2000) Diabetes and bariatric surgery. *Obes Surg* **10**:285.

Dietel M, Jones BA, Petrov I *et al.* (1986) Vertical banded gastroplasty: results in 233 patients. *Can J Surg* **29**:322–4.

Dixon JB and O'Brien PE (2002) Health outcomes of severely obese type 2 diabetic subjects 1 year after laparoscopic adjustable gastric banding. *Diabetes Care* **25**:358–63.

Dolan K, Bryant R and Fielding G (2003) Treating diabetes in the morbidly obese by laparoscopic gastric banding. *Obes Surg* **13**:439–43.

Elton CW, Tapscott EB, Pories WJ *et al.* (1994) Effect of moderate obesity on glucose transport in human muscle. *Horm Metab Res* **26**:181–3.

Favretti F, Cadiere GB, Segato G *et al.* (1995) Laparoscopic placement of adjustable silicone gastric banding: early experience. *Obes Surg* **5**:71–3.

Feng JJ and Gagner M (2002) Laparoscopic biliopancreatic diversion with duodenal switch. *Semin Laparosc Surg* **9**:125–9.

Fielding GA, Rhodes M and Nathanson LK (1999) Laparoscopic gastric banding for morbid obesity: surgical outcome in 335 cases. *Surg Endosc* **13**:550–4.

Fobi MAL and Fleming AW (1986) Vertical banded gastroplasty vs gastric bypass in the treatment of obesity. *J Natl Med Assoc* **78**:1091–6.

Fukuda M, Tahara Y, Yamamoto Y *et al.* (1989) Effects of very low calorie diet weight reduction on glucose tolerance, insulin secretin, and insulin resistance in obese non-insulin dependent diabetics. *Diabetes Res Clin Pract* **7**:61–9.

Gagner M, Garcia-Ruiz A, Arca MJ *et al.* (1999) Laparoscopic isolated gastric bypass for morbid obesity. *Surg Endosc* **S19**:6.

Gleysteen JJ, Barboriak JJ and Sasse EA (1990) Sustained coronary risk factor reduction after gastric bypass surgery for morbid obesity. *Am J Clin Nutr* **51**:774–8.

Greco Av, Mingrove G, Giancaterini A *et al.* (2002) Insulin resistance in morbid obesity: reversal with intramyocellular fat depletion. *Diabetes* **51**:144–51.

Gutnaik M, Orskov C, Holst JJ *et al.* (1992) Antidiabetogenic effect of glucagon-like peptide-1 (7–36) amide in normal subjects and patients with diabetes mellitus. *N Engl J Med* **326**:1316–22.

Hell E and Miller KA (2000) Comparison of vertical banded gastroplasty and adjustable silicone gastric banding. In Deitel M and Cowan SM Jr (eds), *Update: Surgery for the Morbidly Obese Patients.* FD Communications Inc, Toronto, pp. 379–86.

Haciyanli M, Erkan N, Bora S *et al.* (2001) Vertical banded gastroplasty in the Aegean region of Turkey. *Obes Surg* **11**:482–6.

Hanefeld M and Weck M (1989) Very low calorie diet therapy in obese non-insulin dependent diabetes patients. *Int J Obes* **13** (suppl 2):33–7.

Hess DS and Hess DW (1998) Biliopancreatic diversion with a duodenal switch. *Obes Surg* **8**:267–82.

Higa KD, Boone KB, Ho T and Davies OG (2000) Laparoscopic Roux-en-Y gastric bypass for morbid obesity: technique and preliminary results in our first 400 patients. *Arch Surg* **135**:1029–33.

Holst JJ (1994) Glucagon-like peptide 1: a newly discovered gastrointestinal hormone. *Gastroenterology* **97**:1848–55.

IFSO (1997) Statement on patient selection for bariatric surgery. *Obes Surg* **7**:41.

Kellum JM, Kuemmerle JF, O'Dorisio TM *et al.* (1990) Gastrointestinal hormone responses to meals before and after gastric bypass and vertical stapled gastroplasty. *Ann Surg* **211**:763–7.

Knowler WC, Barrett-Connor E, Fowler SE *et al.* (2002) Reduction in the incidence of type 2 diabetes with lifestyle intervention or metformin. *N Engl J Med* **346**:393–403.

Kral JG (1985) Morbid obesity and related health risks. *Ann Intern Med* **103**:1043.

Kral J (2001) Morbidity of severe obesity. *Surg Clin N Am* **81**:1039–61.

Lean MEJ, Powrie JK, Anderson AS *et al.* (1990) Obesity, weight loss and prognosis in type 2 diabetes. *Diabet Med* **7**:228–33.

MacDonald KG, Long SD, Swanson MS *et al.* (1997) The gastric bypass operation reduces the progression and mortality of non-insulin-dependent diabetes mellitus. *J Gastrointest Surg* **1**:213–20.

MacLean LD, Rhode BM and Forse RA (1990) Late results of vertical banded gastroplasty for morbid and superobesity. *Surgery* **107**:20–7.

MacLean LD, Rhode BM and Nohr CW (2000) Late outcome of isolated gastric bypass. *Ann Surg* **231**:524–8.

MacLean LD, Rhode B and Shizgal HM (1987) Nutrition after vertical banded gastroplasty. *Ann Surg* 555–63.

Marceau P, Hould FS, Potvin M *et al.* (1999) Biliopancreatic diversion (duodenal switch procedure). *Eur J Gastroenterol Hepatol* **11**:99–103.

Marceau P, Hould FS, Simard S *et al*. (1998) Biliopancreatic diversion with duodenal switch. *World J Surg* **22**:947–54.

Mason EE (1999) Ilial transposition and enteroglucagon/GLP-1 in obesity (and diabetic?) surgery. *Obes Surg* **9**:223–8.

Mason EE, Renquist K and Jiang D (1992) Predictors of two obesity complications: diabetes and hypertension. *Obes Surg* **2**:231–7.

Mingrove G, De Gaetano A, Greco AV *et al*. (1997) Reversibility of insulin resistance in obese diabetic patients: role of plasma lipids. *Diabetologia* **40**:599–605.

Mittermair RP, Weiss H, Nehoda H *et al*. (2003) Laparoscopic Swedish adjustable gastric banding: 6-year follow-up and comparison to other laparoscopic bariatric procedures. *Obes Surg* **13**:412–17.

Naslund E, Backman L, Holst JJ *et al*. (1998) Importance of small bowel peptides for the improved glucose metabolism 20 years after jejunoileal bypass for obesity. *Obes Surg* **8**:253–60.

Noya G, Cossu ML, Coppola M *et al*. (1998) Biliopancreatic diversion for treatment of morbid obesity: experience in 50 cases. *Obes Surg* **8**:61–6.

Noya G, Cossu ML, Coppola M *et al*. (1998) Biliopancreatic diversion preserving the stomach and pylorus in the treatment of hypercholesterolaemia and diabetes type II: results in the first 10 cases. *Obes Surg* **8**:67–72.

O'Brien PE, Brown WA, Smith A *et al*. (1999) Prospective study of a laparoscopically placed, adjustable gastric band in the treatment of morbid obesity. *Br J Surg* **85**:113–18.

O'Brien PE, Dixon JB, Brown W *et al*. (2002) The laparoscopic adjustable gastric band (Lap-Band): a prospective study of medium-term effects on weight, health and quality of life. *Obes Surg* **12**:652–60.

Paiva D, Bernardes L and Suretti L (2002) Laparoscopic biliopancreatic diversion: technique and initial results. *Obes Surg* **12**:358–61.

Perry IJ, Wannamethee SG, Walker MK *et al*. (1995) Prospective study of risk factors for development of non-insulin dependant diabetes in middle-aged British men. *Br Med J* **310**:560–4.

Pi-Sunyer FX (1993) Medical hazards of obesity. *Ann Intern Med* **119**:655–660.

Pies WJ and Albrecht RJ (2001) Etiology of type II diabetes mellitus: role of the foregut. *World J Surg* **25**:527–31.

Pories WJ, MacDonald KG Jr, Flickinger EG *et al*. (1992) Is type II diabetes mellitus (NIDDM) a surgical disease? *Ann Surg* **215**:633–42.

Pories WJ, Swanson MS, MacDonald KG *et al*. (1995) Who would have thought it? An operation proves to be the most effective therapy for adult-onset diabetes mellitus. *Ann Surg* **222**:339–52.

Rabkin RA, Rabkin JM, Metcalf B *et al*. (2003) Laparoscopic technique for performing duodenal switch with gastric reduction. *Obes Surg* **13**:263–8.

Randle PJ, Garland PB, Newsholme EA *et al*. (1965) The glucose fatty acid cycle in obesity and maturity onset diabetes mellitus. *Ann N Y Acad Sci* **31**:324–33.

Rotella CM, Cresci B, Mannucci E *et al*. (1994) Short cycles of very low calorie diet in the therapy of obese type 2 diabetes mellitus. *J Endocrinol Invest* **17**:171–9.

Rubino F and Gagner M (2002) Potential of surgery for curing type 2 diabetes mellitus. *Ann Surg* **236**:554–9.

Sarson DL, Scopinaro N and Bloom SR (1981) Gut hormone changes after jejunoileal (JIB) or biliopancreatic (BPB) bypass surgery for morbid obesity. *Int J Obes* **5**:471–80.

Schauer PR, Ikramuddin S, Gourash W *et al*. (2000) Outcomes after laparoscopic Roux-en-Y gastric bypass for morbid obesity. *Ann Surg* **232**:515–29.

Scopinaro N, Adami GF, Marinari GM *et al*. (1998) Biliopancreatic diversion. *World J Surg* **22**:936–46.

Scopinaro N, Adami GF, Marinari GM *et al.* (2000) Biliopancreatic diversion: Two decades of experience. In Deitel M and Cowan SM Jr (eds), *Update: Surgery for the Morbidly Obese Patients.* FD Communications Inc, Toronto pp. 227–58.

Scopinaro N, Gianetta E, Adami GF *et al.* (1996) Biliopancreatic diversion for obesity at eighteen years. *Surgery* **119**:261–8.

Scopinaro N, Marinari GM and Camerini G (2002) Laparoscopic standard biliopancreatic diversion: technique and preliminary results. *Obes Surg* **12**:362–5.

Sjostrom CD, Lissner L, Wedel H *et al.* (1999) *Obes Res* **7**:477–84.

Sjostrom CD, Peltonen M, Wedel H *et al.* (2000) Differentiated long-term effects of intentional weight loss on diabetes and hypertension. *Hypertension* **36**:20–5.

Skroubis G, Sakellaropoulos G, Pouggouras K *et al.* (2002) Comparison of nutritional deficiencies after Roux-en-Y gastric bypass and after biliopancreatic diversion with Roux-en-Y gastric bypass. *Obes Surg* **12**:551–8.

Smith SC, Edwards CB and Goodman GN (1996) Changes in diabetic management after Roux-en-Y gastric bypass. *Obes Surg* **6**:345–8.

Stromblad G and Bjorntorp P (1986) Reduced hepatic insulin clearance in rats with dietary-induced obesity. *Metabolism* **35**:323–7.

Sugarman HJ, Kellum JM, Engle KM *et al.* (1992) Gastric bypass for treating severe obesity. *Am J Clin Nutr* **55**:560S–566S.

Svenheden K, Akesson L, Holmdahl C *et al.* (1997) Staple disruption in vertical banded gastroplasty. *Obes Surg* **7**:136–8.

Toppino M, Morino M, Capuzzi P *et al.* (1999) Outcome of vertical banded gastroplasty. *Obes Surg* **9**:51–4.

Tuomilehto J, Lindstrom J, Eriksson JG *et al.* (2001) Prevention of type 2 diabetes mellitus by changes in lifestyle among subjects with impaired glucose tolerance. *N Engl J Med* **344**:1390–2.

Weiner MF (1980) Rapid weight gain due to overinsulinisation. *Obes Bariatric Med* **9**:118–19.

Williams KV, Mullen ML, Kelley DE and Wing RR (1998) The effect of short periods of caloric restriction on weight loss and glycemic control in type 2 diabetes. *Diabetes Care* **21**:2–8.

Wing RR, Blair E, Marcus M *et al.* (1994) Year-long weight loss treatment for obese patients with type II diabetes: does including an intermittent very low calorie diet improve outcomes? *Am J Med* **97**:354–62.

Wing RR, Epstein LH, Paternostro-Bayles M *et al.* (1988) Exercise in a behavioral weight control programme for obese patients with type-2 (non-insulin dependent diabetes). *Diabetologia* **31**:902–9.

Wing RR, Marcus RD, Salata R *et al.* (1991) Effects of a very low calorie diet on long term glycaemic control in obese type 2 diabetic subjects. *Arch Intern Med* **151**:1334–40.

Wittgrove AC and Clark W (1999) Laparoscopic gastric bypass: a five-year prospective study of 500 patients followed from 3–60 months. *Obes Surg* **9**:123–43.

Wittgrove AC, Clark W, Schubert KR *et al.* (1996) Laparoscopic gastric bypass, Roux en Y: technique and results in 75 patients with 3–30 months follow-up. *Obes Surg* **6**:500–4.

Woods WC, Decke E and Vaselli JR (1974) Metabolic hormones and regulation of body weight. *Physiol Rev* **81**:26–43.

Zilli FCM, Croci M, Tufano A and Caviezel F (2000) The compliance of hypocaloric diet in type 2 diabetic obese patients: a brief term study. *Eat Weight Disord* **5**:217–22.

12
Childhood Obesity and Type 2 Diabetes

Krystyna A. Matyka and **Timothy Barrett**

Introduction

In the last 10–20 years childhood obesity has emerged as a disease of major public health significance. It has implications for the physical and emotional well-being of affected children as well as having potential longterm consequences on adult health. The aetiology is complex and attempts at both prevention and intervention have proved extremely challenging. This chapter aims to explore some of the issues surrounding obesity in childhood based on currently available evidence.

Childhood is a time of change

The scope of this chapter cannot cover childhood evolution in any great detail. However, some background is essential as there are implications for the definition, aetiology, potential consequences as well as management of this complex disorder in children of different ages.

The first years of life can be divided into three distinct periods: infancy, childhood and adolescence. Growth and body mass during these periods are determined by genetic, intra-uterine, nutritional, environmental and endocrine influences which vary in importance depending on the developmental stage of the child. Growth velocity is at its greatest during infancy, decelerates during childhood and increases again during the pubertal growth spurt (Clayton and Gill, 2001). During infancy, growth is predominantly nutritionally driven but

Obesity and Diabetes. Edited by Anthony H. Barnett and Sudhesh Kumar
© 2004 John Wiley & Sons, Ltd   ISBN: 0-470-84898-7

by the third year of life the endocrine system becomes more important. Growth hormone is the main mediator of growth during childhood and during puberty the actions of growth hormone are augmented by sex steroids, testosterone and oestrogen.

Body mass index changes dramatically during this time. Body fat increases steeply during the first year of life leading to an increase in body mass index (BMI), falls to a nadir in mid-childhood and then starts to rise again after about 7 years of age (Cole *et al.*, 1995). It has been suggested that the timing of this so-called 'adiposity rebound' is critical to the development of later obesity with children at greater risk if the timing is early, before 5.5 years of age (Dietz, 1997). During puberty BMI increases further and there are gender dependent differences with girls accumulating more fat mass and boys more lean muscle mass during this time (Hergenroeder and Klisch, 1990).

Caloric requirements of growing children are extremely high. Average caloric requirements during the first few months of life are around 110 kcal/kg/day compared to approximately 90 kcal/kg/day during childhood and 50 kcal/kg/day during puberty. These calories are used to promote normal growth as well as cover energy expenditure through activity. The composition of this diet changes considerably throughout the early years. The almost exclusively milk-based diet during infancy is high in both fat and sugar, breast milk has approximately 60 per cent fat, but this changes to a more adult type of diet by adolescence. As a result of all these changes, assessing the aetiology and predicting the consequences and hence the significance of obesity in children at different stages of development is very difficult.

It is also important to remember environmental influences. Infants and children will be totally dependent on their parents for food provision. Even adolescents who are striving for independence will still rely on their parents to do the shopping and make the family food choices. When considering an approach to the assessment and management of obese and overweight children the developmental stage of the child should always be considered and the importance of the family never underestimated.

The problem of size

The definition of childhood obesity should be based on a measure that not only reflects body fatness but also delineates those who are at risk of increased morbidity and mortality. This measure should be easy to perform, be reproducible and population specific normative data should be available. This is a problematic area in childhood for a number of reasons. Tremendous changes occur in body habitus during normal growth and maturation as already described, suggesting that one measure may not be adequate for all stages of development. In addition, although the metabolic complications of obesity can be seen in childhood they are uncommon and the greatest risks of childhood obesity occur in adult life. Finally, although paediatric centile charts are available for a number of growth parameters in many countries no centile charts are available for minority ethnic groups who appear to be at special risk of the complications of obesity in childhood (Whincup *et al.*, 2002).

A variety of measures for the assessment of childhood obesity have been proposed (Cole and Rolland-Cachera, 2002). Skinfold thickness is an assessment of subcutaneous fat and can be measured along the trunk, subscapular and iliac regions, or in the extremities, triceps region. Skinfold thickness correlates reasonably well with total body adiposity and an adverse cardiovascular risk profile. Studies have demonstrated a link between skinfold thickness and adverse lipid and insulin profiles (Freedman *et al.*, 1999a) however these associations do vary with age and gender (Morrison *et al.*, 1999a, b). The assessment of skinfold thickness is relatively easy but is poorly reproducible and as a result it is not routinely used in clinical practice.

The measurement of waist circumference is gaining interest. Waist circumference is easy to measure, reproducible and centile charts are available. Waist and hip circumference are good predictors of abdominal fat and are often expressed as a ratio, waist–hip ratio (WHR; Goran *et al.*, 1998). Abdominal fat is related to adverse health outcomes such as dislipidaemia and glucose intolerance in obese children (Caprio *et al.*, 1995, 1996a). Studies suggest that waist circumference alone is a more powerful predictor of an adverse cardiovascular risk profile than WHR in children (Freedman *et al.*, 1999a). This may be due to the fact that there is a proportionately greater increase in hip circumference during normal childhood growth than waist circumference (Weststrate *et al.*, 1989).

BMI is currently the measure of choice for defining overweight and obesity in children over two years of age (Barlow and Dietz, 1998; Cole *et al.*, 2000). It is easy to measure, reproducible and centile charts are available. Definitions for both overweight and obesity have been proposed based on centiles but there has been little consensus internationally. In the United States the definitions are based on a weight over the 85th centile for overweight and 98th centile for obesity, but the 85th centile is not plotted on United Kingdom centile charts. Recently, the International Obesity Task Force has provided BMI cut-offs based on the adult definition of $25 \, kg/m^2$ for overweight and $30 \, kg/m^2$ for obesity (Cole *et al.*, 2000). Although these measures are not ideal they do provide some international consensus and provide some continuity when moving from paediatric to adult care.

The *clinical* relevance of these BMI cut-offs in childhood is not clear. There are data showing a correlation between BMI and an increased cardiovascular risk profile but the validity of any of these cut-offs in terms of adverse health outcomes in childhood is not described (Freedman *et al.*, 1999b). Currently these criteria are used to highlight those children that *may* be at risk and who may benefit from evaluation and possible intervention. There appears to be no consensus on a definition of 'morbid' obesity in childhood.

The size of the problem

Given the difficulties of defining obesity it is not surprising that attempts to compare prevalence of childhood obesity internationally have been problematic. In addition, pre-school children, children and adolescents are assessed separately making it difficult to generalize across countries. What is clear however is that the prevalence has been increasing steeply with studies showing an increase in the prevalence of obesity of up to 5 fold over the last 10 years (see Table 12.1; Ebbeling *et al.*, 2002). This is true of countries in both the developed and developing world. Recent data from North America suggest that 21.5 per cent of African-Americans, 21.8 per cent of Hispanics and 12.3 per cent of non-Hispanic whites are overweight and this prevalence rapidly increased between 1986 and 1998 (Strauss and Pollack, 2001). In Australia the estimates are that 16.1–16.9 per cent of boys and 17.4–20.4 per cent of girls are overweight (Booth *et al.*, 2001), and again the prevalence has been rising (Lazarus *et al.*, 2000).

What causes obesity in childhood?

Pathological causes of obesity

Genetic and endocrine abnormalities are rare causes of obesity in childhood. However, they are important to mention as many parents of obese children are convinced that their child has an underlying 'hormonal' problem and this belief can be a significant barrier to the lifestyle changes that need to be made when tackling childhood obesity. The clinical features of these genetic and endocrine disorders are highlighted in Table 12.2. Children with simple obesity tend to be tall for their age as excess nutrition supplements the growth hormone drive to growth. They are also more likely to develop early puberty. Obese children with short stature, poor growth or delayed puberty should raise concern as they are more likely to have an underlying disorder for which they should be screened.

Single gene defects, including leptin deficiency, leptin receptor deficiency, melanocortin-4 receptor deficiency and pro-opiomelanocortin deficiency, have been described in children but are extremely rare (Farooqi and O'Rahilly, 2000). These children develop severe early-onset obesity in the first 2 years of life. Although these conditions are rare they have enabled us to gain valuable insight in to the potential mechanisms involved in human weight control with potential implications for the development of effective pharmacological interventions in obesity management.

Environmental causes of obesity

Simple obesity is caused by a long-standing imbalance between calories consumed and calories expended. This does not necessarily imply that an

Table 12.1 Worldwide rate of increase in prevalence of childhood obesity (from Ebbeling *et al.*, 2002)

Country	Measure of obesity	Duration of change	Age (years)	Rate of increase in prevalence
USA	BMI ≥ 95th percentile	1971–74 to 1999	6–11	3.3
			12–19	2.3
England	Age adjusted BMI linked to adult value of 30 kg/m^2	1984 to 1994	4–11	Boys: 2.8 Girls: 2.0
Scotland	Age adjusted BMI linked to adult value of 30 kg/m^2	1984 to 1994	4–11	Boys: 2.3 Girls: 1.8
China	Age adjusted BMI linked to adult value of 25 kg/m^2	1991 to 1997	6–9	1.1
			10–18	1.4
Japan	≥120% of standard weight	1970 to 1996	10	Boys: 2.5 Girls: 2.3
Egypt	Weight for height > 2SD from median	1978 to 1995–6	0–5	3.9
Australia	Age adjusted BMI linked to adult value of 30 kg/m^2	1985 to 1995	7–15	Boys: 3.4 Girls: 4.6
Ghana	Weight for height > 2SD from median	1988 to 1993–94	0–3	3.8
Morocco	Weight for height > 2SD from median	1987 to 1992	0–5	2.5
Brazil	Age adjusted BMI linked to adult value of 25 kg/m^2	1974 to 1997	6–9	3.6
			10–18	3.4
Chile	Weight for height > 2SD from median	1985 to 1995	0–6	1.6
Costa Rica	Weight for height > 2SD from median	1982 to 1996	0–7	2.7
Haiti	Weight for height > 2SD from median	1978 to 1994–95	0–5	3.5

Reprinted with permission from Elsevier (The Lancet, 2002, 360, 473–82).

individual is eating vast quantities of food. Eating an extra packet of potato crisps (approximately 150 calories) every day for one year will lead to the accumulation of just under 8 kg of weight if there is no compensatory increase in caloric expenditure.

Data regarding eating habits in children do suggest that patterns have changed considerably over the last twenty to thirty years. Some healthy eating advice has been accepted. The UK National Food Survey has collected information on household food consumption since the 1940s (National Food Survey, 2000).

Table 12.2   Pathological causes of obesity in childhood

	Clinical findings
Genetic disorders	
Prader–Willi	Short stature
	Hypotonia in early infancy
	Hypogonadotrophic hypogonadism
Bardet–Biedl	Mental deficiency
	Polydactyly
	Retinitis pigmentosa
	Hypogonadism
Alstrom	Retinitis pigmentosa
	Type 2 diabetes
	Cardiomyopathy
	Deafness
Cohen	Hypotonia
	Mental deficiency
	Prominent incisors
Single gene defects	Early onset severe obesity (<2 years)
	Uncontrollable appetite
Endocrine disorders	
Hypothyroidism	Goitre
	Poor linear growth
Growth hormone deficiency	Short stature
	Poor linear growth
	Cherubic facies
Hypothalamic damage due to tumour	History of intracranial tumour
Cushing's syndrome	Moon facies
	Hirsutism
	Violaceous striae
	Hypertension
	Poor linear growth
Pseudohypoparathyroidism	Hypocalcaemia
	Hyperphosphataemia
	Short fourth metacarpal

This shows that there has been a decrease in the purchase of high-fat dairy products, such as full-fat milk and butter, as well as a trend away from frying food in animal fat. However, there is now a trend towards the purchase of calorie-dense, high-fat, convenience foods which are often eaten outside of the house (National Food Survey, 2000). Fast food restaurants appear to fulfil a need in our society and it is unfortunate that there do not appear to be any fast food outlets that provide exclusively 'healthy' options. In addition children are consuming more calories in the form of snacks and carbonated drinks (Harnack *et al.*, 1999; Jahns *et al.*, 2001). As already mentioned these 'added' calories eaten outside of standard mealtimes may provide a considerable number of extra calories that add up over time.

Although it would be easy to blame the obesity epidemic on fast food outlets this is by no means the only reason. Children in recent years have become much less active. There are few objective measures of activity in childhood and there appear to be no studies which have examined changes in physical activity over time. Instead, surrogate markers are used. These have included data regarding TV and video viewing and the purchase of computer games (Dietz, 1996; Andersen *et al.*, 1998). Data do show that life has become much more sedentary for young people with the great majority of 8–15-year-olds in the UK spending at least 3 hours per day in sedentary activities, watching TV or videos for at least 2 hours of this (National Survey of Time Use, 2000). On an average day 25 per cent of these individuals do no physical activity lasting more than 5 min (National Survey of Time Use, 2000). Concerns about child safety have also led to more children being driven to school – 36 per cent of prepubertal children and 20 per cent of adolescents in the UK are driven to school, which is considerably more than 15 years ago (Social Trends, 2000). It is likely that the epidemic of childhood obesity can be blamed on a *combination* of excess calories with decreased expenditure in predisposed individuals.

Does obesity in childhood matter?

Obese children appear to be at risk of the same complications of obesity as are obese adults (Table 12.3). However, no data exist which correlate definitions of childhood obesity based on BMI cut-offs with the risk of adverse health outcomes in childhood. Instead BMI criteria are used to highlight those who may be at greater risk and who would benefit from assessment and intervention. Currently the greatest concern is the development of type 2 diabetes, the emergence of which has changed the face of paediatric diabetes practice over the last 5–10 years.

Gastrointestinal

Non-alcoholic steatotic hepatitis (NASH), is increasingly recognized as a metabolic complication of obesity and is associated with insulin resistance. Studies have suggested that 12–47 per cent of children with clinical obesity have the biochemical and radiological markers of hepatic fatty infiltration (Kinugasa *et al.*, 1984; Guzzaloni *et al.*, 2000). Children may present with abdominal pain and will have raised aminotransferases on biochemical testing. The ideal plan of investigation for obese children with raised liver transaminases remains unclear. A liver biopsy is the only way to accurately differentiate this condition from other hepatic inflammation, but can be a hazardous procedure especially in

Table 12.3   Consequences of obesity

	Consequence	Clinical features
Metabolic	Insulin resistance	Acanthosis nigricans
	Type 2 diabetes	Polyuria
		Polydipsia
		Glycosuria $+/-$ ketonuria
	Hypertension	
	Dislipidaemia	
Gynaecological	Polycystic ovary syndrome	Menstrual irregularity
		Hirsutism
Respiratory	Obesity hypoventilation syndrome	Sleep apnoea
		Snoring
		Burning headaches
		Daytime sleepiness
Gastrointestinal	Non-alcoholic steatotic hepatitis	Abdominal pain
		Raised serum transaminases
	Gallstones	Abdominal pain
Orthopaedic	Slipped femoral epiphysis	Limp
		Joint pain
		Limitation of abduction/internal rotation
Neurological	Benign intracranial hypertension	Headache
		Vomiting
		Papilloedema
Psychological	School bullying	
	Depression	
	Low self esteem	

an obese individual. Even ultrasonography can be practically difficult and is unlikely to be diagnostic. At the very least children should be screened for autoimmune hepatitis and Wilson's disease as these are potentially treatable conditions. The natural history of this condition is not known. On the whole it is felt to be a benign condition although a small number of adults with NASH go on to develop cirrhosis necessitating liver transplantation (James and Day, 1998; Shiva Kumar and Malet, 2000). Results of exercise interventions in adults with NASH have been promising but there are no paediatric data available at the current time (Ueno *et al.*, 1997). Insulin sensitizers such as metformin have been used with some benefit but their use in clinical paediatric practice is also to be defined (Marchesini *et al.*, 2001).

Gynaecological

Polycystic ovarian syndrome (PCOS) involves a triad of symptoms: obesity, menstrual irregularity and hirsutism. The precise aetiology of this complex disorder and whether obesity is a primary or secondary phenomenon is not known (Franks, 1995). However, hyperinsulinaemia, such as occurs during puberty, has been suggested as being a prerequisite for the development of PCOS (Utiger, 1996). Recognized therapeutic options exist making it an important condition to diagnose and treat (Iuorno and Nestler, 1999). Metformin is beneficial in improving menstrual irregularities although the data regarding the effects on weight loss or hirsutism are inconsistent.

Orthopaedic

Slipped upper femoral epiphysis is a recognized complication of obesity and presents as a limp or joint pain, often knee pain (Loder *et al.*, 1993). Clinical findings include limitation of abduction and internal rotation at the hip joint. Referral to an orthopaedic surgeon is necessary. Blount's disease, involving bowing of the tibia, and flat feet have also been described in childhood obesity (Dietz *et al.*, 1982).

Neurological

Benign intracranial hypertension is an uncommon complication of obesity, particularly in children (Grant, 1971; Balcer *et al.*, 1999). Patients present with symptoms of raised intracranial pressure and may need therapeutic lumbar puncture. Symptoms are said to improve with weight loss, but ongoing ophthalmological assessment is important as some children may have residual visual problems.

Psychological

It is beyond the scope of this chapter to provide a comprehensive overview of the psychological consequences of obesity in childhood. Psychological issues may be an aetiological factor in the development of obesity and can be significant barriers to successful intervention (Erikson *et al.*, 2000). Bullying at school is almost universal and needs to be addressed as school often provides the only source of physical activity for these children. Professional help may be necessary and is likely to involve the entire family.

Respiratory

Sleep-disordered breathing is a well-described complication of obesity in adults. It may be more of a problem in childhood than previously thought (Redline *et al.*, 1999), but there do not appear to have been any studies of the prevalence of sleep problems in unselected groups of overweight or obese children. Studies of children attending specialized weight management clinics suggest that obstructive sleep apnoea may affect as many as 40 per cent of these children (Mallory *et al.*, 1989; de la Eva *et al.*, 2002). Snoring is a non-specific symptom but those children with a history of sleep apnoea, burning headaches or excessive daytime sleepiness should be referred for further evaluation (Gaultier, 1995).

Renal

Renal complications are also included in the list of obesity-related problems. One study reported seven African-American children with severe obesity and proteinuria who were found to have focal segmental glomerulosclerosis on renal biopsy (Adelman *et al.*, 2000). One child improved with weight reduction whilst another progressed to end stage renal disease.

Cardiovascular disease risk factors

A number of cohort studies have examined cardiovascular disease (CVD) risk profiles in children (Daniels *et al.*, 1999; Freedman *et al.*, 1999b; Morrison *et al.*, 1999a, b; Sinaiko *et al.*, 1999). One impressive study is the Bogalusa Heart Study which began in 1973 and is a cross-sectional and longitudinal study of the early natural history of atherosclerosis (Berenson *et al.*, 1980). The survey has included school age children and young adults in a biracial (one-third African-American) cohort. This study has published a number of papers that have highlighted the link between overweight and obesity and an abnormal CVD risk profile even in young children. This includes changes in lipid, blood pressure and insulin profiles (Bao *et al.*, 1996; Freedman *et al.*, 1999b). The Bogalusa Heart Study demonstrated that insulin resistance tracked strongly from childhood to adulthood and resulted in a 36-fold increase in the prevalence of obesity, a 2.5-fold increase in hypertension and a 3-fold increase in dislipidaemia in those with persistently elevated fasting insulin (Bao *et al.*, 1996). Childhood obesity *per se* is also a powerful predictor of the metabolic syndrome in young adulthood and this relationship remains significant even after adjusting for fasting insulin values (Srinivasan *et al.*, 2002). An autopsy study of children who died during the course of the survey has confirmed this link with early histological changes in coronary artery architecture (Berenson *et al.*, 1998). Despite these findings the majority of CVD risk prevention programmes are targeted almost exclusively at adults. However, in North America the concerns are so great that the American Heart Association has recently published a consensus statement on cardiovascular health in childhood highlighting childhood obesity as a significant risk factor for adult cardiovascular disease (Williams *et al.*, 2002).

Type 2 diabetes

Type 2 diabetes has always been regarded as a disease of adults. However, in the late 1970s it was recognized that some children of the Pima Indians in North

America had diabetes presenting as a mild and chronic disease associated with obesity. Since that time children with type 2 diabetes have been reported from many countries around the world. The prevalence is increasing and probably relates to the rise in childhood obesity seen in many western and developing countries. This section reviews the recent emergence of type 2 diabetes as a disease of childhood. More extensive reviews are referenced (Libman and Arslanian, 1999; Rosenbloom *et al.*, 1999).

An emerging epidemic

Type 2 diabetes in children has been reported with increasing frequency over the last 20 years, associated with increasing prevalence of obesity in children and young people, and initially from North America (Glaser, 1997). The first reports came from the Pima Indian population, in whom over 1 per cent of those 15–24 years of age had diabetes associated with obesity and long-term diabetes complications (Savage *et al.*, 1979). In the 1990s, type 2 diabetes was reported in 5–14-year-old children among ethnic minority populations (Native American Indians, in Manitoba; Dean *et al.*, 1992; Dean, 1998). Similar findings were seen in Ontario in young people under 16 years, but with a higher prevalence (Harris *et al.*, 1996). In all these reports, females were more often affected than males, with a female to male ratio of 4–6:1. In Cincinnati, Ohio, one-third of all new young people with diabetes aged 10–19 years were classified as type 2 diabetes, with an age-specific incidence of 7.2:100 000 per year (Pinhas Hamiel *et al.*, 1996). Before 1992 type 2 diabetes made up 2–4 per cent of all childhood diabetes however, by 1994, accounted for 16 per cent of all new cases in children. African-Americans accounted for 70–75 per cent of type 2 diabetes patients. In 2000 Fagot-Campagna reported that between 8 and 45 per cent of newly diagnosed children with diabetes in North America had type 2 diabetes, and that this coincided with the rising prevalence of overweight and physical inactivity in young people (Fagot-Campagna *et al.*, 2000). In response to this emerging problem, the American Diabetes Association and the American Academy of Pediatrics issued a joint consensus statement on type 2 diabetes in childhood (American Diabetes Association, 2000). The same phenomenon of a rapidly accelerating incidence of childhood type 2 diabetes has been reported across the globe: in Libyan Arabs (Kadiki *et al.*, 1996), Japanese schoolchildren (Kitagawa *et al.*, 1994), New Zealand Maori children (McGrath *et al.*, 1999), and Singaporese children (Lee, 2000).

The first report from the UK, in 2000, described eight girls with type 2 diabetes, aged 9–16 years, who were of Pakistani, Indian or Arabic origin (Ehtisham *et al.*, 2000). They were all overweight or obese, and had a family history of diabetes in at least two generations. Four had acanthosis nigricans, a marker of insulin resistance, and the others had high plasma concentrations of fasting insulin or C-peptide. Since then there has been a report of type 2 diabetes in four white UK teenagers (Drake *et al.*, 2002). In a UK national survey of non-type 1 diabetes in children, 24 children had type 2, giving a crude minimum prevalence of type 2 diabetes under 16 years as 0.21 per 100 000 (Ehtisham *et al.*, submitted). South Asian children had a relative risk of type 2 diabetes of 13.7 compared to Caucasian UK children.

Pathophysiology

Does childhood obesity predispose to type 2 diabetes? Although the great majority of children with type 2 diabetes are overweight or obese (Fagot-Campagna *et al.*, 2000) there have been no systematic studies of the prevalence of impaired glucose tolerance or type 2 diabetes in cohorts of overweight or obese children. Hyperinsulinaemic, euglycaemic clamp studies suggest that per cent body fat is a primary correlate of insulin sensitivity in both prepubertal and pubertal normal weight children (Arslanian and Suprasongin, 1996). Studies have also demonstrated defects in insulin-stimulated glucose uptake and a reduction in lipid oxidation even in young prepubertal children with short duration of obesity (Caprio *et al.*, 1996b). An important study from Yale has suggested that this insulin resistance is an important risk factor for impaired glucose tolerance in obese children (Sinha *et al.*, 2002). Oral glucose tolerance tests were performed in 55 prepubertal children and 112 adolescents attending the Yale paediatric weight management clinic. Twenty-five per cent of children and 21 per cent of adolescents had impaired glucose tolerance. Four per cent of adolescents had asymptomatic type 2 diabetes suggesting that type 2 diabetes may be an 'iceberg' disease in childhood as well as in adulthood. Insulin resistance as judged by the fasting insulin concentration was a significant predictor for impaired glucose tolerance in these children (Sinha *et al.*, 2002).

The emergence of type 2 diabetes in many societies as rates of obesity increase, and the strong familial tendency, indicate there may have been some advantage to the metabolic phenotype that is now detrimental (Rosenbloom *et al.*, 1999). One hypothesis is that β-cell capacity and insulin resistance might be programmed *in utero*. This is known as the 'thrifty phenotype' hypothesis. This proposes that maternal-fetal under nutrition results in long-term change or 'programming' in metabolic or hormonal activity in the offspring (Hales *et al.*, 1991). An alternative hypothesis is the 'thrifty genotype' hypothesis. This was originally proposed to explain the high prevalence of type 2 diabetes in recently westernized, previously undernourished, communities (Neel, 1962). Neel proposed that a genetic predisposition to type 2 diabetes may have also carried some selective advantage during earlier times of under-nutrition, and would be over-represented in these populations. The rise in prevalence of type 2 diabetes in ethnic minority populations probably represents unfavourable environmental causes of insulin resistance (obesity, over-nutrition and lack of exercise) on an insulin-resistant genetic background. Asian migration to the west has been associated with a deterioration in insulin sensitivity and pancreatic β-cell function, but insulin sensitivity is also impaired in the residents of the Punjab compared to white UK residents. (Bhatnagar *et al.*, 1995). Thus a naturally determined risk factor – an insulin resistance genotype – can be nurtured into a more potent phenotype by westernization.

This difference in insulin resistance is present in childhood (Whincup *et al.*, 2002). British south Asian children show higher average levels of insulin and insulin resistance than Caucasian children. These ethnic differences in insulin resistance are not associated with corresponding differences in adiposity, particularly central adiposity. Insulin metabolism seems to be more sensitive to a given degree of adiposity among the south Asian children compared with Caucasian children.

Clinical findings and differential diagnosis

Most children who present with type 2 diabetes are in puberty. This is most likely to be due to the temporary insulin resistance during pubertal maturation in which a 30 per cent reduction in insulin action compared with prepubertal children or adults has been reported (Amiel *et al.*, 1986). Children and young people with type 2 diabetes may present on a spectrum from being an incidental finding to severe diabetic ketoacidosis. The child may have symptoms suggestive of type 1 diabetes, including thirst, polyuria, hyperventilation, weight loss, vomiting and dehydration. Episodes of ketonuria may occur intermittently with intercurrent illnesses. However, the majority of children are probably relatively asymptomatic. In one reported series, 50 per cent of children with type 2 diabetes were referred only because of glycosuria noted during routine tests for other reasons; 39 per cent initially had polyuria, polydipsia, and weight loss, and only 11 per cent had mild ketoacidosis (Glaser and Jones, 1996). Acanthosis nigricans, a cutaneous manifestation of insulin resistance or hyperinsulinism, has been reported to be present in 60–80 per cent of patients in North America (Libman and Arslanian, 1999). It consists of hyperpigmentation with thickening of the skin into velvety, irregular folds in the axillae, groin and neck.

Type 2 diabetes has also been confused with maturity onset diabetes of the young (MODY). Children with MODY have a single gene disorder resulting in β-cell dysfunction and do not need to be insulin resistant or obese to develop diabetes (Tattersall, 1974). The diagnostic criteria have recently been reviewed (Owen and Hattersley, 2001). These patients have endogenous insulin secretion, are usually not insulin dependent or prone to ketoacidosis, and are not known to be insulin resistant. MODY is now known to be a heterogeneous group of single gene disorders with mutations in at least five genes, with more than 80 per cent of MODY patients having a recognized mutation in a MODY gene.

We recently identified 24 children with type 2 diabetes, and 17 with MODY, as defined by the presence of a MODY mutation. (Ehtisham *et al.*, submitted). Of the 24 children with type 2 diabetes (see Table 12.4), there were 17 females

Table 12.4 Comparison of type 1, type 2 and MODY

	Type 2 diabetes	MODY	Type 1 DUK audit	Type 1 Local data	Type 2 versus type 1	Type 2 versus MODY	MODY versus type 1
n	24	17	7545	50			
Mean age at diagnosis (SD)	12.2 (2.8)	9.7 (3.7)	7.1 (4.0)	8.8 (4.3)	$P < 0.001^*$	$P < 0.001$	$P < 0.01^*$
Female	74%	69%	49%	60%	$P < 0.001^*$	NS	NS*
Ethnic minority	54%	0%	9%	22%	$P < 0.001^*$	$P < 0.001$	NS*
First degree family history of diabetes	54%	100%	–	20%	$P < 0.005$	$P < 0.001$	$P < 0.001$
Obese	75%	14%	–	6%	$P < 0.001$	$P < 0.001$	NS
Ketones at diagnosis	25%	0%	–	74%	$P < 0.001$	$P < 0.05$	$P < 0.001$

*Compared to Diabetes UK (DUK) National Audit data.

and 6 males, presenting mainly in puberty. The majority (13/24) were of ethnic minority origin. Thirteen (54 per cent) had a positive family history of type 2 diabetes in a parent or sibling, but a further seven had a positive family history in other relatives as well (overall 80 per cent had a positive family history). Eighteen were obese and all except one were overweight. Five children had ketonuria at presentation. There were 17 children with mutations identified in MODY genes (nine in glucokinase, seven in HNF1α, one not recorded). All of these children had a positive family history of diabetes in a first-degree relative and 16 (94 per cent) in at least two generations. All were of white UK origin. Seven children were lean, five overweight and two obese. None had acanthosis nigricans, ketones at presentation, or autoantibodies.

The differences in family history between these groups, was that in MODY, diabetes only ran down one side of the family, whereas in type 2 diabetes it was often present in both parents and three out of four grandparents. The characteristics of children with type 2 diabetes and children with MODY were then compared with children with type 2 diabetes from the National Paediatric Diabetes Audit and data from the last 50 children diagnosed with type 1 diabetes at Birmingham Children's Hospital. (See Table 12.4) The characteristics of children with type 2 diabetes are significantly different when compared with children with type 1 diabetes or MODY. Children with type 2 diabetes are significantly more overweight or obese than both type 1 and MODY children. A higher proportion of children with type 2 diabetes come from ethnic minority backgrounds.

There are few data examining the biochemical findings in children with type 2 diabetes. However, in general terms, in comparison with type 1 diabetes, children with type 2 diabetes present with lesser degrees of hyperglycaemia, have significantly higher concentrations of insulin and C-peptide, are less frequently ketonuric, and have milder degrees of acidosis (Libman and Arslanian 1999). Children with type 2 diabetes do not usually have evidence of pancreatic autoimmunity, but this is not absolute, and latent autoimmune diabetes has been described in adults (Tuomi *et al.*, 1999).

There are few long-term follow-up data on children with type 2 diabetes but there is an emerging literature on young adults, 18–44 years, who are the fastest growing group with diabetes (Mokdad *et al.*, 2000). In a comparison of 1616 young adults with type 2 diabetes and 6254 adults diagnosed over the age of 44 years, young adults were more likely to develop macrovascular disease in the first years after diagnosis although incident microvascular complication rates were similar between the two groups (Hillier and Pedula, 2002). Adults with early onset type 2 diabetes were 11 times more likely to develop a myocardial infarction compared to non-diabetic controls. In contrast, adults with later onset diabetes only had three times the risk compared to normal controls. Similarly, incident stroke rates were much higher in adults with early onset type 2 diabetes compared to normal controls (OR 5.1, $P < 0.001$), than with later onset type 2 diabetes compared to non-diabetic controls (OR 2.5, $P < 0.001$).

What is the long-term future for children diagnosed with Type 2 diabetes? A report from Winnipeg, Canada, described a database maintained since 1986 on all 86 children diagnosed with type 2 diabetes under 17 years of age in Manitoba and northwest Ontario (Dean and Flett, 2002). There were two deaths on dialysis, both females aged 25 and 31 years. One female aged 26 years had a toe amputation. Three females aged 26, 28 and 29 years had been on dialysis for 2 months, 1 year and 6 years, respectively. One of these females was also blind at 26 years of age. Of 30 patients with an HbA1c assessment, 5/30 had an HbA1c under 7 per cent, but 19/30 had an HbA1c over 10 per cent. There have been 56 pregnancies with 35 live offspring. The high mortality rate (9 per cent), morbidity (6.3 per cent on dialysis), pregnancy loss (38 per cent) and poor glycaemic control in young adults with type 2 diabetes diagnosed before age 18 years is extremely alarming.

Persistence in to adult life

Longitudinal studies of children followed in to adulthood suggest that many overweight children will become overweight adults (Serdula et al., 1993; Power et al., 1997). The occurrence of parental obesity more than doubles the risk of adult obesity among both obese and non-obese children less than 10 years of age (Whitaker et al., 1997). However the presence of obesity during adolescence is an independent risk factor for adult obesity (Whitaker et al., 1997).

Only a few studies have examined the long-term effects of childhood or adolescent obesity on adult morbidity and mortality. These have shown that coronary heart disease, atherosclerosis and diabetes are increased in adults who were obese in childhood (Sinaiko et al., 1999; Srinivasan et al., 2002). Furthermore, systolic blood pressure, plasma lipids and insulin and obesity tend to cluster and track with age (Bao et al., 1996). This suggests that cardiovascular disease risk factors will persist as obese children become young adults who then want to have children of their own. The implications for future public health could be devastating.

Management of childhood obesity

Prevention

A recent Cochrane review has examined the efficacy of obesity prevention strategies in childhood (Campbell et al., 2002). The authors commented that 'the mismatch between the prevalence and significance of the condition and the knowledge base from which to inform preventive activity, is remarkable and an outstanding feature of this review'. Only seven 'long-term' randomized controlled studies, lasting 12 months, were identified and three short-term studies of 3 months' duration were therefore included. The studies used a number of interventions and it was difficult to generalize the findings. One study examined the effect of dietary education aimed at young children, 3–9 years old. A significant reduction in prevalence of overweight and obesity was reported in the group of children who were given 'multimedia' information regarding healthy eating which included the use of qualified staff to underline health messages (Simonettei *et al.*, 1986). No significant changes were seen in the control group and also in a group of children who were given written information only. Four long-term studies examined the effect of a combination of dietary education and physical activity interventions. The results of these have been disappointing. The APPLES study in the UK assessed the impact of a school-based intervention including teacher training, modification of school meals and action plans tackling physical activity in the school curriculum (Sahota *et al.*, 2001). Six hundred and thirty four children aged 7–11 years old took part. Although the programme had a beneficial effect on changing the healthy living ethos of the schools involved it had little impact on children's behaviour, other than a small increase in the consumption of vegetables. Children, especially young children, have a limited amount of influence on the family food and activity choices and a programme aimed exclusively at children rather than involving the whole family may be of limited success. Another group did examine the effect of behavioural and educational messages regarding diet and activity given to 1640 children aged 5–7 years *and* their parents (Mueller *et al.*, 2001). At one year there were no changes in BMI although there were significant differences in body fat mass, as assessed by skinfold thickness, in the intervention group.

The results from these studies are disappointing. However, given the complexity of the aetiology of the current epidemic of obesity it seems unlikely that a focused approach aimed exclusively at children is likely to succeed, especially in the short term. Instead, the approach to the prevention of obesity in childhood should be seen as part of a bigger picture of social and environmental change which can only be achieved by governments. Changes will need to be accomplished in collaboration with the public health service, the food industry, advertisers and public transport providers, to name but a few, with the aims of changing the behaviour of the general population (Crawford, 2002). The epidemic has evolved over a prolonged period of time and realistic long-term goals need to be developed to protect the health of nations.

Intervention

Aims

North American guidelines recommend that interventions for childhood obesity should begin early (Barlow *et al.*, 1998). Yet data suggest that overweight children are referred less aggressively than underweight children (Miller *et al.*, 2002). Childhood is a time of constant growth and development and any childhood obesity intervention must not compromise this process. The aims of obesity interventions in growing children will therefore be different to those for adults and adolescents who have achieved final adult height (Barlow and Dietz, 1998). Adequate nutritional intake to maintain normal linear growth is essential and severe caloric restriction is inappropriate in young children. Weight loss is difficult to achieve in a growing child and instead the focus should be on a reduction in BMI. This can be achieved by weight maintenance or a reduction in rate of weight gain whilst allowing normal linear growth.

Diet and exercise

There have been a number of childhood obesity intervention studies (Epstein *et al.*, 1998). Almost exclusively the main outcome measure has been weight change: either weight loss or reduction in weight for height. The great majority of studies have involved only a small number of children and have been of relatively short duration. Furthermore most studies have been performed in specialized child obesity centres, mainly in North America, and the appropriateness of generalizing the results to other clinical contexts remains unclear. Although a large number of studies have been performed only randomized controlled studies will be considered in this section.

Few randomized controlled studies have been performed and these have recently been reviewed for the Cochrane Collaboration (Summerbell *et al.*, 2004). Only one study examined the effect of dietary counselling and found no significant difference between a group of 50 prepubertal children who were given dietary counselling and a group who were 'untreated' controls (Flodmark *et al.*, 1993). Other studies focused on physical activity as a means of weight change. In these studies a variety of methods were employed. In one of a number of studies by Epstein, prepubertal children were assigned to either diet alone or diet plus exercise which was provided in the form of an 8-week intensive programme followed by 10 monthly maintenance sessions (Epstein *et al.*, 1985a). Per cent overweight, described as per cent weight for height, was reduced in both intervention groups but was only significantly different at 6 months but not at 12 months following initiation of the intervention.

Epstein has also examined the benefit of a reduction in sedentary behaviour versus an increase in physical activity (Epstein *et al.*, 1985b). The rationale for this approach, often called 'lifestyle activity', is that increasing energy expenditure through normal daily living is potentially a more sustainable form of physical activity than participating in more structured exercise programmes. Statistically significant differences in per cent overweight were found in children in both groups at both 6 and 12 months of treatment. However at 24 months the lifestyle group had maintained their relative weight changes whereas children in the physical activity group had returned to baseline levels (Epstein *et al.*, 1985b).

Behavioural interventions have also been examined. A variety of techniques have been employed and have been shown to be effective compared to conventional treatment, usually dietary advice and medical follow up. Cognitive behavioural therapy, relaxation therapy and family therapy all appear to be effective (Warschburger *et al.*, 2001; Duffy and Spence, 1993; Epstein *et al.*, 1985c; Senediak and Spence, 1985). There is also the suggestion that therapies involving the parents as the main motivators of change are more effective than treatments which are predominantly child focused. However, it is important to note that the great majority of these studies have involved younger children and it is uncertain whether these results could be extrapolated to emotionally challenging adolescents with weight problems.

It would appear from these studies that weight loss is both difficult to achieve and to sustain. It is therefore important to know if weight loss, or even a physical activity intervention *per se*, may have health benefits in children as in adults. A weight reduction of 10 per cent from baseline in adults has been shown to have significant benefits on cardiovascular morbidity (Krebs *et al.*, 2002). Recent studies have also shown a dramatic impact of weight loss on the risk of diabetes. The Finnish Diabetes Prevention Study and the American Diabetes Prevention Program have both shown that intensive lifestyle intervention in obese patients with impaired glucose tolerance (IGT) led to a reduction in the risk of progression to type 2 diabetes of 58 per cent (Tuomilehto *et al.*, 2001; Diabetes Prevention Program, 2002). This was achieved with an average reduction in weight of only 4 kg over the 3–4 year period of the studies. Unfortunately, none of the randomized controlled studies quoted above appear to have examined the health benefits of weight loss in childhood. Smaller studies have suggested that weight management in children does provide some health benefits especially with respect to CVD risk factors. One small study in children has demonstrated a potentially significant benefit of exercise irrespective of weight loss (Ferguson *et al.*, 1999). Four months of exercise training led to a reduction in fasting insulin concentrations suggesting that activity may have beneficial effects on insulin sensitivity in children as in adults. However, these benefits of exercise training were lost when children became less active again, underlining the importance that any intervention needs to be sustainable. Other studies have shown a significant improvement in blood pressure and lipid profiles (Becque *et al.*, 1988; Rocchini *et al.*, 1988; Epstein *et al.*, 1989; Knip and Nuutinen, 1993) with obesity interventions which were more pronounced if exercise was included as part of the weight management strategy (Becque *et al.*, 1988; Rocchini *et al.*, 1988).

Pharmacological therapy

None of the anti-obesity medications available for use in obese adults are currently licensed for use in children. Few studies have been performed of their effectiveness in children. One study has reported that orlistat is well tolerated in the short term (3 months) by adolescents in the context of a multidisciplinary behavioural programme but further studies are awaited to demonstrate its true effect on weight loss (McDuffie *et al.*, 2002).

Surgery

Bariatric surgery is not universally available for children but some operations have been performed. There do not appear to have been any formal studies of the effectiveness of surgery on weight loss and maintenance but there are a number of case reports and series in the literature. One recent report of 10 morbidly obese adolescents who underwent gastric bypass surgery found that nine did achieve significant weight loss although weight did appear to slowly reaccumulate over the period of follow-up (Strauss *et al.*, 2001). Complications were felt to be minimal, although five had clinically significant malabsorption of iron and folate and four had late complications including intestinal obstruction and gallstones. The authors concluded that although the procedure was successful this really was a last resort but did not suggest which patients may benefit from such an intervention (Strauss and Pollack, 2001).

Summary

Although the data for the effectiveness of obesity interventions for childhood are poor there are some suggestions that family based approaches to changes in diet and physical activity may be beneficial. The main goals of management will depend on the age of the child and an age-based, step-wise approach should be pursued. Advice needs to be given on an individual basis but the aim should be to introduce small but sustainable lifestyle changes in diet and physical activity to achieve a gradual improvement in BMI (Barlow and Dietz, 2000). The whole family should be involved and needs to provide support for their child during this process.

Management of Complications

Guardian drugs

The use of 'guardian' drugs to decrease the risk of cardiovascular complications in patients with obesity and/or type 2 diabetes is commonplace. In patients with type 2 diabetes the management of CVD risk factors has been thought to significantly improve the life expectancy of these patients (HOPE, 2000). Although children with obesity have been shown to have abnormal CVD risk profiles no studies exist which have examined the benefits of antihypertensive therapy or lipid lowering agents in children. Given the difficulties of finding a successful intervention to treat childhood obesity it is possible that the use of these drugs may become more common in paediatric practice as an adjunct to lifestyle advice.

Management of type 2 diabetes

Type 2 diabetes is still a relatively novel phenomenon in paediatric practice and as a result the ideal approach to the management of children remains unclear. Paediatric data regarding pharmacological interventions are scarce and currently the adult experience is used. Standard treatment for type 2 diabetes in adults includes advice on healthy eating and overweight patients are encouraged to lose weight. The first line of pharmacological intervention for overweight patients is metformin. In the UKPDS, overweight patients allocated metformin had risk reductions of 32 per cent for any diabetes-related endpoint, 42 per cent for diabetes-related death, and 36 per cent for all-cause mortality (UKPDS, 1998a, b). Metformin showed a greater effect than either sulphonylureas or insulin and was associated with less weight gain and fewer hypoglycaemic episodes than insulin or sulphonylureas. Metformin improves glycaemic control by reducing hepatic glucose production, increasing insulin sensitivity, and reducing intestinal glucose absorption, without increasing insulin secretion (Bailey, 1992). Lee Jones and colleagues have evaluated the safety and efficacy of metformin in doses of up to 1000 mg twice daily in 82 children aged 10–16 years in a randomized double-blind controlled trial (Lee Jones *et al.*, 2002). They showed that metformin significantly improved glycaemic control with mean HbA1c concentrations lower than for placebo (7.5 versus 8.6 per cent respectively, $P < 0.001$). Improvements in fasting blood glucose were seen in both sexes and in all race subgroups. Metformin did not cause weight gain, or have a negative impact on lipid profile. Adverse events were similar to those reported in adults treated with metformin.

Conclusions

Obesity is common in childhood and can lead to significant morbidity as well as premature adult mortality. Of greatest concern is the spectre of juvenile onset type 2 diabetes with its devastating consequences on cardiovascular health. Primary prevention has to be the key aim but this cannot be achieved without a huge investment of public and political will. In the meantime overweight and obese children need to be managed by a dedicated multidisciplinary team, which ideally would span both the hospital and community health networks. Greater investment of resources for both treatment and prevention of childhood obesity need to be made if a public health disaster is to be avoided.

References

Adelman RD, Restaino IG, Alon US and Blowey DL (2001) Proteinuria and focal segmental glomerulosclerosis in severely obese adolescents. *J Pediatr* **138**:481–85.

American Diabetes Association (2000) Type 2 diabetes in children and adolescents. *Diabetes Care* **23**:381–9.

Amiel S, Sherwin R, Simonson D *et al.* (1986) Impaired insulin action in puberty: a contributing factor to poor glycemic control in adolescents with diabetes. *N Engl J Med* **315**:215–19.

Andersen RE, Crespo CJ, Bartlett SJ *et al.* (1988) Relationship of physical activity and television watching with body weight and level of fatness among children. *JAMA* **279**:938–42.

Arslanian S and Suprasongin C (1996) Insulin sensitivity, lipids and body composition in childhood: is 'syndrome X' present? *J Clin Endocrinol Metab* **81**:1058–62.

Bailey C (1992) Biguanides and NIDDM. *Diabetes Care* **15**:755–72.

Balcer LJ, Liu GT, Forman S *et al.* (1999) Idiopathic intracranial hypertension: relation of age and obesity in children. *Neurology* **52**:870–72.

Bao W, Sathanur R, Srinivasan SR and Berenson GS (1996) Persistent elevation of plasma insulin levels is associated with increased cardiovascular risk in children and young adults. The Bogalusa Heart Study. *Circulation* **93**:54–9.

Barlow SE and Dietz WH (1998) Obesity evaluation and treatment: Expert Committee Recommendations. *Pediatrics* **102**(3):E29.

Becque MD, Katch VL, Rocchini AP *et al.* (1988) Coronary risk incidence of obese adolescents: reduction by exercise plus diet intervention. *Pediatrics* **81**:605–12.

Berenson GS, McMahan CA, Voors AW *et al.* (1980) *Cardiovascular Risk Factors in Children: the Early Natural History of Atherosclerosis and Essential Hypertension.* Oxford University Press, New York, NY.

Berenson GS, Srinivasan SR, Bao W *et al.* (1998) Association between multiple cardiovascular risk factors and atherosclerosis in children and young adults. *N Engl J Med* **338**:1650–8.

Bhatnagar D, Anand IS, Durrington PN *et al.* (1995) Coronary risk factors in people from the Indian subcontinent living in West London and their siblings in India. *Lancet* **345**:405–9.

Booth M, Wake M, Armstrong T *et al.* (2001) The epidemiology of overweight and obesity among Australian children and adolescents. *Aust N Z J Public Health* **25**:162–9.

Campbell K, Waters E, O'Meara S *et al.* (2002) Interventions for preventing obesity in children (Cochrane Review). In: The Cochrane Library, Issue 4, Oxford: Update Software.

Caprio S, Hyman LD, Limb C *et al.* (1995) Central adiposity and its metabolic correlates in obese adolescent girls. *Am J Physiol* **269**:E118–E126.

Caprio S, Hyman LD, McCarthy S *et al.* (1996a) Fat distribution and cardiovascular risk factors in obese adolescent girls: importance of the intra-abdominal fat depot. *Am J Clin Nutr* **64**:12–17.

Caprio S, Bronson M, Sherwin RS *et al.* (1996b) Co-existence of severe insulin resistance and hyperinsulinaemia in pre-adolescent obese children. *Diabetologia* **39**:1489–97.

Clayton PE and Gill MS (2001) Normal growth and its endocrine control. In Brook CGD and Hindmarsh PC *Clinical Paediatric Endocrinology.* Blackwell Science, Oxford.

Cole TJ, Freeman JV and Preece MA (1995) Body mass index reference curves for the UK 1990. *Arch Dis Child* **73**:25–9.

Cole TJ, Bellizzi MC, Flegal KM and Dietz WH (2000) Establishing a standard definition for child overweight and obesity worldwide: international survey. *Br Med J* **320**:1240–3.

Cole TJ and Rolland-Cachera MF (2002) Measurement and definition. In Burniat W, Cole T, Lissau I and Poskitt E *Child and Adolescent Obesity.* Cambridge University Press, Cambridge.

Crawford D (2002) Population strategies to prevent obesity. *Br Med J* **325**:728–9.

Daniels SR, Morrison JA, Sprecher DL *et al.* (1999) Association of fat distribution and cardiovascular risk factors in children and adolescents. *Circulation* **99**:541–5.

Dean H (1998) NIDDM-Y in First Nation Children in Canada. *Clin Pediatr* **39**:89–96.

Dean H and Flett B (2002) Natural history of Type 2 diabetes diagnosed in childhood: long term follow-up in young adult years. *Diabetes* **51**(suppl):A24 (99-OR).

Dean HE, Mundy RL and Moffatt M (1992) Non-insulin-dependent diabetes mellitus in Indian children in Manitoba. *Can Med Assoc J* **147**:52–7.

de la Eva R, Baur LA, Donaghue KC and Walters KA (2002) Metabolic correlates with obstructive sleep apnea in obese subjects. *J Pediatr* **140**:654–9.

Diabetes Prevention Program Research Group (2002) Reduction in the incidence of Type 2 diabetes with lifestyle intervention or metformin. *N Engl J Med* **346**:393–403.

Dietz WH (1996) The role of lifestyle in health: the epidemiology and consequences of inactivity. *Proc Nutr Soc* **55**:829–40.

Dietz WH (1997) Periods of risk in childhood for the development of adult obesity – what do we need to learn? *J Nutr* **127**:1884S–1886S.

Dietz WH Jr, Gross WL and Kirkpatrick JA Jr (1982) Blount disease (tibia vara): another skeletal disorder associated with childhood obesity. *J Pediatr* **101**:735–7.

Drake A, Smith A, Betts P *et al.* (2002) Type 2 diabetes in obese white children. *Arch Dis Child* **86**:207–8.

Duffy G and Spence SH (1993) The effectiveness of cognitive self management as an adjunct to a behavioural intervention for childhood obesity: a research note. *J Child Psychol Psychiatry* **34**:1043–50.

Ebbeling CB, Pawlak DB and Ludwig DS (2002) Childhood obesity: public-health crisis, common sense cure. *Lancet* **360**:473–82.

Ehtisham S, Barrett TG and Shaw NJ (2000) Type 2 diabetes mellitus in UK children – an emerging problem. *Diabet Med* **17**:867–71.

Ehtisham S, Hattersley A, Dunger D and Barrett T (2004) Clinical characteristics and prevalence of Type 2 diabetes and MODY in UK children. *Arch Dis Child* in Press.

[1]Epstein LH, Wing RR, Penner BC and Kress MJ (1985a) Effect of diet and controlled exercise on weight loss in obese children. *J Pediatr* **107**:358–61.

[2]Epstein LH, Wing RR, Koeske R and Valoski A (1985b) A comparison of lifestyle exercise, aerobic exercise and callisthenics on weight loss in obese children. *Behav Ther* **16**:345–56.

[3]Epstein LH, Wing RR, Woodall K *et al.* (1985c) Effects of family-based behavioural treatment on obese 5–8 year old children. *Behav Ther* **16**:205–12.

Epstein LH, Kuller LH, Wing RR *et al.* (1989) The effect of weight control on lipid changes in obese children. *Am J Dis Child* **143**:454–7.

Epstein LH, Myers MD, Raynor HA and Saelens BE (1998) Treatment of pediatric obesity. *Pediatrics* **101**:554–70.

Erikson SJ, Robinson TN, Haydel KF and Killen JD (2000) Are overweight children unhappy? Body mass index, depressive symptoms, and overweight concern in elementary school children. *Arch Pediatr Adolesc Med* **154**:931–5.

Fagot-Campagna A, Pettitt D, Engelgau M *et al.* (2000) Type 2 diabetes among North American children and adolescents: an epidemiological review and a public health perspective. *J Pediatr* **136**:664–72.

Farooqi IS and O'Rahilly S. Recent advances in the genetics of severe childhood obesity. *Arch Dis Child* **83**:31–4.

Ferguson MA, Gutin B, Le N-A *et al.* (1999) Effects of exercise training and its cessation on components of the insulin resistance syndrome in obese children. *Int J Obes* **22**:889–95.

Flodmark CE, Ohlsson T, Ryden O and Sveger T (1993) Prevention of progression to severe obesity in a group of obese schoolchildren treated with family therapy. *Pediatrics* **91**:880–4.

Franks S (1995) Polycystic ovary syndrome. *N Engl J Med* **333**:853–61.

Freedman DS, Serdula MK, Srinivasan SR and Berenson GS (1999a) Relation of circumferences and skinfold thicknesses to lipid and insulin concentrations in children and adolescents: the Bogalusa Heart Study. *Am J Clin Nutr* **69**:308–17.

Freedman DS, Dietz WH, Srinivasan SR and Berenson GS (1999b) The relation of overweight to cardiovascular risk factors in children and adolescents: the Bogalusa Heart Study. *Pediatrics* **103**:1175–82.

Gaultier C (1995) Obstructive sleep apnoea syndrome in infants and children: established facts and unsettled issues. *Thorax* **50**:1204–10.

Glaser NS (1997) Non-insulin-dependent diabetes in childhood and adolescence. *Pediatr Clin N Am* **44**:307–37.

Glaser N and Jones KL (1996) Non-insulin dependent diabetes mellitus in children and adolescents. *Adv Paediatr* **43**:359–96.

Goran MI, Gower BA, Treuth M and Nagy TR (1998) Prediction of intra-abdominal and subcutaneous abdominal adipose tissue in healthy prepubertal children. *Int J Obes* **22**:549–58.

Grant DN (1971) Benign intracranial hypertension; a review of 79 cases in infancy and childhood. *Arch Dis Child* **46**:651–5.

Guzzaloni G, Grugni G, Minocci A *et al.* (2000) Liver steatosis in juvenile obesity: correlations with lipid profile, hepatic biochemical parameters and glycemic and insulinemic responses to an oral glucose tolerance test. *Int J Obes* **24**:772–6.

Hales C, Barker D, Clark P *et al.* (1991) Fetal and infant growth and impaired glucose tolerance at age 64. *Br Med J* **303**:1019–22.

Harnack L, Stang J and Story M (1999) Soft drink consumption among US children and adolescents: nutritional consequences. *J Am Diet Assoc* **4**:436–41.

Harris SB, Perkins BA and Whalen-Brough E (1996) Non-insulin dependent diabetes mellitus among First Nations children: new entity among First Nations people of north-western Ontario. *Can Fam Phys* **42**:869–76.

Heart Outcomes Prevention Evaluation Study Investigators (2000) Effects of ramipril on cardiovascular and microvascular outcomes in people with diabetes mellitus: results of the HOPE study and MICRO-HOPE substudy. *Lancet* **355**:253–9.

Hergenroeder AC and Klisch WJ (1990) Body composition in adolescent athletes. *Pediatr Clin N Am* **37**:1057–80.

Hillier T and Pedula K (2002) Are adults with early onset type 2 diabetes a different clinical phenotype? *Diabetes Care* **51**:A228.

Iuorno MJ and Nestler JE (1999) The polycystic ovary syndrome: treatment with insulin sensitizing agents. *Diabetes Obes Metab* **1**:127–36.

Jahns L, Siega-Riz AM and Popkin BM (2001) The increasing prevalence of snacking among US children from 1977 to 1996. *J Pediatr* **138**:493–8.

James OFW and Day CP (1998) Non-alcoholic steatohepatitis (NASH): a disease of emerging identity and importance. *J Hepatol* **29**:495–501.

Kadiki O, Reddy M and Marzouk A (1996) Incidence of insulin-dependent diabetes (IDDM) and non-insulin-dependent diabetes (NIDDM) (0–34 years at onset) in Benghazi, Libya. *Diabetes Res Clin Pract* **32**:165–73.

Kinugasa A, Tsunamoto K, Furakawa N *et al.* (1984) Fatty liver and its fibrous changes found in simple obesity of children. *J Pediatr Gastroenterol Nutr* **3**:408–14.

Kitagawa T, Owada M, Urakami T and Tajima N (1994) Epidemiology of Type 1 (insulin-dependent) and Type 2 (non-insulin-dependent) diabetes mellitus in Japanese children. *Diabetes Res Clin Pract* **24** (Suppl.):S7–S13.

Knip M and Nuutinen O (1993) Long-term effects of weight reduction on serum lipids and plasma insulin in obese children. *Am J Clin Nutr* **57**:490–3.

Krebs JD, Evans S, Cooney L *et al.* (2002) Changes in risk factors for cardiovascular disease with body fat loss in obese women. *Diabetes Obes Metab* **4**:379–87.

Lazarus R, Wake M, Hesketh K and Waters E (2000) Change in body mass index in Australian primary school children, 1985–1997. *Int J Obes* **24**:679–84.

Lee W (2000) The changing demography of diabetes mellitus in Singapore. *Diabetes Res Clin Pract* **50** (Suppl 2):S35–S39.

Lee Jones K, Arslanian S, Peterokova V *et al.* (2002) Effect of metformin in pediatric patients with type 2 diabetes. *Diabetes Care* **25**:89–94.

Libman I and Arslanian S (1999) Type 2 diabetes mellitus: no longer just adults. *Pediatr Ann* **28**:589–93.

Loder RT, Aronson DD and Greenfield ML (1993) The epidemiology of bilateral slipped capital femoral epiphysis. *J Bone Joint Surg* **75**:1141–7.

McDuffie JR, Calis KA, Uwaifo GI *et al.* (2002) Three month tolerability of orlistat in adolescents with obesity-related comorbid conditions. *Obes Res* **10**:642–50.

McGrath N, Parker G and Dawson P (1999) Early presentation of Type 2 diabetes mellitus in young New Zealand Maori. *Diabetes Res Clin Pract* **43**:205–9.

Mallory GB Jr, Fiser DH and Jackson R (1989) Sleep-associated breathing disorders in morbidly obese children and adolescents. *J Pediatr* **115**:892–7.

Marchesini G, Brizi M, Bianchi G *et al.* (2001) Metformin in non-alcoholic steatohepatitis. *Lancet* **358**:893–4.

Miller LA, Grunwald GK, Johnson SL and Krebs NF (2002) Disease severity at time of referral for paediatric failure to thrive and obesity: Time for a paradigm shift? *J Pediatr* **141**:121–124.

Mokdad AH, Ford ES, Bowman BA, Nelson DE, Engelgau MM, Vinicor F and Marks JS (2000) Diabetes trends in the U.S.: 1990–1998. *Diabetes Care* **23**:1278–83.

[1]Morrison JA, Barton BA, Biro FM *et al.* (1999a) Overweight, fat patterning and cardiovascular disease risk factors in black and white boys. *J Pediatr* **135**:451–457.

[2]Morrison JA, Sprecher DL, Barton BA *et al.* (1999b) Overweight, fat patterning and cardiovascular disease risk factors in black and white girls: the National Heart, Lung and Blood Institute Growth and Health Study. *J Pediatr* **135**:458–64.

Mueller MJ, Asbeck I, Mast M *et al.* (2001) Prevention of obesity – more than an intention. Concept and first results of the Kiel Obesity Prevention Study (KOPS). *Int J Obes* **25** (suppl 1):S66–S74.

National Food Survey, 2000. Office for National Statistics (www.statistics.gov.uk)

National Survey of Time Use, 2000. Office for National Statistics (www.statistics.gov.uk)

Neel JV (1962) Diabetes Mellitus: a thrifty genotype rendered detrimental by 'progress'. *Am J Hum Genet* **14**:353–62.

Owen K and Hattersley A (2001) Maturity-onset diabetes of the young: from clinical description to molecular genetic characterisation. *Best Pract Rese Clin Endocrinol Metab* **15**:309–23. Baillière Tindall, London.

Pinhas-Hamiel O, Dolan L, Daniels S *et al.* (1996) Increased incidence of non-insulin-dependent diabetes mellitus among adolescents. *J Pediatr* **128**:608–15.

Power C, Lake JK and Cole TJ (1997) Measurement and long-term health risks of child and adolescent fatness. *Int J Obes* **21**:507–26.

Redline S, Tishler PV, Schluchter M *et al.* (1999) Risk factors for sleep disordered breathing in children: associations with obesity, race and respiratory problems. *Am J Resp Crit Care Med* **159**:1527–32.

Rocchini AP, Katch V, Anderson J *et al.* (1988) Blood pressure in obese adolescents: effect of weight loss. *Pediatrics* **82**:16–23.

Rosenbloom AL, Joe JR, Young RS and Winter WE (1999) Emerging epidemic of type 2 diabetes in youth. *Diabetes Care* **22**:345–54.

Sahota P, Rudolf MCJ, Dixey R *et al.* (2001) Randomised controlled trial of primary school based intervention to reduce risk factors for obesity. *Br Med J* **323**:1029–32.

Savage PJ, Bennett PH, Senter RG and Miller M (1979) High prevalence of diabetes in young Pima Indians. *Diabetes* **28**:937–42.

Senediak C and Spence SH (1985) Rapid versus gradual scheduling of therapeutic contact in a family based behavioural weight control programme for children. *Behav Psychother* **13**:265–87.

Serdula MK, Ivery D, Coates RJ *et al.* (1993) Do obese children become obese adults? A review of the literature. *Prevent Med* **22**:167–77.

Shiva Kumar K and Malet PF (2000) Non-alcoholic steatohepatitis. *Mayo Clin Proc* **75**:733–9.

Simonettei D'Arca A, Tarsitani G, Cairella M *et al.* (1986) Prevention of obesity in elementary and nursery school children. *Public Health* **100**:166–73.

Sinaiko AR, Donahue RP, Jacobs DR and Prineas RJ (1999) Relation of weight and rate of increase in weight during childhood and adolescence to body size, blood pressure, fasting insulin, and lipids in young adults. *Circulation* **99**:1471–6.

Sinha R, Fisch G, Teague B *et al.* (2002) Prevalence of impaired glucose tolerance among children and adolescents with marked obesity. *N Engl J Med* **346**:802–10.

Social Trends, 2000. Office for National Statistics (www.statistics.gov.uk)

Srinivasan SR, Myers L and Berenson GS (2002) Predictability of childhood adiposity and insulin for developing insulin resistance syndrome (syndrome X) in young adulthood. The Bogalusa Heart Study. *Diabetes* **51**:204–9.

Strauss RS and Pollack HA (2001) Epidemic increase in childhood overweight, 1986–1998. *J Am Med Assoc* **286**:2845–8.

Strauss RS, Bradley LJ and Brolin RE (2001) Gastric bypass surgery in adolescents with morbid obesity. *J Pediatr* **138**:499–504.

Summerbell CD, Ashton V, Campbell KJ *et al.* (2004) Interventions for treating obesity in children. In *The Cochrane Library, Issue 1*. John Wiley & Sons, Chichester, UK.

Tattersall R (1974) Mild familial diabetes with dominant inheritance. *Q J Med* **43**:339–57.

Tuomi T, Carlsson A, Li H *et al.* (1999) Clinical and genetic characteristics of type 2 diabetes with and without GAD antibodies. *Diabetes* **48**:150–7.

Tuomilehto J, Lindstrom J, Eriksson JG *et al.* (2001) Prevention of Type 2 diabetes mellitus by changes in lifestyle among subjects with impaired glucose tolerance. *N Engl J Med* **344**:1343–50.

Ueno T, Sugawara H, Sujaku K *et al.* (1997) Therapeutic effects of restricted diet and exercise in obese patients with fatty liver. *J Hepatol* **27**:103–7.

UK Prospective Diabetes Study (UKPDS) Group (1998a) Intensive blood-glucose control with sulphonylureas or insulin compared with conventional treatment and risk of complications in patients with type 2 diabetes (UKPDS 33). *Lancet* **352**:837–53.

UK Prospective Diabetes Study (UKPDS) Group (1998b) Effect of intensive blood-glucose control with metformin on complications in overweight patients with type 2 diabetes (UKPDS 34). *Lancet* **352**:854–65.

Utiger RD (1996) Insulin and the polycystic ovary syndrome. *N Engl J Med* **335**:657–8.

Warschburger P, Fromme C, Petermann F *et al.* (2001) Conceptualisation and evaluation of a cognitive-behavioural training programme for children and adolescents with obesity. *Int J Obes* **25** (suppl 1):S93–S95.

Weststrate JA, Deurenberg P and van Tinteren H (1989) Indices of body fat distribution and adiposity in Dutch children from birth to 18 years of age. *Int J Obes* **13**:456–77.

Whincup P. Gilg J, Papacosta O *et al.* (2002) Early evidence of ethnic differences in cardiovascular risk: cross-sectional comparison of British South Asian and white children. *Br Med J* **324**:635–8.

Whitaker RC, Wright JA, Pepe MS *et al.* (1997) Predicting obesity in young adulthood from childhood and parental obesity. *N Engl J Med* **337**:869–73.

Williams CL, Hayman LL, Daniels SR *et al.* (2002) Cardiovascular health in childhood. A statement for professionals from the Committee on Atherosclerosis, Hypertension, and Obesity in the Young of the Council on Cardiovascular disease in the Young, American Heart Association. *Circulation* **106**:143–60.

13
Obesity and Polycystic Ovary Syndrome

Diana Raskauskiene and **Richard N. Clayton**

Definition of the syndrome

Polycystic ovary syndrome (PCOS) is a commonly diagnosed female endocrinopathy and it is the commonest cause of anovulatory infertility affecting 1–5 per cent of women in the reproductive age group. It is considered to be a *syndrome* not a disease that manifests with heterogeneous clinical features. The most common features of PCOS are irregular menstrual cycles (oligomenorrhoea or amenorrhoea), signs of androgen excess (hirsutism, acne, alopecia), and often obesity. However, only 5–10 per cent of women with PCOS express all the typical clinical features of the syndrome (Balen, 1999; Franks, 1999). At present the diagnosis of PCOS is usually based on the criteria derived from 1990 NIH-NICHHD (National Institutes of Health–National Institutes of Child Health and Human Development) conference, which are ovulatory dysfunction, clinical evidence of hyperandrogenism and/or hyperandrogenaemia and exclusion of related disorders such as congenital adrenal hyperplasia, hyperprolactinaemia, or Cushing's syndrome (Zawadzki and Dunail, 1992). Therefore presence of polycystic ovaries on ultrasound scan, which is defined by presence of eight or more subcapsular follicular cysts ≤10 mm in diameter and increased ovarian stroma, in the absence of clinical features is not sufficient to diagnose PCOS. Polycystic ovaries are present in 20–25 per cent of randomly selected women (Farquhar *et al.*, 1994). Thus, this feature is neither *sufficient nor necessary* to make the clinical diagnosis of PCOS.

Several studies have suggested that PCOS is a familial disorder and various features of the syndrome may be differentially inherited (Franks *et al.*, 1997).

Obesity and Diabetes. Edited by Anthony H. Barnett and Sudhesh Kumar
© 2004 John Wiley & Sons, Ltd   ISBN: 0-470-84898-7

It is further suggested that the morphological appearance of polycystic ovaries is inherited as an autosomal dominant trait, though no single gene has been identified as causal. However, the heterogeneous clinical characteristics of this syndrome indicate the complex interaction between genetic and environmental factors to be causal (Legro, 1995).

Obesity is a feature in between 35 to 60 per cent of women with PCOS and associated with a greater severity of clinical manifestations than non-obese women with the syndrome. Increased insulin resistance is a cardinal feature of obesity and overweight in PCOS and may play a pathogenetic role (Dunaif, 1997). Present data strongly support an association between PCOS and several long-term diseases such as type 2 diabetes, dyslipidaemia, hypertension, and cardiovascular disease. This emphasizes the need for early diagnosis of the syndrome and adequate treatment strategies.

This review will analyse the pathogenetic mechanisms underlying the relationship between obesity and PCOS and survey clinical features of obese women with the syndrome and their management.

Pathogenetic mechanisms underlying the relationship between obesity and PCOS (Table 13.1)

Insulin/insulin resistance

The observation of insulin resistance and hyperinsulinaemia in a subset of women with PCOS has added a new dimension to the understanding of the pathogenesis of PCOS, as well as recognition that the syndrome has

Table 13.1   Main Pathogenic Mechanisms in PCOS

Genetic predisposition	Familial clustering of syndrome
	PCO morphology may be inherited in autosomal dominant manner
Abnormal feedback/regulation of gonadotropin secretion	Altered GnRH pulse frequency/amplitude
	Increased bio/immuno ratio of LH
	Chronic hyperoestrogenaemia inhibits FSH secretion
Increased androgen production	Increased ovarian response to LH (dysregulation of 17–20 lyase)
	Increased adrenal androgens (11β hydroxysteroid dehydrogenase dysregulation leading to ACTH)
	High intraovarian androgens inhibit folliculogenesis
Insulin resistance/hyperinsulinaemia	Amplifies LH stimulated androgen production in ovary and ACTH action in adrenals
	Reduces SHBG levels leading to high free androgen index
	Associated with metabolic complications, and dyslipidaemia

substantial metabolic as well as reproductive implications. Burghen *et al.* (1980) first reported the presence of hyperinsulinaemia in a group of obese PCOS subjects and showed significant correlation with raised serum testosterone, androstendione and insulin. Since then, there have been many reports confirming the presence of insulin resistance and consequent hyperinsulinaemia in obese and non-obese subjects with PCOS. Studies have demonstrated insulin resistance in PCOS unrelated to body weight and composition, though obese PCOS women have consistently been shown to have a greater degree of insulin resistance compared to weight-matched controls. Interestingly, euglycaemic glucose clamp studies have shown significant and substantial decreases ($\sim$35–40 per cent) in insulin-mediated glucose disposal in PCOS which is of similar magnitude to that to seen in patients with type 2 diabetes (Dunaif *et al.*, 1989, 1992). As mentioned above, insulin resistance is consistently accompanied by hyperinsulinaemia. Barbieri *et al.* (1986) first reported the effect of insulin and insulin-like growth factors on ovarian androgen production in ovarian tissue obtained from hyperandrogenic and normal cycling women. At the ovarian level, insulin is able to stimulate steroidogenesis both in granulosa and thecal cells by increasing 17α-hydroxylase and 17–20 lyase activity (both components of the P450c17 enzyme system) (Nestler *et al.*, 1996) and stimulates the expression of 3β-hydroxysteroid dehydrogenase in human luteinized granulosa cells (McGee *et al.*, 1995). In addition, insulin appears to increase the sensitivity of pituitary gonadotropes to gonadotropin-releasing hormone (GnRH) action and potentiate the ovarian steroidogenic response to gonadotropins, by mechanisms probably related to an increase of the luteinizing hormone (LH) receptor number (Poretsky *et al.*, 1999). It has been shown that insulin lowers sex hormone-binding globulin (SHBG) levels thus increasing the circulating, biologically available, androgens particularly free testosterone which by inhibiting follicular maturation, may initiate the sequence of events leading to PCOS (Rajkhowa *et al.*, 1994). Moreover, insulin is able to inhibit both hepatic and ovarian IGF binding protein-1 (IGFBP-1) to regulate ovarian growth and cyst formation (Poretsky *et al.*, 1999). *In vitro* studies have shown that insulin may also increase 17α-hydroxylase and 17–20 lyase activity in the adrenal gland directly (L'Allemand *et al.*, 1996) or potentiates the responsitivity of the enzymes to adrenocorticotropic-hormone (ACTH) stimulation (Moghetti *et al.*, 1996a).

Some aspects of insulin action in obesity are similar to those seen in PCOS. Obesity, especially the abdominal type of the disorder, has a strong relationship to insulin resistance and hyperinsulinaemia. The mechanisms by which obesity may induce insulin resistance have been extensively investigated over last two decades. To sum up, enlargement of adipose tissue increases availability of several metabolites such as free fatty acids, lactate, which can affect insulin secretion and its peripheral action (Vettor *et al.*, 2000). Obesity can be related to insulin resistance by increased production of leptin and tumour necrosis factor-α

(TNF-α) in adipose tissue. TNF-α mediates serine phophorylation of insulin receptor substrate-1, which then interferes with insulin action by inhibiting insulin receptor and type 1 insulin growth factor (IGF) receptor tyrosine kinases and by stimulating IGF binding protein production (Hotamisiligil *et al.*, 1996). TNF-α can also inhibit signalling through peroxisome proliferator-activated receptor-γ (PRAR-γ). Leptin may contribute to insulin resistance of obesity via mechanisms similar to TNF-α (Poretsky *et al.*, 1999). Therefore, obesity is an important factor, and it appears that this has a more pronounced effect on insulin action in PCOS than in control women. In PCOS women the degree of insulin resistance and hyperinsulinaemia is greater than accounted for by obesity alone (Holte *et al.*, 1994a).

Genetic basis of obesity in PCOS

Several studies have shown that PCOS is a familial disorder and various features of the syndrome may be differentially inherited (Franks *et al.*, 1997). However, the genetic basis of the syndrome remains controversial. Since then, many studies have revealed that most women with PCOS, both obese and lean, have a degree of insulin resistance and compensatory hyperinsulinaemia, and genes involved in the secretion and action of insulin have been investigated. Molecular studies of the insulin receptor gene in women with PCOS have shown a large number of polymorphisms, which are common in normal subjects and do not lead to any disturbance of receptor function (Talbot *et al.*, 1996). The observation that although insulin resistance is largely reversible by weight reduction in obese women with PCOS, an abnormality of first-phase insulin secretion from β-cells of pancreas still exists, led to investigation of the insulin gene in the pathogenesis of PCOS. Waterworth *et al.* reported an association between PCOS and allelic variation at the INS VNTR (insulin gene variable number of tandem repeats) locus in three different populations. They showed that class III alleles and especially III/III genotypes are associated with PCOS and are most strongly associated with anovulatory PCOS. The group of women with one or two class III alleles had significantly higher fasting insulin levels and higher mean body mass index (BMI) than women with I/I genotype (Waterworth *et al.*, 1997). At the same time, there is increasing evidence for genetic predisposition to obesity in the general population. Studies in adopted children showed a strong correlation between weight classes and BMI of the biological parents, but no correlation with the BMI of their adoptive parents (Stunkard *et al.*, 1986). Genetic factors are estimated to explain 30–50 per cent of the heritability of obesity. The human obesity map is now complex and currently identified are: six single mutations, 25 Mendelian disorders with map location, 48 candidate genes, 33 human quantitative trait loci and 48 other human linkages (Rankinen *et al.*, 2002). Since there is evidence that insulin gene VNTR class III alleles were found to be associated with type 2 diabetes, the conclusion was that this genotype can be related to anovulatory PCOS as well as the concomitant risk for development of type 2 diabetes mellitus (Ong *et al.*, 1999). Recently it was confirmed that among women with polycystic ovaries, increasing severity of clinical phenotype was associated with decreasing insulin sensitivity and related to paternally transmitted insulin gene VNTR class III alleles (Michelmore *et al.*, 2001).

Growth hormone/IGF

Abnormalities of growth hormone (GH) secretion and/or altered IGF-I concentrations may play a pathogenetic role in PCOS as *in vitro* and *in vivo* evidence supports a stimulatory role of GH in early and later stages of folliculogenesis and ovulation (Hull and Harvey, 2001). Therefore, reduced GH secretion may contribute to impaired follicular development and anovulation in PCOS. Abdominal obesity, which can exacerbate insulin resistance and reproductive features of the PCOS is associated with profoundly reduced and disorderly GH secretion (Pijl *et al.*, 2001). Plasma GH concentrations in PCOS have been reported as reduced, normal or increased (Katz *et al.*, 1993). The majority of studies in PCOS have evaluated the status of the somatotropic axis on the basis of acute secretagogue-stimulated GH release and reported a blunted GH response in women with PCOS compared with weight-matched controls (Wu *et al.*, 2000; Villa *et al.*, 2001). Recently, a profound reduction of daily basal (62 per cent) and pulsatile (76 per cent) GH release in obese women with PCOS compared to healthy lean controls was reported but none of these parameters differed from those in the body mass index-matched controls. Total GH secretion in obese PCOS, lean and obese control women correlated strongly and negatively with percent body fat. The conclusion is therefore that altered GH secretory dynamics are related to obesity and not PCOS *per se*. Serum concentrations of IGF-I and IGF-binding protein-3 were higher in patients with PCOS than in obese controls, but IGF-I/IGF-binding globulin-3 ratio was equivalent in obese PCOS, lean and obese control groups. This observation probably represents that reduced and irregular GH release in obese women with PCOS is related to body fat accumulation and not with PCOS *per se* (Van Dam *et al.*, 2002a).

The effects of IGF-I and IGF-II on ovarian function are well known. They exert their action through activation of two types of receptors, I and II, which are present in granulosa, thecal and stromal cells of ovary (Volitainen *et al.*, 1996). Both IGF's are able to stimulate ovarian progesterone and oestradiol secretion and increase aromatase activity and androgen production in granulosa-luteal and thecal cells (Nahum *et al.*, 1995). Activation of IGF receptors has also been associated with a reduction of IGF binding proteins which may be related to an increase bioavailability of IGF. Insulin regulates IGF and IGF binding proteins system by increasing number of IGF type I receptors and by inhibiting IGF binding protein-I production. Thus, hyperinsulinaemia may lead to a self-perpetuating cycle of events resulting in exaggeration of the effects of both insulin and IGF at an ovarian level. No differences in serum IGF-I and IGF-II levels between PCOS and control women have been found, regardless of body weight, but obese PCOS women have lower serum IGF binding protein-1 level than lean PCOS women. This probably represents an insulin-related effect, as a negative correlation between insulin and IGF binding protein-1 has been found (Poretsky et al., 1999).

In summary, IGF-I and IGF-II may be involved in the pathogenesis of hyperandrogenism in PCOS. In normal-weight PCOS women IGF bioavailability seems to be increased by various mechanisms such as insulin-induced hepatic and ovary IGF binding protein-1 suppression and GH-induced stimulation (Brismar et al., 1994). Conversely, in obese PCOS IGF-1 bioavailability seems to be reduced in comparison to normal-weight PCOS but relatively higher than in non-affected women because of combination of low GH and high insulin levels. Therefore, the IGF/IGF binding protein system in obese PCOS women seems to be differently expressed compared to normal-weight PCOS women, suggesting a different pathogenetic impact.

SHBG

SHBG is a glycoprotein produced in the liver as a carrier for different sex hormones with high binding affinity for testosterone and dihydrotestosterone (DHT) and a lower affinity for oestradiol (Hautanen, 2000). The concentrations of SHBG are stimulated by various factors such as oestrogens, cortisol, iodothyronines, and GH, and decreased by androgens, insulin, prolactin and IGF-I. Decreased basal concentrations are detected in PCOS, with a more significant reduction in obese PCOS women, and insulin is thought to lower serum SHBG levels by acting directly to reduce hepatic SHBG synthesis. An inverse correlation between insulin sensitivity and free testosterone index in obese PCOS women has been found and it is probably secondary to the inverse correlation of SHBG and serum insulin. Furthermore, a significant inverse correlation of SHBG with BMI in both obese PCOS women and obese controls also was shown. This indicates that hyperinsulinaemia in obese PCOS lowers the SHBG levels and hence enhances the expression of hyperandrogenaemia (Rajkhowa et al., 1994). Recently, a prospective study has proposed that measurement of serum SHBG concentration is useful and adequate to identify women with PCOS. They even proposed threshold SHBG level <37 nmol/l which had a sensitivity of 87.5 per cent, a specificity of 86.8 per cent, a positive likelihood ratio 6.63 and negative likelihood ratio 0.14 for the diagnosis of PCOS (Escobar-Morreale et al., 2001). In summary, obesity may directly worsen hyperandrogenism in women with PCOS by reducing SHBG concentration and therefore increasing levels of free androgens.

Androgens

Polycystic ovary syndrome is characterized by chronic anovulation. Raised androgens (testosterone and/or androstendione) is the most consistent biochemical abnormality in PCOS. This supports the hypothesis that, despite the multifactoral and multiorgan nature of the syndrome, it appears that an underlying disorder in androgen biosynthesis or metabolism may be the central event suppressing ovarian folliculogenesis and giving rise to the disorder. The exact nature of this abnormality in androgen secretion/metabolism is, however, still unknown. An important stage of androgen synthesis is activity of P450c17 enzyme which is located in the ovarian theca-interstitial cells and in the adrenal zona reticularis. Expression and activation of P450c17 gene in ovary and/or adrenal cortex is regulated by a number of hormones and growth factors such as LH, ACTH, insulin and IGF. Hyperactivity of P451c17 enzyme represents a major mechanism leading to ovarian hyperandrogenism (Rosenfield, 1999). Whether hyperactivity of P450c17 enzyme system is a primary event or secondary to other central or peripheral factors is unclear. Interestingly, phosphorylation of serine residues of the insulin receptor, which may be a factor leading to insulin resistance and compensatory hyperinsulinaemia in PCOS has been suggested as increasing the activity of the P450c17 enzyme system. Therefore, the serine phosphorylation of both the P450c17 enzymes and the insulin receptor may represent a single primary disorder which could explain the association between insulin resistance and hyperandrogenism in women with PCOS (Dunaif, 1997).

Other factors, such as the follicule stimulating hormone (FSH)-inducible inhibin–follistatin–activin system, produced by the granulosa cell acting on the theca cell, may be implied in the dysregulation of ovarian steroidogenesis in PCOS because some *in vitro* studies have demonstrated that inhibin stimulates ovarian androgen production (Barner, 1998).

Increased secretion of androgens by the adrenal gland often coexist with ovarian hyperandrogenism. The secretion of dehydroepiandrosterone sulphate, an exclusive adrenal steroid, is increased in up to 50 per cent of subjects with PCOS, both basally and in response to ACTH. As adrenal androgen production is ACTH-dependent, central factors may induce a pituitary hyper-responsiveness to corticotropin-releasing hormone. Several peripheral factors have been considered as enhancing adrenal androgen production. As was mentioned, insulin may increase the activity of 17α-hydroxylase and 17–20 lyase in the adrenal both directly and through ACTH stimulation. Interleukin-6 has also been proposed to modulate intra-adrenal steroidogenesis by the ability of this cytokine to increase dihydroepiandrostendione secretion (Rosenfield, 1999). Rodin *et al.* demonstrated dysregulation of 11β-hydroxysteroid dehydrogenase, either primary or secondary, leading to increased ACTH stimulated androgen production in some women with PCOS (Rodin *et al.*, 1994). The increased oxidation of cortisol to cortisone (an inactive metabolite) in PCOS may result in compensatory overstimulation of the hypothalamic–pituitary–adrenal axis which can lead to increased adrenal androgen secretion. Similar altered cortisol metabolism has been reported in obese patients (Pasquali and Vicennati, 2000). Obesity especially abdominal type of the disorder seems to amplify the degree of hyperandrogenism in PCOS. Previous studies reported that obese PCOS women have higher total and free testosterone levels compared with non-obese PCOS (Holte *et al.*, 1994b).

Hyperandrogenism *per se* may enhance insulin resistance and lead to hyperinsulinaemia, which plays a role in development of abdominal type of obesity in PCOS women. In fact, androgens may induce insulin resistance through the activation of the lipolytic cascade, leading to increase free fatty acid release, and this phenomenon has been mainly observed in the visceral fat depot due to the high androgen receptor density present at this site (Björntorp, 1996).

Oestrogens

Elevated levels of oestrone and of free oestradiol have been detected in women with PCOS and it may be a result of reduced concentration of SHBG. Moreover, since androstendione is aromatized to oestrone in fat tissue, this is more marked in obese PCOS subjects. Therefore PCOS women are not oestrogen-deficient, but rather are oestrogen-replete and are not at risk of osteoporosis despite oligo/amenorrhoea. Increased oestrogen concentrations may lead to positive feedback on LH secretion and a negative feedback on FSH secretion and therefore may impact on the LH/FSH ratio. The elevated levels of LH substantially contribute to the development of hyperplasia of the ovarian stroma and thecal cells, further increasing androgen production and in turn providing more substrate for extraglandular aromatization and chronic anovulation. Obesity is a condition of hyperoestrogenaemia and oestrogen production correlates with body weight and amount of body fat (Diamanti-Kadarakis *et al.*, 1995). Oestrogen metabolism is also altered in obese women. There is less formation of inactive oestradiol metabolites, such as 2-hydroxyoestrogens, and a higher production of oestrone sulphate, with concomitant increase in active oestrogens levels in obese women (Diamanti-Kadarakis *et al.*, 1995).

Neuroendocrine factors

Perturbations of gonadotropin secretion are one of the hallmarks of PCOS. The most commonly described abnormality is an elevated serum LH or an elevated LH/FSH ratio, an increased LH pulse frequency and increased LH pulse amplitude, an exaggerated response of LH to GnRH, and altered diurnal LH pulse frequency (Morales *et al.*, 1996; Taylor *et al.*, 1997). However, serum LH levels may be normal in up to 40 per cent of women with PCOS (Conway *et al.*,

1990). On the other hand, Lobo *et al.* reported that bioactive/immunoreactive LH ratio is elevated in PCOS, which means that increased LH bioactivity may be responsible for enhanced androgen production in the ovary of women with the syndrome (Lobo *et al.*, 2002). It is a matter of debate whether the increase of gonadotropins, when present, is a primary abnormality of hypothalamic–pituitary axis or the cause is dysregulation of the feedback signalling. Recent studies have revealed decreased sensitivity of the GnRH pulse generator to inhibition by ovarian steroids, particularly progesterone. This abnormality is reversed by the androgen receptor antagonist flutamide suggesting that elevated androgen levels may alter the sensitivity of the hypothalamic GnRH pulse generator to steroid inhibition and lead to enhanced LH secretion. As such, women with PCOS require higher levels of progesterone to slow the frequency of GnRH pulsatility, resulting in inadequate FSH synthesis and persistent LH stimulation of ovarian androgens (McCartney *et al.*, 2002). In fact, both spontaneous ovulation or exogenous progesterone administration are associated with normalization of LH secretion in PCOS women (Taylor *et al.*, 1997). Obesity may to some extent exaggerate the abnormal LH secretory pattern. A negative correlation between LH and body weight in PCOS has been found and obese PCOS women are characterized by significantly lower LH concentrations than non-obese PCOS women. Interestingly, in very obese PCOS women LH concentrations frequently resemble the normal range (Morales *et al.*, 1996). Potential factors involved in the different LH secretion between obese and non-obese PCOS women may be elevated insulin concentrations, since significant correlations between LH and insulin has been found in PCOS women.

Obesity, as well as PCOS, is also characterized by increased opioid system activity, and studies *in vitro* and *in vivo* have shown that β-endorphin is able to stimulate insulin secretion (Feldman *et al.*, 1983; Pasquali and Casimirri, 1993). Moreover, an inhibition of opioid tone may induce a decreased hyperinsulinaemia in PCOS women as a consequence of reduced insulin secretion and improved hepatic clearance (Fulghesu *et al.*, 1993). In addition, β-endorphin administration reduces LH release in normal women but not in PCOS women, suggesting a condition of β-endorphin resistance in PCOS.

Dietary factors

There are theoretical possibilities that dietary composition may play a role in the development of the obesity in PCOS since there are data suggesting that women eating vegetarian-rich and fibre-rich diet may have lower serum androgen concentrations compared to those following typical Western diets (Hill *et al.*, 1980). Moreover, a very high lipid intake has been described in PCOS and significant negative correlation has been found between lipid intake and SHBG values (Wild *et al.*, 1985).

Clinical features of obese PCOS women

Insulin resistance/impaired β-cell function

PCOS is characterized by several metabolic abnormalities, which are strongly influenced by presence of obesity. Insulin resistance is a common co-morbidity in women with PCOS and is associated with increased risk for hypertension and cardiovascular disease (Figure 13.1). Studies have shown that 25–35 per cent of obese women with PCOS, by 30 years of age, will have either impaired glucose tolerance or type 2 diabetes (Ehrmann, 1997). The studies examining insulin resistance in obese and non-obese women with PCOS have shown that obese PCOS women had significantly lower insulin sensitivity than non-obese women with PCOS. On the other hand, non-obese women with PCOS may demonstrate insulin resistance in the presence of completely normal glucose tolerance. Nevertheless, both fasting and glucose-stimulated insulin concentrations are in fact significantly higher in obese than non-obese PCOS women (Morin-Papunen *et al.*, 2000). Acanthosis nigricans (AN) is a common sign of severe insulin resistance and often occurs in patients with insulin receptor defects. Mild to moderate AN is commonly present in obese PCOS women, but it is not a clinical feature of non-obese counterparts. Moreover, it has been shown that there is no significant difference in prevalence of AN in obese PCOS women compared with weight-matched controls (Rajkhowa and Clayton, 1995).

The percentage of obese women with PCOS is high and this subgroup of PCOS affected women is characterized by increased prevalence of glucose intolerance ranging from 20–40 per cent. In contrast, impaired glucose tolerance in non-obese women with PCOS has been found only occasionally, consistent

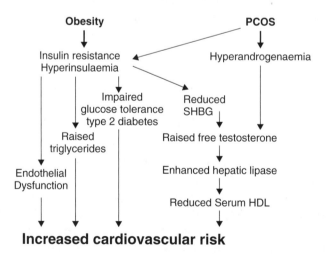

Figure 13.1 Mechanisms of increased cardiovascular risk associated with obesity and PCOS.

with the synergistic negative effect of obesity and PCOS on glucose tolerance (Dunaif, 1997). It has been reported that postmenopausal women with
history of PCOS has a 15 per cent prevalence of type 2 diabetes which is much
higher than in the general population (Dalhgren *et al.*, 1992). In the presence
of peripheral insulin resistance, pancreatic β-cell insulin secretion increases but
impaired glucose tolerance and type 2 diabetes mellitus develops when the compensatory increase in insulin secretion is no longer able to maintain euglycaemia.
Ehrmann *et al.* (1999) recently documented that insulin secretory dysfunction
in women with PCOS contributed significantly to the observed glucose intolerance with up to 40 per cent of women demonstrating either IGT or type 2
diabetes mellitus. Recently Norman *et al.* (2001) performed a follow-up study
of women with PCOS seeking to establish the frequency of change of IGT
and type 2 diabetes over an average period of 6.2 years. They reported 9 per
cent of normoglycaemic women at baseline developed IGT and 8 per cent were
diagnosed having diabetes, and 54 per cent of women with IGT at baseline
had diabetes at follow-up. In the group converting to IGT or diabetes, there
was significantly greater BMI, weight, waist circumference and waist–hip ratio
gain compared with those who remained normoglycaemic. This observation may
indicate that obesity and further weight gain play a crucial role in developing
IGT and diabetes in PCOS.

Dyslipidaemia and vascular risk

Women with PCOS would be predicted to be at high risk for dyslipidaemia
because they are often obese and have elevated androgen levels (Wild, 1995).
Moreover, insulin resistance and hyperinsulinaemia tend to increase risks for
dyslipidaemia associated with insulin resistance. A number of studies have
shown that obese women with PCOS have lower high-density lipoprotein (HDL)
and/or HDL2 levels as well as higher levels of cholesterol, triglyceride, apolipoprotein B and free fatty acids than their lean counterparts and BMI proved to
be the best predictor of these alterations on multiple regression analysis (Robinson *et al.*, 1996; Rajkhowa *et al.*, 1997). Recently it has been reported that PCOS
women have higher concentration and proportion of small, dense low-density
lipoprotein (LDL III) cholesterol (Dejager *et al.*, 2001; Pirwani *et al.*, 2001).
These findings indicate that women with PCOS accompanied by increased concentration of LDL III are at increased risk for cardiovascular morbidity and
mortality, independent of total LDL concentration (Gardner *et al.*, 1996). PCOS
women also have impaired fibrinolytic activity with significantly increased tissue plasminogen activator antigen (t-PA) compared to weight-matched control
women and t-PA correlated with BMI and inversely correlated with insulin sensitivity index in both PCOS and controls. These findings suggest that elevated
t-PA and dysfibrinolysis may be a factor in increased cardiovascular morbidity
seen in PCOS (Kelly *et al.*, 2002a).

The largest retrospective survey of PCOS in the UK (Wild *et al.*, 2000) could not confirm an increased mortality and morbidity from coronary heart disease among women with PCOS. One explanation might be that the number of deaths was quite small (70 out of 700) and longer follow-up might be required to show the effects of increased vascular risk factor prevalence on mortality. Nevertheless, even this study has confirmed that women with PCOS had higher levels of several cardiovascular risk factors such as diabetes, hypertension, hypercholesterolaemia, hypertriglyceridaemia and increased waist to hip ratio and more prevalent history of cerebrovascular disease (Wild *et al.*, 2000).

Other studies have investigated subclinical atherosclerosis among women with PCOS by ultrasound examination of carotid arteries. A significantly higher mean carotid intima–media wall thickness (IMT) and plaque number has been shown in affected women compared to controls. It has also been shown that in the total cohort and in the age group <45 years several cardiovascular risk factors such as age, BMI, blood pressure, waist–hip ratio, and triglycerides are significantly associated with IMT. Conversely, in women ≥45 years PCOS was a highly significant predictor of IMT but BMI, LDL, insulin, systolic blood pressure, and triglycerides were also significant predictors (Talbott *et al.*, 2000). Recently another study investigated macrovascular and microvascular function in PCOS women. Pulse wave velocity (PWV) at the level of the brachial artery was found to be significant by elevated in the PCOS group but PWV measured in the aorta did not differ from controls. Microvascular function was studied by wire myography, by measuring the concentration responses to norepinephrine (NE) before and after incubation with insulin (100 and 1000 pM). In vessels from control subjects, insulin reduced the contraction response to NE but there was no change in maximum contraction in the PCOS group using different doses of insulin. This study demonstrated an increased vascular stiffness and a functional defect in the vascular action of the insulin *ex vivo* in patients with PCOS (Kelly *et al.*, 2002b).

Endothelial function in PCOS

Obesity and insulin resistance are associated with blunted endothelium-dependent but not endothelium-independent vasodilation (Arcaro *et al.*, 1999), with failure of hyperinsulinaemia to augment endothelium-dependent vasodilation (Steinbergs *et al.*, 1996). This indicates that obesity is associated with endothelial dysfunction and endothelial resistance to the enhancing effect of insulin on endothelium-dependent vasodilation. Endothelial dysfunction might therefore contribute to the increased risk of atherosclerosis in obese insulin-resistant subjects, such as those with PCOS (Dunaif, 1997; Wild *et al.*, 2000). Insulin resistance has been proposed as a central metabolic basis for the clustering of risk factors in the multiple cardiovascular risk syndrome (syndrome X). However, Pinkney *et al.* (1997) have argued that the central problem may be endothelial dysfunction rather than insulin resistance. In resistance vessels, the endothelium regulates blood flow and blood pressure through the production of powerful vasoactive substance such as NO, endothelin-1 and thromboxane A2 (Vane et al., 1990). Endothelial dysfunction can lead to defective vasodilation and disturbance of the balance of vasoactive substances favouring vasoconstriction and development of hypertension. The vascular endothelium is a key regulator of haemostasis and fibrinolysis, controlling the activities of the intrinsic pathway, the fibrinolytic and protein-C anticoagulant pathways, as well as influencing platelet activation and adhesion. Endothelial dysfunction can account for the increased levels of plasminogen activator inhibitor-1 observed in patients with the 'insulin resistance syndrome'. Insulin-resistant subjects have reduced skeletal muscle capillarization (Lithell et al., 1981; Lillioja et al., 1987), which, together with failure of the endothelial vasodilator response to insulin, results in delayed delivery of insulin to the interstitial fluid (Jansson et al., 1993; Castillo, 1994). Although the interstitial insulin concentration is not the main determinant of insulin action, in the dynamic state transendothelial insulin transport is a rate-limiting step before insulin binding to tissue receptors (Miles et al., 1995). Thus, the IRS is a marker of peripheral small-vessel endothelial dysfunction.

Central large-vessel endothelial dysfunction plays a major role in atherogenesis. The presence of systemic endothelial dysfunction (large and small vessel) is a plausible explanation for the observed association between atherosclerotic macrovascular disease and IRS. Nevertheless Mather et al. (2000) recently reported normal endothelium-dependent vasodilatation in women with PCOS despite insulin resistance and obesity. In contrast, impairment in metacholine-induced (endothelium-dependent) leg blood flow in obese PCOS women compared with obese controls was recently reported (Paradisi et al., 2001), as was a reduced vasodilator response to insulin. Endothelium-dependent vasodilation was inversely correlated with free testosterone concentration, which was an independent predictor of leg blood flow, as well as with BMI.

Abnormalities of menstrual cycle and infertility

PCOS is the commonest cause (78 per cent) of anovulatory in infertility (Hull, 1987). It was demonstrated that menstrual abnormalities are more frequent in obese than non-obese PCOS women (Kiddy et al., 1990). In addition, it was shown that a reduced incidence of pregnancy and inadequate response to pharmacological treatments to induce ovulation may be more common in obese PCOS women (Galtier-Dereure et al., 1997). Insulin resistance and accompanying hyperinsulinaemia, which can increase amount of body fat, can be directly related to impaired ovulation in obese PCOS women since treatment with insulin-sensitizing agents leads to improvement of menstrual cycles. It has been found that obese PCOS women tend to have lower ovulation response to pulsatile GhRH analogue administration than non-obese counterparts (Filicori *et al.*, 1994). In the recent studies of PCOS women conceiving after *in vitro* fertilization or intracytoplasmic sperm injection, it was observed that those with obesity had a higher gonadotropin requirement during stimulation (Fedorsak *et al.*, 2001). In conclusion, obese women with PCOS demonstrate more pronounced irregularity of menstrual cycles and infertility, which requires a special approach for their treatment.

Treatment of obese women with PCOS (Table 13.2)

Weight reduction by lifestyle modification

There is long-standing clinical evidence concerning the efficacy of weight reduction on clinical and endocrinological features of obese women presenting with PCOS. It has been reported that weight loss may improve menstrual abnormalities and both ovulation and fertility rate. Moreover, it was confirmed that hirsutism and acanthosis nigricans were significantly improved in most patients following weight loss. Reduction of hyperandrogenaemia appears to be the key factor responsible for these effects, since peripheral testosterone, androstendione and dehydroepiandrostendione sulphate values were significantly reduced after weight loss in obese PCOS women (Pasquali *et al.*, 1989). These findings were subsequently confirmed by Kiddy *et al.* (1992) in women who obtained even moderate weight loss after long-term calorie restriction. They reported an improvement in menstrual pattern, endocrine profile and fertility in obese women (BMI > 25) with PCOS if they lost more than 5 per cent of their body weight. Conversely, no significant benefit was observed in women who lost less, maintained their excess body weight or increased it. An important beneficial effect of weight loss is the subsequent reduction of the degree of hyperinsulinaemia and insulin resistance state. Changes in testosterone and insulin (basal and glucose-stimulated) concentrations may be significantly correlated, regardless of body weight variations (Pasquali *et al.*, 1990). Diet-induced reduction of insulin levels has been shown to decrease P450c17α enzyme activity and consequently ovarian androgen production (Jacubowitz and Nestler, 1997). A

Table 13.2   Principal Elements in the Treatment of PCOS

1. Lifestyle modifications of weight reduction and exercise
2. Drugs to reduce insulin resistance, e.g.: metformin, thiazolidinediones, ? D-chiro-inositol
3. Treatment of specific clinical/metabolic features as required:
    hirsutism/acne/alopecia
    anovulation/subfertility
    dyslipidaemia
    IGT/type 2 diabetes

IGT, impaired glucose tolerance.

lifestyle modification program for obese PCOS women was performed in one recent study and included a diet and exercise programme for 6 months. Obese women with PCOS were classified as responders to the intervention if they regained ovulation during the study. As a result of intervention, responders showed 11 per cent reduction in central fat, 71 per cent improvement in insulin sensitivity index, a 33 per cent fall in fasting insulin levels, and a 39 per cent reduction in LH levels, but none of these parameters changed significantly in obese PCOS who failed to restore ovulation pattern (Huber-Buchholz *et al.*, 1999). An interventional study of 12 weeks of energy restriction and followed by 4 weeks of weight maintenance prescribing high protein or low protein diets for obese PCOS women was performed by Moran *et al.* (2003). They reported that pregnancies, improvements in menstrual cyclicity, lipid profile, and insulin resistance as well as decrease in weight (7.5 per cent) and abdominal fat (12.5 per cent) occurred independently of diet composition. Improvements in menstrual cyclicity were associated with greater decreases in insulin resistance and fasting insulin. On the low protein diet, HDL decreased 10 per cent and free androgen index increased 44 per cent, which could suggest that a high-protein weight loss diet may result in minor differential metabolic improvements. Recently, it was reported that a short-term (7 days) very low calorie restriction diet (4.2 MJ/day) prescribed for obese PCOS women reduced plasma glucose (18 per cent), insulin (75 per cent), total testosterone (23 per cent) and leptin (50 per cent) whereas serum oestrogens, SHBG and androstendione concentrations remained unchanged. Contrary to expectation, calorie restriction enhanced basal and pulsatile LH secretion further pointing to anomalous feedback control of pituitary LH release in PCOS (Van Dam *et al.*, 2002b). To summarize, the principal effects of weight loss on both clinical and endocrinological features in women with obesity and PCOS include not only reduction of total and particularly visceral fat, but also improve menstrual cycles and fertility rate, reduced androgen and insulin concentrations, and improved insulin sensitivity.

Insulin-lowering medications

Agents that lower insulin levels by improving insulin sensitivity may provide a new therapeutic modality for obese PCOS women. Metformin acts mainly by suppressing hepatic glucose production, and its insulin-sensitizing actions are primarily mediated through the weight loss that frequently occurs during therapy. Velasquez *et al.* (1994) first demonstrated that metformin administration to obese PCOS women was not only able to significantly improve insulin levels, but also to decrease LH and testosterone concentrations, regardless of changes in body weight, with a significant improvement in menstrual abnormalities in most patients. Glueck *et al.* (1999) reported that following metformin treatment 91 per cent of previously amenorrhoeic women with PCOS resumed normal menses independently of metformin dose and duration of treatment.

They also observed a significant decrease of BMI, fasting insulin, testosterone and increased oestradiol in metformin treated PCOS women. Another study has demonstrated an improvement in insulin action and significant increases in levels of SHBG and decreased testosterone and androstendione in obese PCOS women following 6 months treatment with metformin. Although no changes were recorded in body weight they observed a significant improvement in menstrual cyclicity (Diamanti-Kadarakis *et al.*, 1998). Further, a study by Moghetti and coworkers (2000) demonstrated long-term efficacy of metformin treatment in obese women with PCOS. Their findings demonstrated marked improvement in menstrual cyclicity and ovulation and a significant reduction in serum androgens and LH. These effects were maintained for the entire 12-month treatment period and suggest that metformin may be appropriate for chronic treatment of this syndrome.

However, there are some studies finding no improvement of insulin sensitivity and hyperandrogenism in women with PCOS who were morbidly obese (BMI as high as $50 \, kg/m^2$) women during metformin treatment (Ehrmann *et al.*, 1997). Recently Fleming *et al.* (2002) presented the results of a placebo-controlled trial assessing ovarian activity and utility of metformin treatment in obese (mean BMI 34.2) PCOS women. There was greater ovulation frequency and the time to first ovulation was significantly shorter compared to the placebo group and the effect of metformin on follicular maturation was rapid, because oestrogen levels increased over the first week of treatment. Also, a significant weight loss and increased HDL levels were recorded only in the metformin-treated group of PCOS women, whereas the placebo group actually gained weight. However, metabolic risk factor benefits of metformin treatment were not observed in the morbidly obese subgroup of patients (BMI > 37), and there was an inverse relationship between body mass and treatment efficacy. The latter finding suggests that women with extreme obesity and overwhelming insulin resistance might not respond to metformin therapy.

Another insulin-sensitizing drug belonging to the class of thiazolidindiones, which are selective ligands for PPARγ, a member of the nuclear receptor superfamily of ligand-activated transcription factors, was investigated for PCOS treatment. Troglitazone has been shown to improve total body insulin sensitivity, lower insulin levels, free testosterone and oestrogens, and increases SHBG in obese PCOS women with no significant changes in BMI (Dunaif *et al.*, 1996). Azziz *et al.* (2001) demonstrated the therapeutic effects of troglitazone in PCOS in a large multicentre (305 patients) double blind trial using different doses of the drug. Ovulatory rates were significantly greater for patients receiving 300 mg and 600 mg of troglitazone than for those receiving placebo. Treatment with 600 mg of troglitazone a day was associated with ovulatory cycles at least 50 per cent of the time compared to a 12 per cent ovulation rate of placebo-treated patients. There was a significant decrease of hirsutism, assessed by modified Ferriman–Gallwey scoring, in the troglitazone 600 mg/day treated group. Free testosterone decreased and SHBG increased in a dose-related fashion with troglitazone treatment and was significantly different from the placebo group, and nearly all glycaemic parameters showed dose-related decreases in the treated group. Recently, Paradisi *et al.* (2003) demonstrated benefits of troglitazone treatment of obese women with PCOS. They have observed that after 3 months treatment with troglitazone (600 mg/day) there was a significant improvement in both hormonal and metabolic features (decreased free testosterone levels and insulin resistance) without significant changes in BMI. Moreover, a significant rise in endothelium-dependent vasodilatation (in response to metacholine chloride and euglycaemic hyperinsulinaemia) was documented in PCOS subjects following the treatment, with no difference from that observed in obese control women. Thus, treatment with troglitazone restored endothelial function and insulin-mediated vasodilatation in obese women with PCOS.

Among other insulin-sensitizing agents, the potential use of D-chiro-inositol in PCOS treatment is currently under investigation. Inositol glycans have been described as mediating insulin action on thecal steroidogenesis. In the placebo-controlled trial by Nestler *et al.*, (1999) D-chiro-inositol was administered to 22 obese women with PCOS for a total of 6–8 weeks. Administration of this drug resulted in a 55 per cent decrease in serum free testosterone and increased ovulation rate up to 86 per cent in women with PCOS. Furthermore, the treatment with D-chiro-inositol significantly reduced insulin levels during oral glucose tests, reduced systolic and diastolic blood pressure and decreased triglyceride levels without side effects or toxicity among treated women. In conclusion, knowing that insulin resistance with accompanying hyperinsulinaemia has a key role in pathogenesis of PCOS, insulin-sensitizing drugs have become first-line therapeutic agents, especially in the management of obese women with PCOS. Use of these drugs may improve menstrual cyclicity and restore ovulation and improve fertility, decrease hyperandrogenaemia, offering metabolic and gynaecological benefits for women with the syndrome.

Antiandrogens

Several studies have demonstrated that antiandrogens may significantly decrease insulin resistance and hyperinsulinaemia in women with PCOS as well as reducing androgen levels. These effects have been observed regardless of the type of drug used, similar results being obtained for spironolactone (Moghetti *et al.*, 1996b), flutamide, and finasteride (Diamanti-Kadarakis *et al.*, 1995). Nevertheless, there is no data investigating the effect of pure antiandrogens on fat distribution or impact on weight reduction in obese women with PCOS.

Oral contraceptives

Over the years oral contraceptives have been used in women with PCOS in order to avoid the risk of developing endometrial hyperplasia. The progestagen component decreases the frequency of GnRH pulses and LH secretion, thus reducing ovarian androgen production, while oestrogen increases SHBG concentration. Investigating the long-term effects of oral contraceptive therapy on metabolism and body composition in women with PCOS Pasquali *et al.* (1999) have found a significant reduction of waist circumference and waist–hip ratio, as well as of basal insulin levels and an improvement of glucose tolerance in some patients. Although controversy still exists regarding benefits of oral contraceptive in treatment of obese PCOS women, these findings indicate a potential benefit in body composition and the glucose–insulin system in PCOS women.

Conclusions

This chapter has briefly reviewed the main data supporting the view that obesity may be an important factor in metabolic and endocrine alterations defining PCOS. Obese women with PCOS are significantly more insulin resistant and have higher insulin levels than weight-matched controls or non-obese affected women. The primary role of insulin resistance and hyperinsulinaemia as a pathogenetic factor is supported by evidence that hyperandrogenism and related clinical features can be improved by reducing insulin levels. Obese women with PCOS have a higher risk for cardiovascular disease, endothelial dysfunction, and impaired glucose tolerance or type 2 diabetes mellitus than non-obese counterparts. Therefore, we emphasize weight loss as a first-line approach in the treatment of obese PCOS women, which significantly improves clinical features, hormonal and metabolic abnormalities of these patients.

References

Arcaro G, *et al.* (1999) Body fat distribution predicts the degree of endothelial dysfunction in uncomplicated obesity. *Int J Obes* **23**:936–42.

Azziz R, Ehrmann D, Legro RS *et al.* (2001) O'Keefe M, Ghazzi MN. Troglitazone improves ovulation and hirsutism in the polycystic ovary syndrome: a multicenter, double blind, placebo-controlled trial. *J Clin Endocrinol Metab* **86**:1626–32.

Balen A (1999). Pathogenesis of polycystic ovary syndrome – the enigma unravels? *Lancet* **354**:966–7.

Barbieri RL, Makris A, Randall RW *et al.* (1986) Insulin stimulates androgen accumulation in incubations of ovarian stroma obtained women with hyperandrogenism. *J Clin Endocrinol Metab* **62**:904–9.

Barner RB (1998) The pathogenesis of polycystic ovary syndrome: lessons from ovarian stimulation studies. *J Endocrinol Invest* **21**:567–79.

Björntorp P (1996) The regulation of adipose tissue distribution in humans. *Int J Obes Relat Metab Disord* **20**:291–302.

Brismar K, Ferqvist-Forbes E, Wahren J and Hall K (1994) Effect of insulin on the hepatic production of insulin-like growth factor binding protein-1 (IGFBP-1), IGFBP-3 and IGF-1 in insulin-dependent diabetes. *J Clin Endocrinol Metab* **79**:872–8.

Burghen GA, Givens JR and Kitabchi AE (1980) Correlation of hyperandrogenism with hyperinsulinism in polycystic ovary disease. *J Clin Endocrinol Metab* **50**:113–16.

Castillo C (1994) Interstitial insulin concentration determines glucose uptake rates but not insulin resistance in lean and obese men. *J Clin Invest* **93**:10–16.

Conway GS, Jacobs HS, Holly JM and Wass JA (1990) Effects of luteinizing hormone, insulin like growth factor, and insulin like growth factor small binding protein in polycystic ovary syndrome. *Clin Endocrinol* **33**:593–603.

Dalhgren E, Johansson S, Lindstedt G *et al.* (1992) Women with polycystic ovary syndrome wedge resected in 1956 to 1965: a long-term follow-up focusing on natural history and circulating hormones. *Fertil Steril* **57**:505–13.

Dejager S, Pichard C, Giral P *et al.* (2001) Smaller LDL particle size in women with polycystic ovary syndrome compared. *Clin Endocrinol* **54**:455–62.

Diamanti-Kadarakis E, Kouli C, Tsianateli T and Bergiele A (1998) Therapeutic effects of metformin on insulin resistance and hyperandrogenism in polycystic ovary syndrome. *Eur J Endocrinol* **138**:269–74.

Diamanti-Kadarakis E, Mitrakou A, Hennes MMI *et al.* (1995) Insulin sensitivity and anti-androgenic therapy in women with polycystic ovary syndrome. *Metabolism* **44**:525–31.

Dunaif A (1997) Insulin resistance and polycystic ovary syndrome: mechanism and implication for pathogenesis. *Endocr Rev* **18**:774–800.

Dunaif A, Futterweit W, Segal KR and Dobrjansky A (1989) Profound peripheral insulin resistance, independent of obesity, in polycystic ovary syndrome. *Diabetes* **38**:1165–74.

Dunaif A, Scott D, Finegood D *et al.* (1996) The insulin-sensitizing agent troglitazone improves metabolic and reproductive abnormalities in the polycystic ovary syndrome. *J Clin Endocrinol Metab* **81**:3299–306.

Dunaif A, Segal KR, Shelley DR *et al.* (1992) Evidence for distinctive and intrinsic defects in insulin action in polycystic ovary syndrome. *Diabetes* **41**:1257–66.

Ehrmann DA (1997) Obesity and glucose intolerance in androgen excess. In: Azziz R, Nestler JE, Dewailly D (eds) *Androgen Excess Disorders in Women.* Lippincott-Raven, Philadelphia, pp. 705–712.

Ehrmann E, Cavaghan MK, Barner RB *et al.* (1999) Prevalence of impaired glucose tolerance and diabetes in women with polycystic ovary syndrome. *Diabetes Care* **22**:141–6.

Ehrmann DA, Cavaghan MK, Imperial J *et al.* (1997) KS. Effects of metformin on insulin secretion, insulin action, and ovarian steroidogenesis in women with polycystic ovary syndrome. *J Clin Endocrinol Metab* **82**:524–30.

Escobar-Morreale HF, Acuncion M, Calvo RM *et al.* (2001) Receiver operating characteristic analysis of the performance of basal serum hormone profiles for the diagnosis of polycystic ovary syndrome in epidemiological studies. *Eur J Endocrinol* **145**:619–24.

Farquhar CM, Birdsall M, Manning P *et al.* (1994) The prevalence of polycystic ovaries on ultrasound scanning in a population of randomly selected women. *Aust N Z J Obstet Gynaecol* **34**:67–72.

Fedorsak P, Dale PO, Storeng R *et al.* (2001) The impact of obesity and insulin resistance on the outcome of IVF or ICSI in women with polycystic ovary syndrome. *Hum Reprod* **16**; 1086–91.

Feldman M, Kiser RS, Unger RH and Li CH (1983) β-endorphin and endocrine pancreas. Studies in healthy and diabetic human beings. *N Engl J Med* **308**:349–53.

Filicori M, Flamingi C and Dellai P (1994) Treatment of ovulation with pulsatile gonadotropin-releasing hormone: prognostic factors and clinical results in 600 cycles. *J Clin Enocrinol Metab* **79**:1215–20.

Fleming R, Hopkinson ZE, Wallace AM *et al.* (2002) Ovarian function and metabolic factors in women with oligomenorrhea treated with metformin in a randomised double blind placebo-controlled trial. *J Clin Endocrinol Metab* **87**:569–74.

Franks S (1999) Polycystic ovary syndrome. *N Engl J Med* **333**:853–61.

Franks S, Gharani N, Waterworth D *et al.* (1997) The genetic basis of polycystic ovary syndrome. *Hum Reprod* **12**:2641–8.

Fulghesu AM, Lanzone A, Cucinelli F *et al.* (1993) Long-term naltrexone treatment reduces the exaggerated insulin secretion in patients with polycystic ovary disease. *Obstet Gynecol* **82**:191–7.

Galtier-Dereure F, Pujol P, Dewailly D and Bringer J (1997) Choice of stimulation in polycystic ovarian syndrome: the influence of obesity. *Hum Reprod* **12**:88–96.

Gardner CD, Fortmann SP and Krauss RM (1996) Association of small LDL particles with the incidence of coronary artery disease in men and women. *JAMA* **276**:875–81.

Glueck CJ, Wang P, Fontaine R *et al.* (1999) Metformin-induced resumption of normal menses in 39 of 43 (91%) previously amenorrheic women with polycystic ovary syndrome. *Metabolism* **48**:511–19.

Hautanen A (2000) Synthesis and regulation of sex hormone-binding globulin in obesity. *Int J Obes Metab Disord* **24**:S64–S70.

Hill P, Garbaczewski L and Helman P (1980) Diet, lifestyle and menstrual activity. *Am J Clin Nutr* **33**:1192–8.

Holte J, Bergh C, Berglund L and Lithell H (1994a) Enhanced early insulin respond to glucose in relation to insulin resistance in women with polycystic ovary syndrome and normal glucose tolerance. *J Clin Endocrinol Metab* **78**:1054–8.

Holte J, Bergh T, Gennarelli G and Wide L (1994b) The independent effects of polycystic ovary syndrome and obesity on serum concentrations of gonadotropins and sex steroids in premenopausal women. *Clin Endocrinol* **41**:473–81.

Hotamisiligil GS, Peraldi P, Budavari A *et al.* (1996) IRS-1 mediated inhibition of insulin receptor tyrosine kinase activity in TNF-α and obesity-induced insulin resistance. *Science* **271**:665–8.

Huber-Buchholz MM, Carey DGP and Norman RJ (1999) Restoration of reproductive potential by lifestyle modification in obese polycystic ovary syndrome: role of insulin sensitivity and luteinizing hormone. *J Clin Endocrinol Metab* **84**:1470–4.

Hull KL and Harvey S (2001) Growth hormone: roles in female reproduction. *J Endocrinol* **168**:1–23.

Hull MG (1987) Epidemiology of infertility and polycystic ovarian disease: endocrinological and demographic studies. *Gynaecol Endocrinol* **1**:235–45.

Jacubowitz DJ and Nestler JE (1997) 17α-Hydroxyprogestrone responses to leuprolide and serum androgens in obese women with and without polycystic ovary syndrome after weight loss. *J Clin Endocrinol Metab* **82**:556–60.

Jansson PA, Fowelin JP, Von Schenck HP *et al.* (1993) Measurement by microdialysis of the insulin concentration in subcutaneous interstitial fluid. *Diabetes* **42**:1469–73.

Katz E Ricciarelli E and Adashi EY (1993) The potential relevance of growth hormone to female reproductive physiology and pathophysiology. *Fertil Steril* **59**:8–34.

Kelly CJG, Lyall H, Petrie JR *et al.* (2002a) A specific elevation in tissue plasminogen activator antigen in women with polycystic ovary syndrome. *J Clin Endocrinol Metab* **87**:3287–90.

Kelly CJG, Speirs A, Gould GW *et al.* (2002b) Altered vascular function in young women with polycystic ovary syndrome. *J Clin Endocrinol Metab* **87**:742–6.

Kiddy DS, Hamilton-Fairley D, Buch A *et al.* (1992) Improvement in endocrine profile and ovarian function during dietary treatment of obese women with polycystic ovary syndrome. *Clin Endocrinol* **36**:105–11.

Kiddy DS, Sharp PS, White DM *et al.* (1990) Differences in clinical and endocrine features between obese and non-obese subject with polycystic ovary syndrome: an analysis of 263 consecutive cases. *Clin Endocrinol* **32**:213–20.

L'Allemand D, Penhoat A, Lebrethon M-C *et al*. (1996) Insulin-like growth factors enhance steroidogenic enzyme and corticotropin receptor messenger ribonucleic acid levels cells. *J Clin Endocrin Metab* **81**:3892–4.

Legro RS (1995) The genetics of polycystic ovary syndrome. *Am J Med* **98**(S1A):9–11.

Lillioja S, Young AA, Culter CL *et al*. (1987) Skeletal muscle capillary density and fiber type are possible determinants of in-vivo insulin resistance in man. *J Clin Invest* **80**:415–24.

Lithell H, Lindegarde F, Hellsing K *et al*. (1981) Body weight skeletal muscle morphology and enzyme activities in relation to fasting serum insulin concentration and glucose tolerance in 48-year-old men. *Diabetes* **30**:19–25.

Lobo RA, Kelzky OA, Campeau JD and Di Zerga GS (1983) Elevated bioactive luteinizing hormone in women with polycystic ovary syndrome. *Fertil Steril* **39**:674–8.

Mather KJ, Verma S, Corenblum B and Anderson TJ (2000) Normal endothelial function despite insulin resistance in healthy women with polycystic ovary syndrome. *J Clin Endocrinol Metab* **85**:1851–6.

McCartney CR, Eagleson CA and Marshall JC (2002) Regulation of gonadotropin secretion: implications of polycystic ovary syndrome. *Semin Reprod Med* **20**(4):317–26.

McGee E, Sawetawan C, Bird I *et al*. (1995) The effects of insulin on 3β-hydroxysteroid dehydrogenase expression in human luteinized granulosa cells. *J Soc Gynecol Invest* **2**:535–41.

Michelmore K, Ong K, Mason S *et al*. (2001) Clinical features in women with polycystic ovaries: relationship to insulin sensitivity, insulin gene VNTR and birth weight. *Clin Endocrinol* **55**:439–46.

Miles PDG, Lerisetti M, Reichart D *et al*. (1995) Kinetics of insulin action *in vivo*: identification of rate limiting steps. *Diabetes* **44**:947–53.

Moghetti P, Castello R, Negri C *et al*. (1996a) Insulin infusion amplifies 17α-hydroxycorticosteroid intermediates to ACTH in hyperandrogenetic women: apparent relative impairment of 17, 20-lyase activity. *J Clin Endocrinol Metab* 1996; **81**: 881–885.

Moghetti P, Tosi F, Castello R *et al*. (1996b) The insulin resistance in women with hyperandrogenism is partially reversed by antiandrogen treatment: evidence that androgen impair insulin action in women. *J Clin Endocrinol Metab* **81**:952–60.

Moghetti P, Castello, Negri C *et al*. (2000) Metformin effects on clinical, endocrine and metabolic profiles, and insulin sensitivity in polycystic ovary syndrome: a randomised, double-blind, placebo-controlled 6-month trial, followed by open, long-term clinical evaluation. *J Clin Endocrinol Metab* **85**:139–46.

Morales AJ, Laughlin GA, Butzow T *et al*. (1996) Insulin, somatotropic, and luteinizing hormone axes in non-obese and obese women with polycystic ovary syndrome: common and distinct features. *J Clin Endocrinol Metab* **81**:2854–64.

Moran LJ, Noakes M, Clifton PM *et al*. (2003) Dietary composition in restoring reproductive and metabolic physiology in overweight women with polycystic ovary syndrome. *J Clin Endocrinol Metab* **88**:812–19.

Morin-Papunen LC, Vauhkonen I, Koivunen RM *et al*. (2000) Insulin sensitivity, insulin secretion, and metabolic and hormonal parameters in healthy women and women with polycystic ovarian syndrome. *Hum Reprod* **15**:1266–74.

Nahum R, Thong KJ and Hillier SG (1995) Metabolic regulation of androgen production by human thecal cells *in vitro*. *Hum Reprod* **10**:75–81.

Nestler JE, Jacubowitz D, Reamer P *et al*. (1999) Ovulatory and metabolic effects of d-chiro-inositol in the polycystic ovary syndrome. *N Engl J Med* **340**:1314–20.

Nestler JE and Jacubowitz DJ (1996) Decrease in ovarian cytochrome P450c17α activity and serum free testosterone after reduction of insulin secretion in polycystic ovary syndrome. *N Engl J Med* **335**:617–23.

Norman RJ, Masters L, Milner CR *et al.* (2001) Relative of conversion from normoglycaemia to impaired glucose tolerance or non-insulin dependent diabetes mellitus in polycystic ovarian syndrome. **16**:1995–8.

Ong KK, Phillips DI, Fall C *et al.* (1999) The insulin gene VNTR, type 2 diabetes and bird weight. *Nat Genet* **21**:262–3.

Paradisi G, Steinberg HO, Hempfling A *et al.* (2001) Polycystic ovary syndrome is associated with endothelial dysfunction. *Circulation* **103**:1410–15.

Paradisi G, Steinberg HO, Shepard MK *et al.* (2003) Troglitazone therapy improves endothelial function to near normal in women with polycystic ovary syndrome. *J Clin Endocrinol Metab* **88**:576–80.

Pasquali R, Antenucci D, Casimirri F *et al.* (1989) Clinical and hormonal characteristics of obese amenorrheic women before and after weight loss. *J Clin Endocrinol Metab* **68**:173–9.

Pasquali R and Casimirri F (1993) The impact of obesity on hyperandrogenism in polycystic ovary syndrome in premenopausal women. *Clin Endocrinol* **39**:1–16.

Pasquali R, Gambineri A, Anconetani B *et al.* (1999) The natural history of the metabolic syndrome in young women with the polycystic ovary syndrome and the effect of long-term oestrogen-progestagen treatment. *Clin Endocrinol* **50**:517–27.

Pasquali R and Vicennati V (2000) The abdominal obesity phenotype and insulin resistance with abnormalities of the hypothalamic–pituitary–adrenal axis in humans. *Horm Metab Res* **32**:521–5.

Pijl H, Langerdonk JG, Burggraaf J *et al.* (2001) Altered neuroregulation of growth hormone secretion in viscerally obese premenopausal women. *J Clin Endocrinol Metab* **86**:5509–15.

Pinkney JH, Stehouwer CD, Coppacle SW and Yudkin S (1997) Endothelial dysfunction: cause of insulin resistance syndrome. *Diabetes* **46** (Suppl 2):S9–S13.

Pirwani IR, Fleming R, Greer IA *et al.* (2001) Lipids and lipoprotein subfractions in women with PCOS: relationship to metabolic and endocrine parameters. *Clin Endocrinol* **54**:447–53.

Poretsky L, Cataldo NA, Rosenwaks Z and Giudice LC (1999) The insulin related ovarian regulatory system in healthy and diseased. *Endocr Rev* **20**:535–82.

Rajkhowa M, Bicknell J, Jones M and Clayton RN (1994) Insulin sensitivity in obese and non-obese women with polycystic ovary syndrome – relationship to hyperandrogenaemia. *Fertil Steril* **61**:605–11.

Rajkhowa M and Clayton RN (1995) Polycystic ovary syndrome. *Curr Obstet Gynaecol* **5**:191–200.

Rajkhowa M, Neary RH, Kumpatla P *et al.* (1997) Clayton RN. Altered composition of high density lipoproteins in women with the polycystic ovary syndrome. *J Clin Endocrinol Metab* **82**:3389–94.

Rankinen T, Perusse L, Weisnagel SJ *et al.* (2002) The human obesity gene map: the 2001 update. Review. *Obes Res* **10**:196–247.

Robinson S, Hederson AD, Gelding SV *et al.* (1996) Dyslipidaemia is associated with insulin resistance in women with polycystic ovaries. *Clin Endocrinol* **44**:277–84.

Rodin A, Thakker H, Taylor N and Clayton RN (1994) Hyperandrogenism in polycystic ovary syndrome. Evidence of dysregulation of 11β hydroxysteroid dehydrogenase. *N Engl J Med* **330**:460–5.

Rosenfield RL (1999) Ovarian and adrenal function in polycystic ovary syndrome. *Endocrinol Metab Clin N Am* **28**:265–93.

Soule AG (1996) Neuroendocrinology of the polycystic ovary syndrome. *Baillière's Clin Endocrinol Metab* **10**:205–19.

Steinberg HO *et al.* (1996) Obesity/insulin resistance is associated with endothelial dysfunction. Implications for the syndrome of insulin resistance. *J Clin Invest* **11**:2601–10.

Stunkard AJ, Sorensen TI, Hanis C *et al.* (1986) An adoption study of human obesity. *N Engl J Med* **314**:193–8.

Talbot JA, Bicknell EJ, Ranjhova M *et al.* (1996) Molecular scanning of the insulin receptor gene in women with polycystic ovary syndrome. *J Clin Endocr Metab* **81**:1979–83.

Talbott EO, Guzick DS, Sutton-Tyrrelli K *et al.* (2000) Evidence for association between polycystic ovary syndrome and premature carotid atherosclerosis in middle-aged women. *Atherosc Thromb Vasc Biol* **20**:2414–18.

Taylor AE, McCourt B, Martin KA *et al.* (1997) Determinants of abnormal gonadotropin secretion in clinically defined women with polycystic ovary syndrome. *J Clin Endocrinol Metab* **83**:2248–56.

Van Dam EW, Roelfsema F, Helmerhorst FH *et al.* (2002a) Low amplitude and disorderly spontaneous growth hormone release in obese women with or without polycystic ovary syndrome. *J Clin Endocrinol Metab* **87**:4225–30.

Van Dam EW, Roelfsema F, Veldhuis JD *et al.* (2002b) Meinders A, Krans HM, Pijl H. Increase in daily LH secretion in response to short-term calorie restriction in obese women with PCOS. *Am J Physiol Endocrinol Metab* **282**:865–72.

Vane JR, Anggard EE and Botting RM (1990) Regulatory functions of vascular endothelium. *N Engl J Med* **323**:27–36.

Velasquez EM, Mendoza S, Hamer T *et al.* (1994) Metformin therapy in polycystic ovary syndrome reduced hyperinsulinemia, insulin resistance, hyperandrogenemia, and systolic blood pressure, while facilitating normal menses and pregnancy. *Metabolism* **43**:647–54.

Vettor R, Lombardi AM, Fabris R *et al.* (2000) Substrate competition and insulin action in animal models. *Int Obes Relat Metab Disord* **24**:S22–S24.

Villa P, Soranna L, Mancini A *et al.* (2001) Effect of feeding on growth hormone response to growth hormone-releasing hormone in polycystic ovary syndrome: relation with body weight and hyperinsulinism. *Hum Reprod* **16**:430–4.

Volitainen R, Franks S, Mason HD and Marticainen H (1996) Expression of insulin-like growth factors (IGF), IGF-binding protein, and IGF receptor messenger ribonucleic acids in normal and polycystic ovaries. *J Clin Endocrinol Metab* **81**:1003–8.

Waterworth DM, Bennett ST, Gharani N *et al.* (1997) Linkage and association of insulin gene VNTR regulatory polymorphism with polycystic ovary syndrome. *Lancet* **349**:986–90.

Wild RA (1995) Obesity, lipids, cardiovascular risk, and androgen excess. *Am J Med* **98**:27S–32S.

Wild RA, Painter PC and Coulson RB (1985) Lipoprotein lipid concentrations and cardiovascular risk in women with polycystic ovary syndrome. *J Clin Endocrinol Metab* **61**:946–51.

Wild S, Pirpoint T, McKeigue Panel Jacobs H (2000) Cardiovascular disease in women with polycystic ovary syndrome at long-term follow-up: a retrospective cohort study. *Clin Endocrinol* **52**:595–600.

Wu X, Sallinen K, Zhou S *et al.* (2000) Androgen excess contributes to altered growth hormone/insulin-like growth factor-1 axis in nonobese women with polycystic ovary syndrome. *Fertil Steril* **73**:730–4.

Zawadzki JK and Dunaif A (1992) Diagnostic criteria for polycystic ovary syndrome: towards a rational approach. In Dunaif A, Givens JR, Haseltine F and Merriam GR *Current issues in Endocrinology and Metabolism. Polycystic Ovary Syndrome*, Blackwell, Boston, MA; pp 377–84.

14

Management of Diabesity in Primary Care: a Multidisciplinary Approach

Ian W. Campbell

Prevalence of obesity in primary care

The prevalence of overweight and obesity in the community, in both adults and children is already at epidemic levels. Half of all adult females and nearly two-thirds of men are overweight. Almost one in five, 17 per cent of men and 21 per cent of women, are clinically obese (body mass index; BMI $\geq$ 30) (National Audit Office, 2001). The implications for primary care, both now and in the future, are immense. Obese patients are 30 per cent more likely to require an appointment with their GP, and will, on average, account for 30 per cent more in prescription costs. A study of the socio-economic costs of obesity reveals a catalogue of social deprivation, increased sick-leave, higher unemployment and earlier retirement through ill-health (National Audit Office, 2001). All this impacts greatly on the ability of primary care to deliver adequate care with limited resources. It is, however, the direct effect of the co-morbidities of obesity that carries the heaviest burden on primary care. A review of the health consequences of excess adiposity leaves one in no doubt that primary care is already deeply involved in treating the complications of obesity. Hypertension, coronary heart disease, hyperlipidaemia, cancer (for example of the colon, breast, prostate), infertility, respiratory and sleep disorders, osteoarthritis and psychological disease can be attributed to some degree, directly or indirectly, to obesity (Jung, 1997). It is, however, the effect of the metabolic syndrome leading to

Obesity and Diabetes. Edited by Anthony H. Barnett and Sudhesh Kumar
© 2004 John Wiley & Sons, Ltd ISBN: 0-470-84898-7

increased insulin resistance and type 2 diabetes that portrays the most tangible and demonstrable effects of obesity into the everyday life of primary care doctors and nurses.

Current approach to diabetes care in primary care

The management of diabetes has, rightly, been given a high priority within general practice in recent years, with marked improvements in the level of pro-active care, reduction in risk factors, and prevention of co-morbidities being observed as a result. However, it is only recently that the direct relationship between type 2 diabetes and obesity has been accepted by the majority of clinicians. This chapter seeks to describe the way in which overweight type 2 diabetics might be managed in primary care. The distinction between type 1 and type 2 diabetics may be made at a very early stage in treatment, and the criteria for deciding when insulin treatment is required is dealt with elsewhere. It is also assumed that the ongoing management of diabetics, including annual reviews and dealing with complications is not within the remit of this chapter and will also be covered elsewhere in the book.

While up to 80 per cent of an individual's predisposition to developing type 2 diabetes is genetic (McCarthy *et al.*, 1994), obesity is now acknowledged as the determining factor in that development, and, conversely, it is quite clear that even a modest reduction in body weight, of between 5 and 10 per cent, can lead to significant improvements in fasting blood glucose and Hba1c (Goldstein, 1992). In newly diagnosed type 2 diabetics a reduction in body weight by 10 per cent would lead to a return to normal fasting glucose in half of all cases, and sustained weight loss of 10 per cent would produce a 30 per cent fall in diabetes-related deaths (see Table 14.1). Faced with this compelling evidence many practitioners now accept that weight management should form an integral part of the management of type 2 diabetes. The difficulty then faced is how to deliver that aspect of care within a primary care setting?

Table 14.1 Benefits of 10% weight loss

Mortality	>20% fall in total mortality
	>30% fall in diabetes related deaths
	>40% fall in obesity related deaths
Blood pressure	fall of 10 mmHg systolic and 20 mmHg diastolic pressure
Diabetes	50% fall in fasting glucose
Lipids	10% dec. total cholesterol
	15% dec. in LDL
	30% dec. in triglycerides
	8% inc. in HDL

World Health Organization. Obesity: Preventing and Managing the Global Epidemic. Geneva: WHO, 1997 with permission.
LDL, low-density lipoprotein; HDL, high-density lipoprotein.

Early treatment with hypoglycaemic agents

In an already pressured general practice setting it is perhaps too easy to reach for the prescription pad and prescribe hypoglycaemics at an early stage in the management of new diabetics. We are, understandably, concerned with reducing glycaemic levels as quickly possible, to improve symptomatology, and prevent potentially serious complications. However, in the early stages of management, treatment with hypoglycaemic agents is often not necessary, and the judicious withholding of such medication can have its own benefits. Sulphonylureas have been used extensively to treat type 2 diabetics. However, they can promote weight gain in an individual of, on average 2–4 kg (up to 10 kg) and therefore will adversely affect the underlying cause of the problem. Metformin does not lead to weight gain but can induce side effects of diarrhoea in 10 per cent of cases. On the other hand, within only a few weeks or months the benefits of weight loss can produce dramatic improvements in diabetic control to rival hypoglycaemic drugs. The clinician needs to ask himself at the outset of treatment whether weight loss should be the mainstay of management, at least for the first 3 to 6 months, before considering the introduction of hypoglycaemics as an adjunctive treatment, or in circumstances where beneficial weight loss has not been achieved.

Integrating obesity management with diabetes

Within primary care there has been a lot of interest in developing distinctive practice-based obesity clinics, often led by one or two enthusiastic members of the practice team and some achieving excellent results. Many others, however, find the prospects of developing such a stand-alone clinic daunting, citing the lack of time, staff, resources or skill-base as their main concerns. When considering the management of diabetes in primary care, however, the need for medical management of overweight is inescapably integral to any serious diabetes treatment plan. It must therefore be within the scope and remit of primary care diabetic clinics to provide for the management of overweight. To do otherwise is to fail to recognize and address the root cause of the disease we are trying to control, and thereby miss the perfect opportunity to develop life-long lifestyle change with all the medical benefits that would confer. This approach does however require an informed and motivated practice team approach, with involvement of a wide variety of professionals to offer the ongoing support and advice necessary for the patient to be encouraged to develop new attitudes to dietary intake and activity levels which are required to produce positive and significant results.

A multidisciplinary approach

In the management of the overweight diabetic, a great strength of primary care is ready access to a multidisciplinary team. The general practitioner, working closely with an enthusiastic practice nurse can, together, deliver high quality care in a familiar and accessible clinical setting. They are ideally placed to take into account the past and present medical history of the patient, and to incorporate proposed lifestyle changes into treatment strategies, tailored to the patient's domestic and employment circumstances. The general practitioner and nurse will often, over several years, have built up a significant and important trusting relationship, not only with the patient, but also their family. For the majority of type 2 diabetics care will be delivered almost exclusively by the general practitioner and the practice nurse. However, management can be greatly enhanced by the involvement of specialists within the primary care setting, both in the early stages of treatment but also when control becomes problematic.

Dietary treatment of diabetes

Dietary advice will form the backbone of a diabetic's future management and it is therefore crucial to get the right message across from the outset. Poor information delivered early in management can have adverse short, and long-term effects, and should be avoided. The aims of dietary advice should be to minimize symptoms of hyperglycaemia, minimize the risk of hypoglycaemia, and to promote weight loss, while ensuring that any proposed changes are tolerable and sustainable (Frost *et al.*, 1991). Remember that in encouraging the patient to make (possibly) substantial changes to their dietary intake you will be asking them to change life-long habits, to stop doing things they enjoy (and perhaps replace with less-well-received alternatives) and will at first appear to be asking them to make changes that will diminish their ability to socialize with family and friends at the dinner table and on special occasions. For most new diabetics, but depending on the severity of their glycaemia, it is perhaps best to keep the message simple at first, to avoid alienation or confusion.

Dietary changes should modify, rather than totally change the patient's eating pattern. Total calorie intake should be restricted to that needed to achieve and maintain an agreed target weight. At least half the energy intake should be made up of carbohydrate, and from mainly complex carbohydrates, with a high fibre content. At least five portions, and preferably more, of fruit and vegetables should be consumed every day (a portion is 80 g but is most simply measured as one handful), refined carbohydrates in the form of sugary food and drinks should be reduced. Total fat intake should be reduced, and saturated (animal) fats replaced with monounsaturated and polyunsaturated fats commonly found in oily fish and green leafy vegetables (Royal College of General Practitioners, 1994). Dietary salt should be reduced, alcohol intake should be in moderation, and special 'diabetic' products which are high in calories are not to be recommended. Much can be achieved from a few simple dietetic changes.

Over the next few appointments, and depending on the symptomatic and glycaemic response, advice can begin to specifically promote weight loss, to include detailed information on reducing portion sizes, reducing calorific intake by 600 kcal (or 20 per cent) daily, calorie calculations for specific and favourite foods, and steps to maximize the potential for a daily intake of at least five portions of fruit and vegetables, an increase in dietary protein and fibre, a reduction of fat intake to less than 10 per cent, and moderation of carbohydrate intake to 50 per cent of calorific intake. Although it may sound rather simplistic, asking the patient to complete a 'food diary' for 1 week can provide both the clinician and the patient with invaluable information. In the absence of a pre-printed diary form, a simple A4 piece of paper, marked off into days of the week will suffice. By the end of the week the patient will usually have begun to make some changes as they confront their previously unrecognized, or unacknowledged habits. Comments such as 'I never realized I ate so much between meals', or 'I wasn't aware that I used so much sugar in my tea over the course of the day' are not unusual when the patient presents the diary. For those patients whose diaries are awash with high sugar, high fat foods, and frequent snacking, it is best to select only a few possible changes to suggest to the patient, the ultimate choice of what to alter resting with the patient. A repeat food diary after a few weeks will present further opportunity assist the patient in refining their intake even further. Some patients will want to become expert in managing their diet, to facilitate weight loss, and to exert maximum control of the diabetes. The general practitioner and nurse can be a useful source of information material to aid patient education, by using published healthy eating leaflets and manuals.

For those general practitioners or nurses who lack experience or confidence to advise new diabetics on dietary matters, referral to a community based dietitian is essential. An experienced dietitian is ideally placed to provide detailed, but pragmatic dietary advice to facilitate an immediate improvement in symptomatology, but also to promote long-term dietary control of diabetes. Community dietitians are unfortunately an uncommon commodity in practice but when available to the primary care team the value of their contribution can be immense.

The role of the practice receptionist is all too often overlooked. Whilst not directly involved in patient care, they are usually closely involved in administering practice-based diabetic clinics and administering annual examination recall systems and encouraging patients to attend. An informed and enthusiastic receptionist can play a significant role in ensuring patients receive the clinical care they require, by being alert to previous non-attendance and under-use of regular diabetic medication, and responding positively to requests for consultations by the patient. The receptionist team can also play a significant part in developing obesity management services in primary care. The National Obesity Forum's annual Award for Excellence in Obesity Management in Primary Care (Lean *et al.*, 1991) receives entries from many excellent practice-based weight-loss programmes (incorporating diabetic management) which have been initiated, and run, by the receptionists, who have then gone on to enthuse and involve the rest of the primary care team in the practice.

Clinical assessment

Clinical assessment of new overweight diabetics need not be arduous. After diagnosis, it is essential, if not already done, to measure the patient's weight and height to calculate body mass index (BMI = weight (kg)/height (m^2)). Waist circumference is also a valuable indicator of excess body fat and is independent of height. Measured just below the umbilicus, a reading of 102 cm or above in males, and 90 cm or above in females (Guidelines on the Management of Adult Obesity, 2000), equates to similar levels of adiposity and increased risk of co-morbities as a BMI of 30+ (see table below). Electronic body fat monitors, often incorporated into weighing scales, provide a useful indication of body fat mass percentage providing yet another baseline measurement to monitor progress during a weight loss programme. Such equipment is no longer prohibitively expensive and can be easily acquired. Urinalysis, for proteinuria, and successive blood pressure readings are, of course, mandatory and easily performed in a primary care setting. Biochemical assessment is straightforward. In the process of diagnosis a fasting blood sugar, and possibly a glucose tolerance test will have been done. Further biochemical assessment as first line investigation should include fasting lipid profile, electrolytes, urea and creatinine, thyroid function and sex hormones (when indicated). These results will not only form a baseline from which to assess future changes as weight loss follows, but will also help to reassure the patient that there are no medical reasons why they might not be able to achieve beneficial weight loss. Second line investigations for obesity, where indicated, might include a chest x-ray, electrocardiogram, and 24-hour cortisol levels (Guidelines on the Management of Adult Obesity, 2000).

Treatment groups

There is still much debate about which obese patients' primary care professionals should invest time and resources to help. However, it should now be beyond any argument that there is a need, indeed an obligation, to assist overweight and obese diabetics to modify their diet, improve their levels of physical activity, and achieve weight loss. Guidelines for obesity management generally advise that medical support and intervention is appropriate in patients with a BMI ≥ 30, in the absence of any co-morbidities, but also in those with a BMI ≥ 27 in the presence of co-morbidities such as diabetes, hypertension, coronary heart disease and hyperlipidaemia. However, it is clear that even a modest increase in weight over desired weight levels confers additional risk both of developing type 2 diabetes, but also impairs management. Any type 2 diabetic whose weight is above the normal BMI range of 18.5–24.9 should be offered an appropriate level of advice and medical support to encourage weight loss. Of course, any weight loss attempts are reliant on patient participation, and so while it is ultimately a patient's choice whether to aim for weight loss, the clinician can be hugely influential by providing positive information concerning the desirability of weight loss, the potential benefit, and the level of support they are able to offer in order to help their patient make their decision. Patient motivation is commonly in direct proportion to the enthusiasm of their general practitioner and practice nurse.

Within primary care, consideration must be given to working with reputable commercial weight loss organizations. These groups can offer patients basic dietary and activity advice to support and encourage a return to a healthier lifestyle and promote weight loss and should be seen as added support, not a threat to primary care workers involved in managing the overweight. They can also offer a valuable psychological focus and social contact, often offer out-of-hours meetings and can ease some of the financial and time constraints of primary care. Practices should make their own assessment of local groups if they wish to 'refer' patients to them. It is important not to rely on patients to inform you of their own additional efforts to lose weight and use of 'over-the-counter' commercial products. Many will not see them as having a bearing on their medical care and clearly this is not the case.

It is important that realistic goals are set. Obese patients often have overly optimistic expectations of what weight loss can be achieved. One study in a hospital-based overweight clinic found that the average weight loss expected by patients was in excess of 30 per cent. The reality is that in a clinical setting, primary or secondary care, medically supported weight loss, over 1 year, is likely to average between 5–10 per cent of body weight. This discrepancy needs to be addressed at the outset of management, as bitter disappointment is likely to follow shortly. Patients should be encouraged to work towards a gradual loss of between 0.5–1 kg weekly, perhaps for the first 3 or 6 months, following which a period stability is likely. For some, weight maintenance at this level will be sufficient, for others, further weight loss might be achievable in later months. Weight loss is never easy, but for diabetics weight loss usually proves to be slower and harder won than for most, and yet in the same group, the benefits of sustained weight loss are more substantial and therefore unquestionably worth the effort of both patient and clinician. Patients should be encouraged to attend the practice at least monthly, and in the early stages 2-weekly appointments can prove highly beneficial. A good practice team can work together to provide continuity of care, the patient often alternating between doctor and nurse, with added dietetic consultations to optimize successful intervention. As management progresses, repeated examination should follow the national recommended guidelines for diabetic care.

Physical activity

The health benefits of regular physical activity are immense and this must be conveyed to the patient from the outset of treatment. Just 30 min of moderate intensity exercise each day can be shown to reduce blood pressure, improve lipid profile, decrease cardiovascular risk, improve energy levels and self esteem, all in addition to aiding weight loss and hence improved diabetic care (Sarvis, 1998). It is recognized that not only does increased activity help produce weight loss, but individuals who exercise regularly are also more likely to maintain their weight loss. Advice on physical activity has not traditionally been seen as the responsibility of the general practitioner, and yet so much can be achieved by a patient motivated to become more active. Before embarking on an exercise campaign, it may be helpful for the health professional to discuss with the individual which type, and what intensity of activity would be appropriate (see Box 14.1). Patients are often resistant to increasing their activity levels for a variety of reasons. They often, wrongly, perceive that to be beneficial exercise must be intense, and involve frequent gym attendance and exhausting sessions on various types of expensive equipment. They may complain that they are too old, too unfit, embarrassed, too busy, unable to afford it, have no-one to go with, or simply that they don't want to make the effort. However, for the majority, a careful explanation of the benefits, and the type of exercise required may quickly alleviate those fears. In those who are disabled, elderly, suffering from concomitant disease such as coronary heart disease, or to whom physical activity is but a distant memory, more specific advice than that available from the general practitioner or nurse might be necessary. For those who are significantly challenged, a community-based physiotherapist might contribute advice and reassurance about resuming activity. For others, and for those to whom the gym is appealing, the reassurance of a qualified fitness instructor (usually at a sports club, or fitness centre) who understands the need to make any new activity accessible and achievable, and who can recognize the particular needs of the overweight, can be worthwhile. However, not everyone has the financial resources, or desire, to make use of such clubs. Some local health trusts have developed 'exercise on prescription' schemes, the aim being to encourage inactive people to take up formalized activity at their local sports centre, either at subsidized rates, or in specific sessions, for example, for the very overweight,

---

Box 14.1 – Choosing the right activity – points to discuss with patients

- What do you want to be able to do?
- How active you've been in the past few months?
- What kind of activity do you enjoy?
- What fits in with your lifestyle?
- What is appropriate for your physical condition?
- What activity is appropriate for your age?
- How quickly do you want to lose weight?
- What activity will you still enjoy in a years time?

or disabled. Organization of such programmes requires the involvement of more than the immediate practice team. Primary Care Trusts (PCTs) need to work closely with local government leisure departments, and may have to put forward strongly the case for increased physical activity as an important contributor to improved health, not just for diabetics, but for everyone. PCTs will have to determine how such schemes can be funded. Experience however has shown that the effectiveness of such schemes varies enormously. Harland *et al.* (1999) found that the most effective form of activity was not formal, sports centre based schemes, but those that encouraged 'home-based' activity, that is, walking! However, for those who are attracted to formal organized exercise such schemes can provide a welcome re-introduction to physical activity. The reality of course is that for any long-term benefit to be achieved exercise must be regular and frequent. In order to facilitate weight loss, promote dietary control, and to improve fitness generally, the patient should be encouraged to find an extra 30 min of activity in their daily routine (for example, three episodes of 10 min each) at least 5 days each week. Patients can therefore be effectively encouraged to increase activity by, for example, leaving the car at home whenever possible, using stairs and avoiding lifts, getting off the bus a stop or two early, and by being more active generally around the house. Some primary care teams have even set up links with local rambling groups to facilitate more creative walking activities. While I would not expect this type of involvement to be embraced by every practice, it does show what can be achieved by those who are motivated to look beyond the confines of the practice to maximize the potential for health through lifestyle change.

Behavioural change

Behavioural change, encouraging and facilitating changes in habits, is a complex subject in its own right, and not something generally taught to primary care clinicians and nurses. However, it should not be seen as a separate form of management, rather as integral to the whole programme of empowering patient control of their diabetes, dietary habits and attitudes activity. Formal behavioural change, by qualified professionals, can produce sustained benefit, but input needs to be long term and the cost is therefore probably prohibitive in a primary care setting. Much can be achieved, however, by an informed and enthusiastic and patient doctor and nurse, using learned techniques as well as employing patient management skills acquired in practice. An increasing number of dietitians are developing expertise in this area, and their skills can be used to great advantage in helping overweight diabetics. The simplest form of support, deliverable from primary care might involve encouragement of the patient to learn to control unhelpful eating patterns. Advice such as to eat only at the table, to savour eating, and avoid distractions such as watching television simultaneously, to chew longer, to put down the fork back on the plate between mouthfuls, to wait for 20 min between courses to avoid over-eating, and so on. Continuous positive reinforcement is required, an absence of negative criticism a must, and a willingness to overlook repeated apparent failure essential.

Use of medication to aid weight loss in primary care

In spite of the best efforts of clinicians and patients, the reality is that many patients will not achieve significant weight loss within the first 6 months of treatment. Many who have achieved a degree of weight loss show a tendency for their weight loss to 'plateau' after 3–6 months, with a subsequent weight regain not unusual. This should not come as a surprise. Obesity should never be regarded as a short-term problem. It is a chronic condition, with even the most radically motivated patients experiencing times of relapse over months, even years, after initial treatment. The use of weight loss medication should be considered as an adjunctive treatment to lifestyle modification after 3–6 months of compliance to dietary, behavioural and activity advice, a failure to achieve 10 per cent body weight loss or significant reductions in HbA1c, to further reduce markers of co-morbidity such as hyperlipidaemia and hypertension, and to reduce symptomatology such as joint pain and breathlessness (Royal College of Physicians, 1998). The role of weight loss medication has often been mis-understood. It should be viewed as an *adjunct* to supported lifestyle change, and as an aid to enhance weight loss, and in so doing help educate patients towards establishing long-term habit change of improved diet and increased physical activity.

There are several agents available and currently used by medical practitioners to aid weight loss. There are, however, only two agents currently recommended and licensed for use, orlistat (Xenical) and sibutramine (Reductil). Orlistat first became available in 1999, is classified as an intestinal lipase inhibitor and prevents absorption of fats from the small intestine. Sibutramine has been available in some parts of Europe and the USA since 1999, and in the UK since 2001, is centrally acting, and is classified as a serotonin and noradrenaline reuptake inhibitor. Both orlistat (Hauptman *et al.*, 2000) and sibutramine (Jones *et al.*, 1996) have been shown to be effective in primary care and to convey significant benefit in the treatment of overweight diabetics (Hollander *et al.*, 1998; Finer *et al.*, 2000). The National Institute of Clinical Excellence has considered both agents and has given its approval to their use within primary care, citing in addition to improved rates of weight loss, significant improvements in glycaemia, lipid levels and blood pressure. Both agents have been used extensively within primary care and can greatly increase the prospects of patients achieving beneficial levels of weight loss. The commonly used hypoglycaemic agent metformin has been shown to have advantageous effects in some diabetics trying to reduce their weight. Its effect on insulin resistance has been utilized in obese non-diabetic subjects to aid weight loss, and in particular in women who are overweight because of polycystic ovarian syndrome (PCO). Some practitioners have tried to use it in combination with orlistat or sibutramine. It does not have any specific licensing arrangements for the treatment of obesity and currently does not have a clearly defined role.

For a detailed review of the currently licensed anti-obesity agents refer to Chapter 10.

Summary

In recent years the increasing prevalence of type 2 diabetes has been accompanied by an increasing willingness, and ability, of the primary health care team to deliver evidence based, best practice in diabetes management from primary care. There is clear evidence, not only that obesity and overweight are implicated in the development of this growing public health threat, but also that medically supported and modest reductions in weight can lead to significantly improved prevention and treatment of diabetes, with a reduction in associated complications. The motivated general practitioner and practice nurse can soon equip themselves with the necessary clinical skills and tools to offer effective weight management services within the practice, and draw on the support of the specialist skills of allied professionals when available and appropriate. Diabesity is a disease of complex aetiology with multi-system pathological results. If we are to continue to offer the best possible care to our patients, it is beholden to the primary care team to embrace each proven effective treatment modality with enthusiasm and dedication. The multidisciplinary, comprehensive approach to disease management in primary care is an ideal environment to incorporate the management of obesity as an integral, and inescapable part of normal diabetes care.

References

Finer N, Bloom SR, Frost GS *et al.* (2000) Sibutramine is effective for weight loss and diabetic control in obesity with type 2 diabetes. *Diabetes, Obes Metab* **2**:105–12.

Frost G, Masters K, King C *et al.* (1991) A new method of energy prescription to improve weight loss. *J Hum Nutr Diet* **4**:369–73.

Goldstein D (1992) Beneficial health effects of modest weight loss. *Int J Obes* **16**:397–415.

Guidelines on the Management of Adult Obesity (2000) National Obesity Forum, Nottingham.

Harland J, White M, Drinkwater C *et al.* (1999) The Newcastle exercise project: a randomised controlled trial of methods to promote physical activity in primary care. *Br Med J* **319**:828–32.

Hauptman J, Lucas C, Boldrin MN *et al.* (2000) Orlistat in the long term treatment of obesity in primary care settings, *Arch Fam Med* **9**:160–7.

Hollander PA, Elbein SC, Hirsch IB *et al.* (1998) Role of orlistat in the treatment of obese patients with type 2 diabetes. *Diabetes Care* **21**:1288–94.

Jones SP, Smith IG, Kelly F and Gray JA (1995) Long term weight loss with sibutramine. *Int J Obes Relat Metab Disord* **19** (Suppl. 2):41.

Jung RT (1997) Obesity as a disease. *Br Med Bull* **53**:307–21.

Lean MEJ, Han TS and Seidell JC (1991) Impairment of health and quality of life in people with large waist circumference. *Lancet* **351**:853–6.

McCarthy MG *et al.* (1994) The development of non insulin dependent diabetes mellitus. *Diabetologia* **37**: 959–68.

National Obesity Forum. PO Box 6625 Nottingham NG2 5 PA

National Audit Office (2001) Tackling Obesity in England. HC 220 Sess. 2000–2001 15 Feb 2001.

Royal College of General Practitioners (1994) Nutrition in General Practice 1 Basic Principles of Nutrition. RCGP, London.

Royal College of Physicians (1998) Clinical Management of Overweight and Obese Patients with Particular Reference to the Use of Drugs. RCP, London.

Sarvis WHM (1998) Physical activity in the treatment of obesity. Symposium on Obesity – The threat ahead. 24–25

Index

Note: Figures and Tables are indicated by *italic page numbers*

Obesity and Diabetes. Edited by Anthony H. Barnett and Sudhesh Kumar
© 2004 John Wiley & Sons, Ltd ISBN: 0-470-84898-7

Index compiled by Paul Nash